Essentials of
Glaucoma Surgery

EDITED BY

Malik Y. Kahook, MD
Professor of Ophthalmology
Director of Clinical and Translational Research
University of Colorado School of Medicine
Denver, Colorado

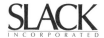

SLACK
INCORPORATED

www.Healio.com/books

ISBN: 978-1-61711-012-2

The procedures and practices described in this publication should be implemented in a manner consistent with the professional standards set for the circumstances that apply in each specific situation. Every effort has been made to confirm the accuracy of the information presented and to correctly relate generally accepted practices. The authors, editors, and publisher cannot accept responsibility for errors or exclusions or for the outcome of the material presented herein. There is no expressed or implied warranty of this book or information imparted by it. Care has been taken to ensure that drug selection and dosages are in accordance with currently accepted/recommended practice. Off-label uses of drugs may be discussed. Due to continuing research, changes in government policy and regulations, and various effects of drug reactions and interactions, it is recommended that the reader carefully review all materials and literature provided for each drug, especially those that are new or not frequently used. Some drugs or devices in this publication have clearance for use in a restricted research setting by the Food and Drug and Administration or FDA. Each professional should determine the FDA status of any drug or device prior to use in their practice.

Any review or mention of specific companies or products is not intended as an endorsement by the author or publisher.

SLACK Incorporated uses a review process to evaluate submitted material. Prior to publication, educators or clinicians provide important feedback on the content that we publish. We welcome feedback on this work.

Published by: SLACK Incorporated
                   6900 Grove Road
                   Thorofare, NJ 08086 USA
                   Telephone: 856-848-1000
                   Fax: 856-848-6091
                   www.Healio.com/books

Contact SLACK Incorporated for more information about other books in this field or about the availability of our books from distributors outside the United States.

Library of Congress Cataloging-in-Publication Data

Essentials of glaucoma surgery / edited by Malik Y. Kahook.
      p. ; cm.
   Includes bibliographical references and index.
   ISBN 978-1-61711-012-2 (pbk. : alk. paper)
   I. Kahook, Malik Y.
   [DNLM: 1. Glaucoma--surgery. WW 290]

   617.7'41059--dc23
                        2012019861

Printed in the United States of America.

Last digit is print number: 10   9   8   7   6   5   4   3   2   1

DEDICATION

We dedicate this book to our families for their tireless support,
our mentors for their valued advice and friendship,
and our patients for the privilege of being entrusted with their care.

Malik Y. Kahook, MD

John P. Berdahl, MD
Jonathan A. Eisengart, MD
Mahmoud A. Khaimi, MD
Nathan M. Radcliffe, MD
Joshua D. Stein, MD, MS
Jeffrey M. Zink, MD

Contents

About the Editor

Malik Y. Kahook, MD is Professor of Ophthalmology and Director of Clinical and Translational Research in the Department of Ophthalmology at the University of Colorado. He also directs the glaucoma service and glaucoma fellowship, and serves as a faculty member in the Department of Bioengineering at the University of Colorado. He specializes in the medical and surgical treatment of glaucoma and cataracts. He is active within the ophthalmology community including memberships in the American Academy of Ophthalmology, American Glaucoma Society, American Society of Refractive and Cataract Surgeons, and the Association for Research in Vision and Ophthalmology. Dr. Kahook has authored more than 180 peer-reviewed manuscripts, abstracts, and book chapters, and is editor of *Chandler and Grant's Glaucoma*. He was awarded an American Glaucoma Society Clinician-Scientist Fellowship Award for 2007 as well as the American Glaucoma Society Compliance Grant for 2006 and was named New Inventor of the Year for the University of Colorado in 2009 and Inventor of the Year for 2010. He has filed for 12 patents, several of which have been licensed by companies for development and commercialization. Dr. Kahook is a consultant to the Food and Drug Administration's Ophthalmic Device Division.

Dr. Kahook completed his residency training at the University of Colorado, Rocky Mountain Lions Eye Institute in Denver, Colorado, where he was named Chief Resident. He then went on to complete his fellowship in glaucoma from the University of Pittsburgh Medical Center in Pittsburgh, Pennsylvania.

ABOUT THE ASSOCIATE EDITORS

John P. Berdahl, MD specializes in advanced cataract, corneal and glaucoma surgery, in addition to refractive surgery. He earned his medical doctorate, graduating with honors, from Mayo Medical School in Rochester, Minnesota and finished his internship at the Mayo Clinic in Scottsdale, Arizona. He completed his ophthalmology residency at Duke University where his published work, research, teaching, and care of patients brought him many honors, including Best Resident and national recognition as the first place winner of the Resident Writers Award. Dr. Berdahl pursued additional advanced surgical training at the most coveted cornea and glaucoma fellowship in the country at Minnesota Eye Consultants. As a fellow he received the Claes H. Dohlman Award from Harvard University, which is given to the top cornea fellow in the country.

Originally from Hills, Minnesota, Dr. Berdahl graduated from Augustana College and taught and coached at Hills-Beaver Creek prior to entering medical school. Dr. Berdahl has published numerous book chapters and peer-reviewed articles, and his extensive research has been presented nationally and internationally. His commitment to those in need is demonstrated by his leadership role in EyeCare America (which provides free eye care to the underserved) and the numerous surgical mission trips he continues to participate in worldwide.

Dr. Berdahl currently lives in Sioux Falls with his wife Tamme, young son Tommy, and daughter Anabel. His main interests include outdoor activities, reading, scuba diving, community involvement, and spending time with his family.

Jonathan A. Eisengart, MD is on the glaucoma staff at the Cleveland Clinic Cole Eye Institute. He completed his residency and glaucoma fellowship at the University of Michigan Kellogg Eye Center before returning to the Cleveland area. His primary research interest focuses on glaucoma surgical outcomes. He is intimately involved in the residency and fellowship programs at the Cole Eye Institute, and maintains a busy glaucoma clinical and surgical practice.

Mahmoud A. Khaimi, MD is a clinical assistant professor at the Dean A. McGee Eye Institute/University of Oklahoma in Oklahoma City, Oklahoma. A native of Detroit, Michigan, he received his undergraduate and medical degrees from Wayne State University in Detroit, graduating Summa Cum Laude with honors, and went on to complete an ophthalmology residency at Henry Ford Hospital also in Detroit. Following his residency, Dr. Khaimi completed a fellowship in glaucoma at the Dean McGee Eye Institute at the University of Oklahoma Health Science Center in Oklahoma City where he was asked to stay on as a faculty member. He now also serves as the Director of Glaucoma Services at the Oklahoma City VA Medical Center and is the Chairman of the Clinical Care Committee at the Dean McGee Eye Institute. Dr. Khaimi's commitment and dedication to residents' education has led him to be the 2010 recipient of the Excellence in Attending at VA award. He has taught several cataract and glaucoma surgical courses to ophthalmology residents throughout the nation. Dr. Khaimi has an active interest in glaucoma-related surgical innovations and is involved in numerous clinical trials. He is the primary investigator for the Primary Trabeculectomy versus Tube study, RiGOR study, and several pharmaceutical research studies. He is co-investigator for the Ex-Press mini shunt versus Trabeculectomy (XVT) study, the COMPASS study, and the Ologen versus Mitomycin C study. As the Associate Lead Ophthalmologist for the NBA Oklahoma City Thunder basketball team, Dr. Khaimi enjoys attending basketball games with his wife. He currently lives in Edmond, Oklahoma with his wife Suzie and his 3 children Maryam, Ahmad, and Zakariya.

Nathan M. Radcliffe, MD is the director of the Glaucoma Service at Weill Cornell Medical College and New York Hospital in New York, New York. Dr. Radcliffe graduated from Temple University School of Medicine and then completed his internship at the University of Hawaii in Honolulu. He was Chief Ophthalmology Resident at New York University and completed his glaucoma fellowship at the New York Eye and Ear Infirmary. Dr. Radcliffe is a dedicated teacher and researcher who is involved in numerous investigations related to the care of glaucoma patients. He is a surgical video competition enthusiast and is proud to have won the American Glaucoma Society's Surgical Video Award in 2011.

Joshua D. Stein, MD, MS is an Assistant Professor on the Glaucoma Service at the University of Michigan Department of Ophthalmology and Visual Sciences. Dr. Stein attended medical school at Jefferson Medical College. He then completed an internship at Abington Memorial Hospital followed by residency in ophthalmology at New York University where he served as Chief Resident. Following residency training, Dr. Stein did a 2-year clinical and research glaucoma fellowship at Duke University. He joined the faculty at the University of Michigan in 2007. Dr. Stein enjoys teaching residents and fellows how to medically and surgically manage patients with various types and complexities of glaucoma. He is also an avid researcher who studies the epidemiology, risk factors, and resource consumption associated with caring for patients with ocular diseases.

Jeffrey M. Zink, MD is a member of the Glaucoma Service at the Cincinnati Eye Institute. He received his medical degree from the University of Pennsylvania School of Medicine where he was inducted into the Alpha Omega Alpha Honor Society. After finishing an internship in Internal Medicine at Pennsylvania Hospital, he completed his residency in Ophthalmology at the Kellogg Eye Center of the University of Michigan, where he served as Chief Resident in his final year. Subsequently, he did a fellowship in glaucoma at the Bascom Palmer Eye Institute. As a member of the Cincinnati Eye Institute, Dr. Zink is involved in resident education at the University of Cincinnati, and he has an interest in the management of complicated glaucomas.

CONTRIBUTING AUTHORS

R. Rand Allingham, MD (Chapter 1)
Richard and Kit Barkhouser
    Professor of Ophthalmology
Director, Glaucoma Service
Duke University Eye Center
Durham, North Carolina

Ramesh S. Ayyala, MD, FRCS,
    FRCOphth (Chapter 49)
Professor of Ophthalmology
Director, Glaucoma Services
Director, Residency Program
Tulane School of Medicine
New Orleans, Louisiana

Amy Badger-Asaravala, MD
    (Chapter 28)
Glaucoma Specialist
Optima Ophthalmic Medical
    Associates
Hayward, California

Gabriel T. Chong, MD (Chapter 9)
Raleigh Ophthalmology
Raleigh, North Carolina

Nathan Congdon, MD, MPH
    (Chapter 45)
Staff Ophthalmologist
North Asia Region
ORBIS International
Professor
Department of Preventive
    Ophthalmology and
    State Key Laboratory
Zhongshan Ophthalmic Center
Sun Yat-sen University
Guangzhou, China

Anna-Maria Demetriades, MD
    (Appendix D)
Assistant Professor of
    Ophthalmology
Department of Ophthalmology
Weill Cornell Medical College
New York-Presbyterian Hospital
New York, New York

David L. Epstein, MD, MMM
    (Chapter 46)
Joseph A. C. Wadsworth Clinical
    Professor of Ophthalmology
Chairman, Department of
    Ophthalmology
Duke University School of Medicine
Durham, North Carolina

Malvina B. Eydelman, MD
    (Chapter 44)
Director
Division of Ophthalmic,
    Neurologic, and Ear, Nose and
    Throat Devices
Office of Device Evaluation
Center of Devices and Radiological
    Health
Food and Drug Administration
Silver Spring, Maryland

Robert D. Fechtner, MD (Chapter 51)
Professor of Ophthalmology
Director, Glaucoma Division
Institute of Ophthalmology and
    Visual Science
New Jersey Medical School
Newark, New Jersey

David Fleischman, MD (Chapter 2)
Department of Ophthalmology
University of North Carolina
     Hospitals
Chapel Hill, North Carolina

James A. Fox, MD (Chapter 4)
Resident Physician
Mason Eye Institute
University of Missouri-Columbia
Columbia, Missouri

Douglas E. Gaasterland, MD
     (Chapter 25)
Retired, Eye Doctors of Washington
Formerly Clinical Professor
     Ophthalmology
Georgetown University and George
     Washington University
Washington, DC

Preeya K. Gupta, MD (Chapters 35
     and 37)
Assistant Professor of
     Ophthalmology
Cornea and Refractive Surgery
     Service
Duke Eye Center
Durham, North Carolina

Ben J. Harvey, MD (Chapter 18)
Clinical Instructor
Bascom Palmer Eye Institute
University of Miami
Miami, Florida

Leon W. Herndon, MD (Chapter 29)
Associate Professor of
     Ophthalmology
Duke University Eye Center
Durham, North Carolina

Michael B. Horsley, MD (Chapter 16)
Private Practice
Phoenix, Arizona

Nauman Imami, MD, MHSA
     (Chapter 27)
Vice-Chair
Senior Staff Physician
Department of Ophthalmology
Henry Ford Hospital
Detroit, Michigan

Denise A. John, MD, FRCSC
     (Chapter 21)
Clinical Instructor of Ophthalmology
     and Visual Sciences
Kellogg Eye Center
University of Michigan
Chief of Ophthalmology VA
Ann Arbor Healthcare Systen
Ann Arbor, Michigan

Suzanne Johnston, MD (Chapter 30)
Instructor in Ophthalmology
Harvard Medical School
Associate in Ophthalmology
Children's Hospital Boston
Boston, Massachusetts

Anup K. Khatana, MD (Chapter 10)
Glaucoma Fellowship Director
Cincinnati Eye Institute
Volunteer Clinical Assistant
     Professor of Ophthalmology
University of Cincinnati College of
     Medicine
Cincinnati, Ohio

R. Lee Kramm, MD (Chapter 44)
Medical Officer
Division of Ophthalmic,
    Neurological and ENT Devices
Center of Devices and Radiological
    Health
Food and Drug Administration
Silver Spring, Maryland

Dennis S. C. Lam, MD(HK),
    FRCS(Edin), FRCOphth(UK),
    FCOphth(HK) (Chapter 24)
Honorary Professor, Department of
    Ophthalmology and Visual
    Sciences
S. H. Ho Professor of Ophthalmology
    and Visual Sciences
The Chinese University of Hong
    Kong
Hong Kong SAR, China

Danielle M. Ledoux, MD (Chapter 30)
Instructor in Ophthalmology
Harvard Medical School
Associate in Ophthalmology
Children's Hospital Boston
Boston, Massachusetts

Richard K. Lee, MD, PhD (Chapter 9)
Associate Professor of
    Ophthalmology, Cell Biology, and
    Neuroscience Graduate Program
Bascom Palmer Eye Institute
University of Miami
Miller School of Medicine
Miami, Florida

Christopher K. S. Leung, MD
    (Chapter 23)
Associate Professor
Department of Ophthalmology and
    Visual Sciences
The Chinese University of Hong
    Kong
Hong Kong, China

Richard A. Lewis, MD (Chapter 48)
Consultant, Private Practice
Sacramento, California

Marlene R. Moster, MD (Chapter 50)
Professor of Ophthalmology
Thomas Jefferson School of Medicine
Wills Eye Institute
Philadelphia, Pennsylvania

Sayoko E. Moroi, MD, PhD
    (Chapter 33)
Professor,
Department of Ophthalmology and
    Visual Sciences
W. K. Kellogg Eye Center
University of Michigan
Ann Arbor, Michigan

David C. Musch, PhD, MPH
    (Chapter 43)
Professor of Ophthalmology and
    Visual Sciences
Associate Research Scientist
Department of Epidemiology
University of Michigan
Ann Arbor, Michigan

Mina Pantcheva, MD (Chapter 41)
Assistant Professor in
    Ophthalmology
University of Colorado School of
    Medicine
Department of Ophthalmology
Aurora, Colorado

*Kathryn L. Pepple, MD, PhD
    (Chapter 1)*
Department of Ophthalmology
Duke University Eye Center
Durham, North Carolina

Marcos Reyes, MD (Chapter 4)
Assistant Professor of Clinical
    Ophthalmology
University of Missouri
Department of Ophthalmology
University Hospital
Columbia, Missouri

Douglas J. Rhee, MD (Chapter 16)
Associate Chief, Operations and
    Practice Development
Massachusetts Eye and Ear
    Infirmary
Associate Professor
Harvard Medical School
Boston, Massachusetts

Robert Ritch, MD (Chapter 24)
Shelley and Steven Einhorn
    Distinguished Chair in
    Ophthalmology
Professor of Clinical Ophthalmology
Chief, Glaucoma Service
Surgeon Director
The New York Eye and Ear Infirmary
New York, New York

Matthew Rouse, MD (Chapter 17)
University Eye Surgeons
University of Tennessee Medical
    Center
Knoxville, Tennessee

Travis C. Rumery, DO (Chapter 43)
Ophthalmology Resident
University of Michigan Kellogg Eye
    Center
Department of Ophthalmology and
    Visual Sciences
Ann Arbor, Michigan

*Sarwat Salim, MD, FACS
    (Chapter 42)*
Associate Professor of
    Ophthalmology
Director, Glaucoma Service
Hamilton Eye Institute
University of Tennessee
Memphis, Tennessee

*Thomas W. Samuelson, MD
    (Chapters 14 and 47)*
Glaucoma and Anterior Segment
    Surgery
Minnesota Eye Consultants
Adjunct Associate Professor
University of Minnesota
Duluth, Minnesota

Fiorella Saponara, MD (Chapter 22)
Resident in Ophthalmology
University of Michigan Health
    Systems
Department of Ophthalmology
Kellogg Eye Center
Ann Arbor, Michigan

Steven R. Sarkisian Jr, MD
(Chapter 15)
Glaucoma Fellowship Director
Clinical Associate Professor
Dean McGee Eye Institute
Department of Ophthalmology
University of Oklahoma College of
 Medicine
Oklahoma City, Oklahoma

Joel S. Schuman, MD, FACS
(Chapter 52)
Eye and Ear Foundation
Professor and Chairman
Department of Ophthalmology
School of Medicine
University of Pittsburgh
Director
University of Pittsburgh Medical
 Center, Eye Center
Professor of Bioengineering
Swanson School of Engineering
University of Pittsburgh
Interim Co-Director
Fox Center for Vision Restoration
Member, The McGowan Institute
 for Regenerative Medicine
Professor, Center for the Neural
 Basis of Cognition
Carnegie Mellon University and
 University of Pittsburgh
Pittsburgh, Pennsylvania

Leonard K. Seibold, MD (Chapter 3)
Instructor of Ophthalmology
University of Colorado, Denver
Department of Ophthalmology
Rocky Mountain Lions Eye Institute
Denver, Colorado

Robert Stamper, MD (Chapter 28)
Professor of Clinical Ophthalmology
Director, Glaucoma Service
University of California,
 San Francisco
Department of Ophthalmology
San Francisco, California

Tiffany N. Szymarek, MD
(Chapter 33)
Clinical Instructor
Department of Ophthalmology and
 Visual Sciences
W. K. Kellogg Eye Center
University of Michigan
Ann Arbor, Michigan

Clement C. Y. Tham,
 FRCS(Glasgow), FCOphth(HK)
 (Chapter 24)
Professor
Department of Ophthalmology and
 Visual Sciences
The Chinese University of Hong
 Kong
Honorary Chief-of-Service
Hong Kong Eye Hospital
Hong Kong SAR, China

Stephen P. Verb, MD, MHSA
(Chapter 27)
Private Practice
Coburn-Kleinfeldt Eye Clinic
Livonia, Michigan

Elizabeth T. Viriya, MD (Chapter 20)
Albert Einstein College of Medicine
Department of Ophthalmology
Bronx Lebanon Hospital Center
Bronx, New York

David S. Walton, MD (Chapter 30)
Professor of Ophthalmology
Harvard Medical School
Department of Ophthalmology
Massachusetts Eye and Ear
   Infirmary
Boston, Massachusetts

*Jennifer Somers Weizer, MD
   (Chapter 21)*
Assistant Professor of
   Ophthalmology and Visual
   Sciences
Kellogg Eye Center
University of Michigan
Ann Arbor, Michigan

Joseph R. Zelefsky, MD (Chapter 20)
Assistant Professor of
   Ophthalmology
Albert Einstein College of Medicine
Department of Ophthalmology
Bronx Lebanon Hospital Center
Bronx, New York

Introduction

Essentials of Glaucoma Surgery was written for both the trainee as well as the experienced glaucoma surgeon. Our intention was to create a reference that provided an introduction to the basics of glaucoma surgery while also introducing pearls for practice that were collectively learned by the authors. The text is divided into sections that cover the "bread and butter" of glaucoma surgery including basic anatomy, trabeculectomy, glaucoma drainage device implants, and combined procedures. We also focus entire sections on how to handle complications of glaucoma surgery, as well as the basics of new and novel approaches recently introduced to our practice. There are specific sections that deal with clinical trials as well as the regulatory pathway for ophthalmic surgical devices. We are particularly excited about the essays from senior surgeons who share their experience and insights (past, present, and future) regarding the art of treating glaucoma patients.

The contributors to this book are experts in their fields and offer many pearls that the reader can use instantly for improving patient care. Each Associate Editor brings a unique skill set to this project including expertise in basic glaucoma surgery, leadership in introducing novel surgeries to the operating room, and proficiency in dealing with the inevitable postoperative challenges.

On a personal note, this project represents a continuation of the lessons and wisdom offered by my teachers Joel S. Schuman and Robert J. Noecker. It is our collective hope that the reader will learn from this text and expand their surgical skills based on the insights provided. Moreover, it is our sincere desire that reading *Essentials of Glaucoma Surgery* results in as much enjoyment as we had during the creative process of collaboration for this project!

Malik Y. Kahook, MD

I

INTRODUCTION TO BASIC CONCEPTS OF GLAUCOMA SURGERY

1

THE SURGICAL
DECISION-MAKING PROCESS

Kathryn L. Pepple, MD, PhD and R. Rand Allingham, MD

Glaucoma is a potentially blinding disease, affecting 2% to 3% of the United States population,[1] that includes a group of diseases with a characteristic optic neuropathy and typical pattern of progressive vision loss.[2] Glaucoma is also a disease that can progress to blindness, even in the treated patient population. Lowering intraocular pressure (IOP) is the only intervention that has proven successful in halting or delaying the rate of visual loss over time.[3-5] Initial therapy for most forms of glaucoma center on medical and/or laser therapy. When these therapies fail to control the disease process, surgical intervention is generally recommended.

Although each patient represents a unique combination of factors that relate to disease process, comorbid conditions, and social and other factors that require individualized care, there are helpful guidelines that can assist the decision-making process regarding when to offer surgery and which procedures to recommend. Surgical techniques have evolved dramatically over the years and, along with new technologies and approaches, promise to improve outcomes. In the following chapter, we will discuss when to pursue surgical intervention and how to choose the most appropriate procedure (Table 1-1).

THE DECISION TO PROCEED TO SURGERY

There is a large body of information that outlines the process for the initial diagnosis of glaucoma, how to establish an appropriate target IOP, and how to initiate management with either medical or laser therapy. Before proceeding with surgery, it is essential to step back and take a fresh look at the patient. One wants to discover that the patient was taking steroid-containing medications, has early angle closure, or has not been adherent

Kahook M.
Essentials of Glaucoma Surgery (pp 3-10).
© 2012 SLACK Incorporated.

TABLE 1-1. FACTORS THAT SHOULD BE EVALUATED IN
TRABECULECTOMY, GLAUCOMA IMPLANTS, OR A CYCLODESTRUCTIVE PROCEDURE

Factor	Trabeculectomy	Glaucoma Implant	Cyclophotocoagulation
Postoperative intraocular pressure requirement	Need for IOP <13 mm Hg	IOP in mid-teens or higher	Reduction of IOP from current level
Need to reduce or eliminate glaucoma medications	Likely to eliminate medications in near term	Likely to reduce need for glaucoma medications, not likely to eliminate	Unpredictable, usually medications required
Long-term risk of postoperative infection	Moderate, 1% per year	Rare	No increased risk
Average period of success	5 years	5 years	Variable
Need for frequent postoperative appointments	High	Moderate	Low
Complexity of postoperative care	High	Moderate	Low
Risk of visual acuity loss	Low to moderate	Low to moderate	Moderate to high
Risk of postoperative complication	Moderate to high	Moderate	Low to moderate

(continued)

TABLE 1-1 (CONTINUED). FACTORS THAT SHOULD BE EVALUATED IN TRABECULECTOMY, GLAUCOMA IMPLANTS, OR A CYCLODESTRUCTIVE PROCEDURE

Factor	Trabeculectomy	Glaucoma Implant	Cyclophotocoagulation
Open angle glaucoma (OAG) or exfoliation glaucoma, pigmentary glaucoma with no prior incisional surgery	Generally first option	Considered if additional factors (eg, difficulty with postoperative care)	Rarely performed
OAG or exfoliation glaucoma, pigmentary glaucoma with prior incisional surgery	Good option if conjunctiva acceptable	Good option in most cases	Rarely performed unless reduced visual acuity or other factors present
Inflammatory glaucomas, neovascular glaucoma, traumatic glaucoma (major ocular trauma)	Poor to fair option, only if conjunctiva acceptable	Good option	Fair option depending on visual acuity, increased risk of hypotony or phthisis with poor aqueous outflow (eg, extensive angle closure)
Glaucoma of infancy or early childhood (after goniotomy or trabeculotomy if indicated)	Poor to fair option, depending on ability to comply with surgical regimen	Good option	Option in cases with poor visual potential or after surgical glaucoma procedures

with medications before performing a major surgical intervention. From this point further, we will assume that a correct diagnosis of glaucoma has been made and that, as part of the patient's ongoing care, there is a need for surgical intervention.

The most common indication for surgery is when, despite maximal medical and laser therapy, visual field loss or optic nerve damage continues. Surgery is also pursued when the likelihood of progression with the current management plan is judged to be high. When maximal medical and laser therapy has failed, patients will frequently fall into 1 of 2 categories: either the patient is seemingly "well" controlled (goal IOP achieved) or "poorly" controlled (goal IOP not achieved). When progression occurs with a presumably therapeutic IOP, this suggests that a lower target IOP is required. In the poorly controlled group, progression indicates a failure of drug and laser therapy to achieve the goal IOP. Surgery may be required for patients who cannot tolerate topical medications or those who are not able to adhere to the prescribed medical regimen. Less commonly, patients may present with previously undiagnosed and advanced glaucoma or an acute glaucomatous condition. Often, these patients will need rapid IOP lowering, which is unlikely to be achieved with medical or laser therapy. However, these modalities will often be attempted over a short-term window to give less invasive therapies a chance to begin the process of IOP lowering and to prepare the patient for the need for surgery.

The Collaborative Initial Glaucoma Treatment Study (CIGTS) was conducted to determine the role for surgery versus medical therapy as initial management for patients with newly diagnosed open-angle glaucoma.[6] The medical arm allowed the use of currently available topical medications, whereas the surgical arm consisted of trabeculectomy with or without 5-fluorouracil (5-FU). Each arm had the intention of lowering IOP to a target IOP that was assigned as a function of the baseline IOP and initial visual field, such that patients with more severe disease had lower target IOPs. After controlling for vision loss from postoperative cataract progression, no difference was found in disease progression between the medical versus surgically managed groups. This result suggests early surgery has a role in glaucoma treatment; however, the risks of serious postoperative complications (eg, endophthalmitis) have historically encouraged a more conservative approach among practitioners.

DISCUSSING SURGERY WITH YOUR PATIENTS

For many patients, understanding the balance between the risks and benefits of surgery is difficult. Many glaucoma patients have excellent central vision, so they understandably feel that there is nothing "wrong" with their vision. In these cases, there is a need to discuss how glaucoma causes vision loss and why surgery is required despite seemingly good vision. Due to the chronic nature of this disease and typically slow rate of progression, most patients will require several visits before surgical procedures are scheduled. Familiarizing patients with their visual field results and how they have progressed over time can be an effective approach to educate patients about vision loss in glaucoma and help them to understand the need for incisional surgery.

Regardless of the type of surgery, it is very important that the patient understands the risks of the procedure so they can be weighed against the benefits. In this era of high-precision cataract and refractive surgery, patients can easily have unrealistic expectations for glaucoma surgery. Specifically, the patient needs to understand that the intent of glaucoma surgery is not to improve vision but rather to prevent continuing vision loss. Patients also need to be cautioned that if they are phakic, glaucoma surgery will likely cause progression of cataract development. In addition, it is important to explain that there may be a need to continue eye drops even after a successful surgery. The most serious risks of glaucoma surgery include infections such as endophthalmitis and blebitis, suprachoroidal hemorrhages, retinal detachment, choroidal effusion, and hypotony with or without maculopathy. The incidence of more serious complications varies in the literature and, although uncommon, they are not rare and carry significant morbidity.[7,8] Therefore, the balance of the risk of long-term vision loss from glaucoma versus the risk of short-term visual loss from surgical complications must be addressed by the treating physician and understood by each patient.

CHOOSING AN OPERATIVE TECHNIQUE

Two main categories of surgery are commonly offered to adults with glaucoma: trabeculectomy and glaucoma implants, sometimes called tube shunts.[9,10] Less commonly performed glaucoma surgeries are goniotomy, trabeculotomy, and laser photocoagulation of the ciliary body.[2] Goniotomy and trabeculectomy are more common in the pediatric glaucoma population, whereas photocoagulation of the ciliary body with endocyclophotocoagulation (ECP) and transscleral diode cycloablation (TDC) are generally utilized in the later stages of the disease or in refractory or end-stage glaucoma patients.

Answering a few questions about your patient can help determine which surgical intervention is most appropriate: (1) What is the target IOP? (2) Has he or she had prior glaucoma surgery? (3) Does the patient have a secondary form of glaucoma such as neovascular glaucoma or uveitis? For maximum IOP lowering, trabeculectomy with mitomycin C (MMC) is usually considered the gold standard for IOP reduction into the teens or upper single digits. However, it is rarely the appropriate choice for patients with secondary forms of glaucoma, such as neovascular glaucoma or uveitis. Glaucoma implant surgery (eg, Baerveldt, Ahmed, or Molteno) is commonly used for eyes that have failed prior trabeculectomy or other ocular incisional surgery or in cases in which trabeculectomy, with or without antifibrotic treatment, has a high probability of failure. However, glaucoma implant surgery is increasing in popularity among surgeons.

This section on Choosing an Operative Technique is a very general framework for the considerations of surgical management, and additional information will generally be required to customize treatment for the individual patient. These considerations will be explored in more detail in the chapters that follow. In general, most patients can be divided into 2 groups. The first consists of patients with open-angle forms of glaucoma, including primary open-angle glaucoma (POAG), normal-tension glaucoma (NTG), and patients with noninflammatory secondary forms of glaucoma, such as pigment dispersion, exfoliation, and adult developmental glaucomas (eg, Axenfeld-Rieger syndrome). For this group, a trabeculectomy with or without antifibrotic agents is most commonly performed as a primary surgical procedure. However, glaucoma implants are increasingly being performed for glaucoma occurring in younger patients, particularly infants, and in patients with higher risk for postoperative inflammation. A variation on the traditional trabeculectomy uses the Ex-Press mini shunt (Alcon, Fort Worth, Texas) to enter the anterior chamber in place of an incisional sclerostomy. The Ex-Press mini shunt is a stainless steel device, that has a flat metal plate positioned under the scleral flap and a 50-μm tip that is inserted into the anterior chamber. The shunt provides a more predictable rate of flow than the traditional sclerostomy, does not require an iridectomy, and the resultant blebs tend to be lower. If a primary trabeculectomy fails, one may consider repeat trabeculectomy or glaucoma implant surgery. In cases in which repeat surgery fails to control IOP within the target range, cyclodestructive procedures such as TDC and ECP are a final option.

Patients with inflammatory forms of secondary glaucoma, such as neovascular glaucoma and uveitic glaucoma, have a high rate of trabeculectomy failure due to scarring and fibrosis of the sclerostomy and bleb. In these cases, glaucoma implants are frequently chosen for primary surgery. In patients with a significant inflammatory component to their disease, some surgeons feel that use of a valved glaucoma implant (eg, the Ahmed glaucoma valve [New World Medical, Inc., Rancho Cucamonga, California]) versus a nonvalved glaucoma implant (eg, the Baerveldt implant [Abbott Medical Optics, Santa Ana, California]) reduces the risk of postoperative hypotony and its attendant complications. If the target IOP is not achieved after trabeculectomy or glaucoma implant surgery, an additional implant or cycloablation type of surgery can be performed.

To avoid the postoperative complications associated with the more common procedures such as trabeculectomy with antimetabolites and tube shunts, newer IOP-lowering technologies continue to be developed.[11] Examples of new technologies include canaloplasty, the Trabeculotome (Katena Eye Instruments, Denville, New Jersey), the iStent (Glaukos Corp., Laguna Hills, California), and the SOLX suprachoroidal shunt (SOLX, Waltham, MA), and their potential uses will be more fully explored in further chapters. Due to their recent emergence, there is limited data on their long-term safety and efficacy, and none have been compared in randomized controlled trials with established surgeries. However, if proven effective, these new technologies could offer the possibility of IOP lowering without the complications associated with blebs or large extraocular implants.

CONCLUSION

Many options for IOP-lowering surgery are available to the glaucoma surgeon. Choosing the course of therapy that offers the greatest likelihood of success and the fewest return trips to the operating room is an important strategic goal. Keeping abreast of new techniques that improve success and/or reduce the risk of complications is key to the optimal management of this chronic disease.

KEY POINTS

1. The decision to proceed to surgery requires balancing the risks and benefits of surgery against the risk of progressive vision loss.

2. The surgical technique you choose should be influenced by each patient's unique disease presentation and his or her prior treatment history.

3. Preoperative patient education is a key factor in establishing appropriate expectations for postsurgical goals and outcomes.

REFERENCES

1. Friedman DS, Wolfs RC, O'Colmain BJ, et al. Prevalence of open-angle glaucoma among adults in the United States. *Arch Ophthalmol.* 2004;122(4):532-538.
2. Shields BM, Cooke DB, eds. *Textbook of Glaucoma.* 4th ed. Baltimore, MD: Lippincott Williams & Wilkins; 1998.
3. The AGIS Investigators. The Advanced Glaucoma Intervention Study (AGIS): 7. The relationship between control of intraocular pressure and visual field deterioration. *Am J Ophthalmol.* 2000;130(4):429-440.

4. Kass MA, Heuer DK, Higginbotham EJ, et al. The Ocular Hypertension Treatment Study: a randomized trial determines that topical ocular hypotensive medication delays or prevents the onset of primary open-angle glaucoma. *Arch Ophthalmol.* 2002;120(6): 701-713.

5. Heijl A, Leske MC, Bengtsson B, et al. Reduction of intraocular pressure and glaucoma progression: results from the Early Manifest Glaucoma Trial. *Arch Ophthalmol.* 2002; 120(10):1268-1279.

6. Lichter PR, Musch DC, Gillespie BW, et al. Interim clinical outcomes in the Collaborative Initial Glaucoma Treatment Study comparing initial treatment randomized to medications or surgery. *Ophthalmology.* 2001;108(11):1943-1953.

7. Gedde SJ, Herndon LW, Brandt JD, Budenz DL, Feuer WJ, Schiffman JC. Surgical complications in the Tube Versus Trabeculectomy Study during the first year of follow-up. *Am J Ophthalmol.* 2007;143(1):23-31.

8. Sarkisian SR Jr. Tube shunt complications and their prevention. *Curr Opin Ophthalmol.* 2009;20(2):126-130.

9. Nguyen QH. Primary surgical management refractory glaucoma: tubes as initial surgery. *Curr Opin Ophthalmol.* 2009;20(2):122-125.

10. Dietlein TS, Hermann MM, Jordan JF. The medical and surgical treatment of glaucoma. *Dtsch Arztebl Int.* 2009;106(37):597-605.

11. Mosaed S, Dustin L, Minckler DS. Comparative outcomes between newer and older surgeries for glaucoma. *Trans Am Ophthalmol Soc.* 2009;107:127-133.

2

SURGICAL ANATOMY

David Fleischman, MD and John P. Berdahl, MD

Successful surgery requires a thorough knowledge of anatomy. All glaucoma-related procedures require a thorough understanding of the terrain of the external eye, as well as an intimate relationship with the contents of the anterior chamber angle. A discussion of the gross and surgical anatomy of the eye follows, with special considerations for the pediatric patient and patients with other less common conditions.

GROSS AND SURGICAL ANATOMY

Knowledge of the boundaries and composition of the anterior chamber angle, in addition to the anatomical and surgical limbus, is critical to determine the location and depth of all incisions (including those with lasers) performed during glaucoma procedures. Appreciation of the ocular anatomy that may be affected or complicated during surgery will also allow the surgeon to remedy a potentially dangerous situation in a timely and efficient manner. Our discussion will follow an "inside-out" approach, first reviewing the anatomy of the angle and surrounding structures, then the surgical anatomy of the eye.

Drainage Angle

The drainage angle is responsible for the outflow of aqueous humor from the anterior chamber, and thus provides the primary resistance against this outflow, contributing to and maintaining intraocular pressure (IOP).

Anatomy of the Angle

The *angle* is an anatomically small yet physiologically indispensible region of the eye. The angle is formed by the intersection of the trabecular meshwork and the attachment of the peripheral iris. It contains the anterior extension of the ciliary muscle, the scleral spur, and Schlemm's canal within its boundaries.

Kahook M.
Essentials of Glaucoma Surgery (pp 11-22).
© 2012 SLACK Incorporated.

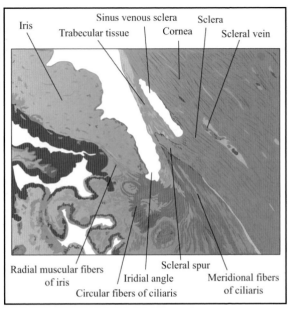

Figure 2-1. Histology image showing the spatial relationship between the iris, ciliary body, trabecular meshwork, and Schlemm's canal.

One way to consider the anatomy of this area is to follow the outflow of aqueous humor through it. After its formation by the ciliary processes in the posterior chamber, the aqueous humor flows around the lens and iris, through the pupil, and into the angle of the anterior chamber. Here, in the anterior chamber, the aqueous first encounters the trabecular meshwork.

The trabecular meshwork is triangular in cross-section, and its base rests on the scleral spur, with a small region abutting the ciliary muscle (Figure 2-1). Its apex is tethered by the most peripheral region of cornea and the termination of Descemet's membrane, known as Schwalbe's line. Aqueous encounters the trabecular meshwork for the first time through the uveal meshwork, a histological subregion of the trabeculum. It proceeds further into the corneoscleral meshwork and, finally, into the juxtacanalicular tissue. The juxtacanalicular tissue is the interface with the inner wall of Schlemm's canal, a primary area of aqueous fluid resistance in the eye, which establishes physiologic and potentially pathologic IOPs.[1-3]

The fluid that traverses the Schlemm's canal's inner endothelial wall flows some distance to reach any of the nearly 25 to 35 collector channels emanating from it. From the aqueous humor collector channels, the fluid continues to the aqueous veins, episcleral veins, orbital veins, and ultimately the intracranial cavernous venous sinus. Approximately 90% of aqueous outflow follows this path. The remaining 10% is drained through the uveoscleral pathway, with the anterior aspect of the ciliary muscle as its interface (Figure 2-2).

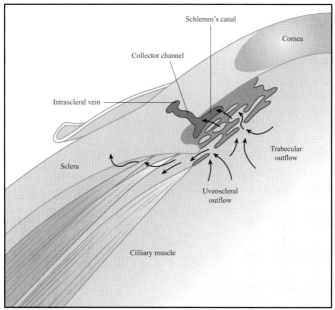

Figure 2-2. Sketch of the traditional and uveoscleral physiologic outflow pathways. (Adapted from Alm A. *Uveoscleral Outflow: Biology and Clinical Aspects.* London, UK: Mosby-Wolfe Medical Communications; 1998.)

Gonioscopic Anatomy of the Angle

Gonioscopy is the most accurate way of examining angle depth and providing a physiologic perspective for inspection of pathology. Its role in determining angle closure from open-angle glaucoma makes it an essential skill for all ophthalmologists. Gonioscopy also allows the ophthalmologist to appreciate the patient's anatomy prior to and during procedures, such as laser trabeculoplasty in the adult and goniotomy in the infant. Keeping in mind the anatomy of the angle as described previously, the gonioscopic view makes sense. In a deep view of the angle, with a flat attachment of the peripheral iris, the following structures should be appreciated from anterior to posterior[4] (Figures 2-3 and 2-4):

- *Schwalbe's line:* This is the demarcation of the final extent of Descemet's membrane and its transition toward the unpigmented trabecular meshwork.

- *Trabecular meshwork:* A fine, granular-appearing structure resembling ground glass is located just posterior to the margin of Schwalbe's line. The anterior portion of the trabecular meshwork is unpigmented, whereas the posterior portion of the trabecular meshwork is pigmented. The majority of aqueous outflow occurs here.

Figure 2-3. Gonioscopic image. 1. Pupil border, 2. Peripheral iris, 3. Ciliary body, 4. Scleral spur, 5. Pigmented and nonpigmented trabecular meshwork, 6. Schwalbe's line.

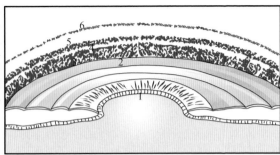

Figure 2-4. Gonioscopic sketch relating to Figure 2-3 that shows the anterior chamber angle structures. 1. Pupil border, 2. Peripheral iris, 3. Ciliary body, 4. Scleral spur, 5. Pigmented and nonpigmented trabecular meshwork, 6. Schwalbe's line.

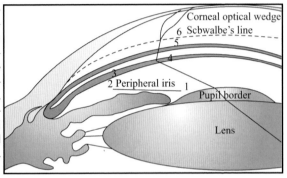

- *Scleral spur:* The posterior attachment of the trabecular meshwork. This is the most prominent structure within the angle.
- *Ciliary body:* The innermost region of the ciliary body is appreciated in the open angle. Located just posterior to the scleral spur, it serves as the aqueous outflow of the uveoscleral pathway.
- *Peripheral iris:* The insertion of the peripheral iris is best seen when the approach is flat.

Iris

The iris should always be examined and its insertion angle, as viewed by gonioscopy, noted. Rubeosis or other iris abnormalities must be identified, if present, through slit-lamp examination or gonioscopy. Rubeotic irides are prone to bleeding during iridectomy or iris manipulation.[1-3]

Ciliary Body and Pars Plana

The ciliary body is the most internal of the angle structures. It is composed of the ciliary muscle and the ciliary processes and draws out from the foundation of the iris. At the ora serrata, the flat part of the anterior

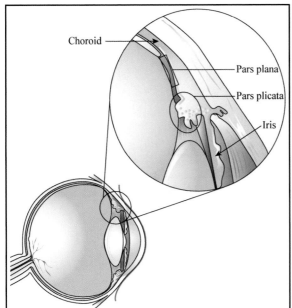

Figure 2-5. Drawing demonstrating the relationship of the choroid, pars plana, pars plicata, lens, and iris.

Labels in figure: Choroid, Pars plana, Pars plicata, Iris

ciliary body—the pars plicata—fuses with the choroid. The posterior portion of the ciliary body is the pars plana, the oft-accessed site for performing procedures, such as vitrectomies, injections, and ultrasonic lensectomies. Figure 2-5 shows the relationship of the ciliary body. The outermost fibers of the ciliary muscle attach to the corneoscleral trabecular meshwork and the scleral spur. Approximately 70 ciliary processes project off the pars plicata in a radial fashion. The ciliary processes are found internal to the ciliary muscle and, with the pars plana, form the lateral wall of the posterior chamber. Underlying the iris, the ciliary processes can occasionally be seen gonioscopically with dramatic mydriasis, aniridia, or a surgical coloboma. Otherwise, they are easily visualized endoscopically.[1-3] Functionally, the ciliary processes are responsible for the production and inflow regulation of the aqueous humor. For this reason, the ciliary body could be ablated to decrease the production of aqueous humor as a means of IOP reduction in refractory cases. With endocyclophotocoagulation, a laser unit attached to a probe is inserted through a scleral or corneal incision and endoscopically delivers a pulsed, continuous wave to the ciliary processes, thereby causing localized destruction. Transscleral cyclophotocoagulation uses a similar concept but is performed externally. The laser's focus is delivered 1 to 1.5 mm behind the limbus. It is offset from the aiming beam for the purpose of delivering the maximal amount of energy at the level of the ciliary body.[5]

Figure 2-6. Photograph of the limbus (inset).

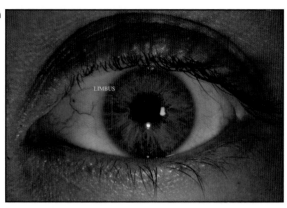

Surgical Anatomy of the Eye

Limbus

The limbus is one of the most important landmarks in glaucoma surgery. This is the junction between the cornea and the sclera. Grossly, it appears as a faint blue ring around the cornea (Figure 2-6). The clear corneal tissue inserts into white sclera. The anterior portion of the limbus represents the clear cornea, and the posterior end is white scleral tissue. This results in the gray and bluish hue of the limbus. Occasionally, conjunctival vessels can obscure this view; however, a scleral dissection clearly identifies the limbus.

The surgical limbus has a degree of dimensionality, and it is more accurate to conceptualize the limbus as having 2 distinct regions, a border between the cornea and limbus and a border between the sclera and limbus. (Worthen[3] uses the analogy of a "river with two banks.") The anatomical limbus is defined by its anterior aspect, which overlies a line composed of the ends of Bowman's layer and Descemet's membrane. Therefore, the surgical limbus lies anterior to the anatomical limbus. The posterior end overlies the conjunctival tissue, which rests in the iris recess; this is clearly seen as the posterior aspect of the blue limbus. The limbus is much broader in the superior and inferior aspects of the eye as compared to the vertical meridians. The average limbus width is 1.2 mm superiorly, 1.1 mm inferiorly, 1.0 mm nasally, and 0.9 mm temporally (Figure 2-7). For this and other reasons, a superior approach is usually taken in filtration procedures, often in the nasal quadrant, to better allow for future glaucoma or cataract surgery.

The limbus overlies the angle recess. In most cases, a full-thickness perpendicular incision on the scleral edge of the limbus will intersect the

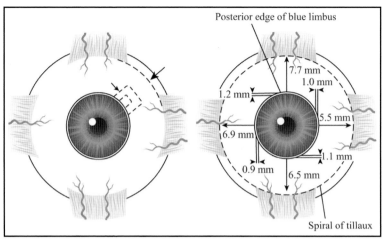

Figure 2-7. Sketch demonstrating the spiral of Tillaux, the width of the limbus, and the insertion of the extraocular muscles.

anterior trabecular meshwork. However, variability in the shape of the eye influences its exact orientation and depth. For example, a small or hyperopic eye may have the limbus lying deeper into the angle, whereas a larger or myopic eye will have more depth within the angle recess below and perpendicular to the posterior limbus (Figure 2-8).

Sclera

Over 80% of the globe is covered by sclera. This structure is often surgically manipulated for filtering procedures and traction sutures. Much like the cornea, its main component is type I collagen. As opposed to the cornea, these fibrils are oriented in random fashion, which is the main difference between the optically transparent cornea and the characteristically white sclera. The tendons of the rectus muscles insert into the sclera posterior to the limbus (see Figure 2-7).

The scleral thickness varies by location, ranging from 300 μm to just over 1 mm. The insertions of the rectus muscles are the thinnest areas of the sclera. The sclera is at its thickest around the optic nerve and the posterior pole—approximately 0.86 mm ± 0.26. The sclera thins as it extends anteriorly towards the cornea to the equator (0.42 mm ± 0.14) and ora serrata (0.42 mm ± 0.13). The sclera again thickens slightly at the limbus (0.50 mm ± 0.10). Trabeculectomies are often performed over the area anterior to the equator and directly over the ora serrata. This undoubtedly increases one's appreciation for the delicate nature of the partial thickness scleral dissection.[6]

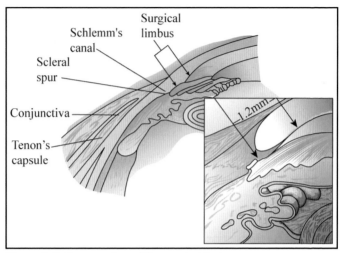

Figure 2-8. Cross-section of the surgical limbus.

Myopes, in particular those who have enlarged axial lengths, have thinner scleras when compared to normal-sized eyes. In comparison to those with normal axial lengths, the sclera is thinner at the equator and posterior pole—a difference of nearly a tenth of a millimeter at the equator and almost three-tenths of a millimeter at the posterior pole.[6]

The sclera is nearly avascular. Two exceptions are the episcleral vessels overlying the sclera, and the intrascleral vascular plexus located posterior to the limbus. Slit-lamp examination will also enable the clinical to identify a number of emissary channels that transmit nerves and vessels.

Conjunctiva

The conjunctiva covers the entirety of the inner eyelid, the fornix, and the external eye up to the limbus. The adequacy of mobility of the conjunctiva should be assessed prior to trabeculectomy or drainage device implantation. Conjunctival hyperemia must always be addressed in the assessment prior to glaucoma surgery. The implications of episcleral vein engorgement or infection are significant, as opposed to irritation from medication or preservative-induced hyperemia.

It is important to appreciate that procedures that violate the conjunctiva may lead to its scarring or reduce its mobility for subsequent procedures. Many times, excessive scarring from prior surgeries will alter the procedure and approach or preclude its utility. Handle the conjunctiva delicately.

Tenon's Capsule

Found between the sclera and conjunctiva, Tenon's capsule is a distinct vascular and elastic connective tissue that arises from the episclera approximately 2 mm posterior to the margin of the cornea and extends across the entire globe to the optic nerve where it fuses with dura mater.

Extraocular Muscles and Their Insertions

Two anterior ciliary arteries mark the insertion of the rectus muscles, with the exception of the lateral rectus muscle, which has one. Underlying the insertion points of the extraocular muscles is the ora serrata internally. A circle can be drawn, with variable distances from the posterior limbus, termed the spiral of Tillaux. The distance of the superior rectus muscle to the posterior limbus is 7.7 mm, 5.5 mm from the medial rectus to the limbus, 6.5 mm at the inferior rectus, and finally 6.9 mm at the lateral rectus (see Figure 2-7).

CONSIDERATIONS OF THE SURGICAL ANATOMY OF THE PEDIATRIC PATIENT

Congenital conditions can cause glaucoma in the infant with distortions of normal anatomy. Apart from pathologic conditions, there are normal developmental anatomic differences of the pediatric patient when compared with the adult. The eye of a newborn is two-thirds the size of an adult's eye, crowding an already tiny area into a smaller space. Landmarks are not necessarily in their adult configuration until 1 year of age. The following list highlights some significant differences:

- *The angle and peripheral iris:* The contents of the angle have not fully developed and oriented themselves in their final locations until 6 to 12 months after birth. On gonioscopy, the most characteristic feature of the angle is the trabecular meshwork in the child of age 1 or younger, as opposed to the scleral spur in adults. The peripheral iris attachment is also thinner and flatter in children.

  In infantile glaucoma, the iris has a more anterior insertion than in a healthy child. Associated with this is a diffuse translucency of the angle structures, creating an obscure view of the ciliary body, trabecular meshwork, and scleral spur. This is known as Barkan's membrane.

- *Ciliary processes:* These structures are much thinner and fingerlike in infants and children.

- *Limbus:* The bluish hue of the limbus is much more difficult to appreciate in the young patient. Other landmarks must then be used. The edge of Bowman's layer, where the corneal and conjunctival epithelia merge, is one alternative.

The texture of the scleral border of the limbus is fragile compared with adults. Procedures in this area must be performed carefully in the pediatric patient for this reason, as it is possible to damage the ciliary body or enter the anterior chamber even with minimal dissection.

- *Tenon's capsule:* Tenon's capsule is more prominent in infants and children compared with adults.

SPECIAL CONSIDERATIONS

A number of operations and postoperative conditions exist that alter the external and internal anatomy of the eye, creating a number of unique anatomical considerations. The following discussion is limited to 2 important procedures that have frequent associations with glaucoma.

Prior Vitrectomy and Silicone Oil Injection

Vitrectomy is a common ophthalmic surgery. Secondary glaucomas are a frequent complication of this procedure.[7] It is increasingly important to recognize the anatomical changes and challenges that arise from these procedures. IOP reduction is helpful in the management of these patients.[8] Late effects of silicone oil tamponade can include pupillary block, anterior synechiae, rubeosis iridis, or migration of silicone oil into the angle.[9] In a situation in which the patient is aphakic and has undergone vitrectomy with silicone oil injection, cohesive forces produce a smooth, rounded surface of the silicone bubble. With a peripheral iridectomy and excess silicone oil, the bubble, abutted against the posterior surface of the superior iris (at the 12 o'clock position), will enter the anterior chamber and produce pupillary block. For this reason, a peripheral iridectomy at 6 o'clock can produce an alternate aqueous outflow pathway.[10]

Scleral Buckle

Scleral buckling is another retinal surgery that can dramatically alter the contour and shape of the eye. The procedure has been frequently associated with glaucoma and typical glaucoma visual field deficits. The most common explanation given for this is the external compression-induced IOP elevation. Some argue that the visual field changes following a buckle are in fact due solely to choroidal vascular compression, impeding disc supply. Experimental evidence points toward mechanisms resulting in angle closure. The venous system emptying toward the vortex veins is occluded by the buckle, causing congestion of the ciliary body. As the ciliary body begins to swell, it pushes the iris anteriorly, resulting in angle closure. Another similar explanation suggests that the obstructed uveoscleral outflow and increased episcleral venous pressure results in elevated IOP.[11]

Because glaucoma can result from or independently develop in an eye operatively treated with a scleral buckle, a filtration or shunting surgery may eventually be needed. Unfortunately, by the very nature of altering the ocular superstructure, excessive crowding and poor conjunctival conditions make tube shunts very difficult to perform procedurally. The anterior chamber tube shunt to an encircling band (ACTEB) procedure developed by Shocket et al[12] has been shown to be efficacious in these cases, as it creates an artificial outflow from the aqueous chamber to an episcleral explant.[12,13]

CONCLUSION

A thorough understanding of the anatomy related to glaucoma surgery is essential. Familiarity with the anatomy of the angle, limbus, ciliary body, iris, and insertions of the extraocular muscles will enable the surgeon to ably and confidently approach the procedure, and adapt accordingly when necessary. Appreciating the anatomical differences in the pediatric patient dictates the type of procedure performed and can potentially prevent complications. The anatomic changes from scleral buckles, vitrectomies, and other retinal salvage procedures can result in secondary glaucomas. As these complications are responsive to surgical intervention, knowledge of these unique conditions can assist the surgeon greatly.

KEY POINTS

- The angle is composed of the anterior extension of the ciliary muscle, the scleral spur, and Schlemm's canal.
- The juxtacanalicular tissue is the interface with the inner wall of Schlemm's canal, the primary area of aqueous fluid resistance.
- Ninety percent of aqueous fluid outflow exits through the trabecular meshwork; the remaining 10% flows through the uveoscleral pathway.
- From anterior to posterior, the gonioscopic appearance of the angle in an adult: Cornea, Schwalbe's line, nonpigmented trabecular meshwork, pigmented trabecular meshwork, scleral spur, ciliary body, and peripheral iris.
- The average limbus width is 1.2 mm superiorly, 1.1 mm inferiorly, 1.0 mm nasally and 0.9 mm temporally.
- Tenon's capsule originates from the episclera 2 mm posterior to the margin of the cornea and extends to the dura mater at the optic nerve.

- The spiral of Tillaux describes the distance of the insertion of the extraocular muscles to the posterior limbus: superior rectus, 7.7 mm; medial rectus, 5.5 mm; inferior rectus, 6.5 mm; and lateral rectus, 6.9 mm.

- The contents of the angle do not orient themselves in their final locations until 6 to 12 months after birth.

- Anatomical changes from surgeries (eg, vitrectomies, silicone oil insertion, and scleral buckles) must be accounted for because they may pose challenges to the treatment of glaucoma.

REFERENCES

1. Mills RP, Weinreb RN. *Glaucoma Surgical Techniques: Ophthalmology Monographs 4.* San Francisco, CA: American Academy of Ophthalmology; 1991.
2. Trope GE. *Glaucoma Surgery.* Boca Raton, FL: Taylor & Francis Group; 2005.
3. Worthen DM. Anatomical landmarks in glaucoma surgery. *Int Ophthalmol Clin.* 1981;21(1):15-28.
4. Choplin NT, Lundy DC. *Atlas of Glaucoma.* 2nd ed. London, UK: Informa UK Limited; 2007.
5. Lin SC. Endoscopic and transscleral cyclophotocoagulation for the treatment of refractory glaucoma. *J Glaucoma.* 2008;17:238-247.
6. Vurgese S, Panda-Jonas S, Jonas JB. Scleral thickness in human eyes. *PLoS ONE.* 2012;7(1):e29692.
7. Gedde SJ. Management of glaucoma after retinal detachment surgery. *Curr Opin Ophthalmol.* 2002;13(2):103-109.
8. Budenz DL, Taba KE, Feuer WJ. Surgical management of secondary glaucoma after pars plana vitrectomy and silicone oil injection for complex retinal detachment. *Ophthalmology.* 2001;108(9):1628-1632.
9. Honavar SG, Goyal M, Majji AB, et al. Glaucoma after pars plana vitrectomy and silicone oil injection for complicated retinal detachments. *Ophthalmology.* 1999;106(1):169-176.
10. Beekhuis WH, Ando F, Zivojnović R, et al. Basal iridectomy at 6 o'clock in the aphakic eye treated with silicone oil: prevention of keratopathy and secondary glaucoma. *Br J Ophthalmol.* 1987;71(3):197-200.
11. Sato EA, Shinoda K, Inoue M, et al. Reduced choroidal blood flow can induce visual field defect in open angle glaucoma patients without intraocular pressure elevation following encircling scleral buckling. *Retina.* 2008;28(3):493-497.
12. Schocket SS, Nirankari VS, Lakhanpal V, et al. Anterior chamber tube shunt to an encircling band in the treatment of neovascular glaucoma and other refractory glaucomas. A long-term study. *Ophthalmology.* 1985;92:553-562.
13. Suh MH, Park KH, Kim TW, Kim DM. The efficacy of a modified ACTSEB (anterior chamber tube shunt to an encircling band) procedure. *J Glaucoma.* 2007;16(7):622-626.

3

WOUND MODULATION AFTER FILTRATION SURGERY

Leonard K. Seibold, MD and Malik Y. Kahook, MD

Filtration surgery for the treatment of glaucoma presents a unique challenge to surgeons. Although most incisional surgeries require adequate and complete wound healing for a successful outcome, filtration surgery relies on an abbreviated and incomplete healing process for long-term success. It is, in fact, a vigorous and robust healing process that accounts for the failure of most surgery in glaucoma.

WOUND HEALING

After the conjunctiva is incised during surgery, a sequential and complex process of wound healing begins. This cascade of events begins with vascular leakage and coagulation. Blood vessels leak platelets, blood cells, plasma proteins, clotting factors, numerous tissue growth factors, and chemokines. The coagulation cascade is stimulated and clot formation begins, augmented by platelet aggregation. This insoluble fibrin-fibronectin matrix serves as the initial scaffold for future inflammatory cells to invade. Cellular migration and proliferation constitute the next phase of wound healing. Within a few days, inflammatory cells such as neutrophils, macrophages, and monocytes migrate to the wound site and begin tissue debridement and control of infection. Macrophages also serve to provide several pro-inflammatory growth factors such as platelet derived growth factor, fibroblast growth factor, and transforming growth factor beta (TGF-β).[1,2]

During the proliferative phase, quiescent fibroblasts differentiate into a more active state—termed myofibroblasts. These activated fibroblasts not only produce loose connective tissue but they begin the process of remodeling existing extracellular matrix with the aid of matrix metalloproteinases. Pro-angiogenic factors, such as vascular endothelial growth factor (VEGF),

Kahook M.
Essentials of Glaucoma Surgery (pp 23–30).
© 2012 SLACK Incorporated.

help to stimulate angiogenesis with the arrival of endothelial cells to create new capillary networks. The resultant primitive granulation tissue is then remodeled into a mature scar in the final phase of healing. Immature collagen fibrils are crosslinked, condensed, and dehydrated, whereas fibroblasts undergo apoptosis and disappear. Primitive vessels are remodeled, and a mature scar is completed.[1,2]

WOUND MODULATION

Successful glaucoma filtration surgery hinges on the incomplete closure of newly created aqueous outflow pathways and the formation of filtration blebs. Therefore, several methods have been used in an attempt to augment or blunt the natural wound healing response during the preoperative, intraoperative, and postoperative periods. This concept of wound modulation is especially valid in patients at high risk for surgical failure, including those with aphakia, pseuodophakia, neovascular glaucoma, uveitic glaucoma, African-American origin, or previous failed filtration surgery.

ANTI-INFLAMMATORIES

The first and most obvious choice for modification of the normal wound healing pathway are anti-inflammatory agents. Glucocorticoids in particular have been shown to successfully inhibit postoperative scarring and increase bleb survival rates. Steroids achieve this through the alteration of several stages in wound healing. Early on, the concentration and migration of neutrophils and macrophages are mitigated through steroidal effect. Resultant phagocytosis and growth factor release is blunted as well. Within the cell, steroids block the production of arachidonic acid and its downstream mediators such as leukotrienes, prostaglandins, and thromboxanes. Due to their broad effects, steroids are frequently used at the operative and postoperative phases with repeatedly proven success.[1,3,4] Preoperative steroidal use has also been found to be beneficial to long-term trabeculectomy success.[5] While not as extensively studies, limited evidence suggests an equivalent benefit with nonsteroidal agents as well.[6]

ANTIFIBROTICS

In clinical practice today, antifibrotic agents such as 5-FU and mitomycin C (MMC) have emerged as the preferred wound modulation agents worldwide.[7] Although steroids and nonsteroidal anti-inflammatory drugs (NSAIDs) inhibit early wound healing, antifibrotic agents help to prevent end-stage scar formation by direct modification of fibroblast proliferation and activity at the wound site.

The antimetabolite 5-FU is a fluorinated pyrimidine analogue that competitively inhibits the further synthesis of thymidine nucleotides. By blocking normal production of the essential nucleotide, DNA synthesis is prevented and cell death results.[1] Experimental studies have illustrated 5-FU's strong inhibition of human Tenon's fibroblast activity and growth, as well as interfering with fibroblast-mediated collagen contraction.[8] This desirable effect in the laboratory quickly translated to clinical use, initially as a series of subconjunctival injections after filtration surgery. The Fluorouracil Filtering Surgery Study (FFSS) was a major National Eye Institute-sponsored multicenter, randomized, prospective clinical study on the use of postoperative 5-FU in patients at high risk for failure. A total of 213 patients who had undergone cataract surgery or had 1 failed filtering surgery were randomized to either trabeculectomy alone or trabeculectomy with 1 week of twice-daily 5-mg 5-FU injections, followed by 1 week of daily injections. At 5 years, the failure rate was significantly less in the 5-FU group (51%) compared with the control group (74%). The greatest benefit of 5-FU injections appears to be within the first 18 months, after which the rate of failure progresses at a similar, steady rate in both groups.[9] Subsequent studies have found similar success with the use of 5-FU intraoperatively, typically applied to the surgical bed for up to 5 minutes with a sponge soaked in 25 to 50 mg/mL of the drug.[10] This method of administration has gained favor due to the 1-time dosing and eliminated need for frequent postoperative injection visits.

The most commonly reported adverse event with the postoperative use of the antimetabolite involves corneal toxicity. Findings include punctuate epitheliopathy, filamentary keratopathy, gross epithelial defects, and melanokeratosis. The frequency of such corneal findings is dependent on the dose and frequency of injection but may exceed 50% in large accumulative doses. The intraoperative use of 5-FU has dramatically reduced this complication rate by reducing or eliminating the need for sunconjunctival injections. More serious complications, such as bleb leaks, were also found to be more common in the FFSS trial (2% in controls, 9% in 5-FU).[1,9,10] Although no randomized trial has shown an increase in endophthalmitis with 5-FU use, the increase in bleb leaks has been shown to be a significant risk factor for infection.

MMC is an antibiotic agent derived from the fungus *Streptomyces caespitosus* that is now commonly utilized during filtration surgery for its antiproliferative actions. The drug acts as a cell cycle, nonspecific alkylating agent that crosslinks DNA, preventing proliferation. As a wound-modulating agent, MMC has been shown to be more potent and durable than 5-FU, requiring only single intraoperative applications at doses approximately 100 times less. Cell culture experiments found that while 5-FU is fairly specific for inhibition of fibroblasts, MMC was toxic to both fibroblasts and endothelial cells.[1,11,12]

The initial success of MMC as a wound-modulating agent in glaucoma surgery was established by Chen et al[13] in 1983, in which they found that the agent prolonged bleb survival in high-risk patients. Subsequent animal and human studies have also shown MMC to be effective at achieving lower intraocular pressure (IOP) after surgery and enhancing bleb survival rates.[1] In primary trabeculectomy, prospective and placebo-controlled studies have found MMC to significantly reduce failure rates at 1 year, but IOP reduction was similar to controls.[13,14] One large review of intermediate long-term results of MMC (0.2 to 0.5 mg/mL) in trabeculectomy found survival rates of 94.2% at 1 year and 88.7% at 3 years.[14] In patients undergoing combined trabeculectomy and phacoemulsification, 2 separate prospective, randomized, placebo-controlled trials found that the MMC group produced significantly lower IOP compared to placebo in the first year of follow-up.[15,16] Filtration blebs were also found to be larger, and patients required fewer medications to achieve target IOP.[15,16] Subgroup analysis from a later, large prospective study found improved outcomes with MMC only in patients with either African-American origin, IOP greater than 20 mm Hg on maximum medical therapy, or using at least 2 medications.[17] Recent publications have also shown the superiority of MMC over 5-FU with regard to efficacy in IOP-lowering and survival rates. However, this applied only to high-risk eyes, as primary or low-risk eyes showed similar outcomes between the 2 antifibrotics.[18,19]

The potency and duration of action of MMC comes at the cost of potentially more complications. The use of MMC has been associated with the development of thin-walled, avascular blebs that have a higher propensity to develop late-onset bleb leaks, over-filtration, hypotony, infection, and endophthalmitis. The infection rate with MMC-augmented surgeries has been found to be as high as 2.1% at 16 months and hypotony rate as high as 14%.[1] Recent reviews of bleb-associated endophthalmitis found more than 80% of the identified cases were after MMC-augmented surgeries.[20]

NEW METHODS OF WOUND MODULATION

Despite the efficacy of current antifibrotic agents, safety concerns have driven the research and development of new methods to modulate the healing process in filtration surgery. Newer agents offer a more targeted and potentially safer approach to impeding wound healing. Several methods have been studied in vitro and in animals, although few have progressed to human use and clinical trials.

A large area of research centers on the blockade of growth factors involved in stimulating the healing process. The anti-VEGF agents, bevacizumab and ranibizumab, have been used in several small series and trials as an intravitreal or subconjunctival adjunct to trabeculectomy. Most reports found good outcomes with the agents, particularly in cases of neovascular glaucoma, without any significant adverse events.[21] TGF-β is a significant catalyst in the scarring process and has become a target for inhibition. A novel monoclonal antibody against TGF-β2, CAT-152, was found to be effective at inhibiting fibroblasts in vitro and prolonging bleb survival in rabbits. However, subsequent human trials failed to show a benefit of the antibody over placebo.[22] Other drugs utilized for their inhibitory effects on growth factors include suramin and tranilast. Both agents have shown good success in vitro and in rabbits. Initial small human trials have been at least as efficacious as MMC, but larger trials are needed.[23,24]

Multiple other approaches have been attempted and are involved in ongoing study. Inside the cell, signal pathway transduction is being targeted to block the effects of pro-inflammatory factors like TGF-β.[25] Gene therapy and siRNA molecules are also being utilized for their ability to selectively impede the proliferation and activity of Tenon's fibroblast cells.[26,27] Serum amyloid P is a naturally occurring protein with the ability to interfere with the monocyte–macrophage response at the site of wound creation. In vitro, the blockade of macrophage action has been found to significantly alter fibroblast activation and proliferation.[28] One alternative to pharmacologic agents is the use of beta radiation at the time of surgery. Initial human studies found no improvement of success over placebo in low-risk cases, but in later work, failure rates did significantly decline with beta radiation in a more high-risk population.[29] Finally, photodynamic therapy (PDT) has been employed as a method to localize treatment to bleb area alone. In the lone human trial, a small group of patients showed good success rates with PDT, but no placebo-controlled trials have been published.[29,30]

Although it is challenging to compare these agents given the wide variability in study design and patient populations, none of these newer methods have been proven as efficacious as the more established antimetabolites. Research is ongoing and more extensive human trials are needed to fully characterize the effectiveness and safety profile of these newer agents.

Key Points

1. The wound healing process after filtration surgery is quite complex, occuring in overlapping and sequential stages.
2. Successful glaucoma surgery depends on modification of normal wound healing to prevent scarring.
3. Steroids are an important agent to prolong bleb survival.
4. The antifibrotic agents 5-FU and MMC can reduce surgical failure rates and may help achieve lower IOP postoperatively.
5. These agents must be used with caution, as they may lead to adverse events such as increased rates of hypotony and bleb-related infections.

6. Multiple new agents are being researched to achieve a safer and more effective wound modulating agent.

REFERENCES

1. Lama PJ, Fechtner RD. Antifibrotics and wound healing in glaucoma surgery. *Surv Ophthalmol.* 2003;48(3):314-346.
2. Skuta GL, Parrish RK II. Wound healing in glaucoma filtering surgery. *Surv Ophthalmol.* 1987;32(3):149-170.
3. Araujo SV, Spaeth GL, Roth SM, Starita RJ. A ten-year follow-up on a prospective, randomized trial of postoperative corticosteroids after trabeculectomy. *Ophthalmology.* 1995;102(12):1753-1759.
4. Starita RJ, Fellman RL, Spaeth GL, et al. Short- and long-term effects of postoperative corticosteroids on trabeculectomy. *Ophthalmology.* 1985;92(7):938-946.
5. Baudouin C, Nordmann JP, Denis P, et al. Efficacy of indomethacin 0.1% and fluorometholone 0.1% on conjunctival inflammation following chronic application of antiglaucomatous drugs. *Graefes Arch Clin Exp Ophthalmol.* 2002;240(11):929-935.
6. Breusegem C, Spielberg L, Van Ginderdeuren R, et al. Preoperative nonsteroidal anti-inflammatory drug or steroid and outcomes after trabeculectomy: a randomized controlled trial. *Ophthalmology.* 2010;117(7):1324-1330.
7. Joshi AB, Parrish RK II, Feuer WF. 2002 survey of the American Glaucoma Society: practice preferences for glaucoma surgery and antifibrotic use. *J Glaucoma.* 2005;14(2):172-174.
8. Khaw PT, Sherwood MB, MacKay SL, et al. Five-minute treatments with fluorouracil, floxuridine, and mitomycin have long-term effects on human Tenon's capsule fibroblasts. *Arch Ophthalmol.* 1992;110(8):1150-1154.
9. Five-year follow-up of the Fluorouracil Filtering Surgery Study. The Fluorouracil Filtering Surgery Study Group. *Am J Ophthalmol.* 1996;121(4):349-366.
10. Smith MF, Sherwood MB, Doyle JW, Khaw PT. Results of intraoperative 5-fluorouracil supplementation on trabeculectomy for open-angle glaucoma. *Am J Ophthalmol.* 1992;114(6):737-741.
11. Jampel HD. Effect of brief exposure to mitomycin C on viability and proliferation of cultured human Tenon's capsule fibroblasts. *Ophthalmology.* 1992;99(9):1471-1476.
12. Smith S, D'Amore PA, Dreyer EB. Comparative toxicity of mitomycin C and 5-fluorouracil in vitro. *Am J Ophthalmol.* 1994;118(3):332-337.
13. Chen CW, Huang HT, Bair JS, Lee CC. Trabeculectomy with simultaneous topical application of mitomycin-C in refractory glaucoma. *J Ocul Pharmacol.* 1990;6(3):175-182.
14. Cheung JC, Wright MM, Murali S, Pederson JE. Intermediate-term outcome of variable dose mitomycin C filtering surgery. *Ophthalmology.* 1997;104(1):143-149.
15. Carlson DW, Alward WL, Barad JP, et al. A randomized study of mitomycin augmentation in combined phacoemulsification and trabeculectomy. *Ophthalmology.* 1997;104(4):719-724.
16. Cohen JS, Greff LJ, Novack GD, Wind BE. A placebo-controlled, double-masked evaluation of mitomycin C in combined glaucoma and cataract procedures. *Ophthalmology.* 1996;103(11):1934-1942.
17. Shin DH, Ren J, Juzych MS, et al. Primary glaucoma triple procedure in patients with primary open-angle glaucoma: the effect of mitomycin C in patients with and without prognostic factors for filtration failure. *Am J Ophthalmol.* 1998;125(3):346-352.
18. Lamping KA, Belkin JK. 5-Fluorouracil and mitomycin C in pseudophakic patients. *Ophthalmology.* 1995;102(1):70-75.
19. Palanca-Capistrano AM, Hall J, Cantor LB, et al. Long-term outcomes of intraoperative 5-fluorouracil versus intraoperative mitomycin C in primary trabeculectomy surgery. *Ophthalmology.* 2009;116(2):185-190.

20. Song A, Scott IU, Flynn HW Jr, Budenz DL. Delayed-onset bleb-associated endophthalmitis: clinical features and visual acuity outcomes. *Ophthalmology.* 2002;109(5):985-991.
21. Horsley MB, Kahook MY. Anti-VEGF therapy for glaucoma. *Curr Opin Ophthalmol.* 2010;21(2):112-117.
22. Siriwardena D, Khaw PT, King AJ, et al. Human antitransforming growth factor beta(2) monoclonal antibody—a new modulator of wound healing in trabeculectomy: a randomized placebo controlled clinical study. *Ophthalmology.* 2002;109(3):427-431.
23. Chihara E, Dong J, Ochiai H, Hamada S. Effects of tranilast on filtering blebs: a pilot study. *J Glaucoma.* 2002;11(2):127-133.
24. Mietz H, Krieglstein GK. Suramin to enhance glaucoma filtering procedures: a clinical comparison with mitomycin. *Ophthalmic Surg Lasers.* 2001;32(5):358-369.
25. Xiao YQ, Liu K, Shen JF, et al. SB-431542 inhibition of scar formation after filtration surgery and its potential mechanism. *Invest Ophthalmol Vis Sci.* 2009;50(4):1698-1706.
26. Perkins TW, Faha B, Ni M, et al. Adenovirus-mediated gene therapy using human p21WAF-1/Cip-1 to prevent wound healing in a rabbit model of glaucoma filtration surgery. *Arch Ophthalmol.* 2002;120(7):941-949.
27. Wang F, Qi LX, Su Y, et al. Inhibition of cell proliferation of Tenon's capsule fibroblast by S-phase kinase-interacting protein 2 targeting SiRNA through increasing p27 protein level. *Invest Ophthalmol Vis Sci.* 2010;51(3):1475-1482.
28. Duffield JS, Lupher ML Jr. PRM-151 (recombinant human serum amyloid P/pentraxin 2) for the treatment of fibrosis. *Drug News Perspect.* 2010;23(5):305-315.
29. Kirwan JF, Cousens S, Venter L, et al. Effect of beta radiation on success of glaucoma drainage surgery in South Africa: randomised controlled trial. *BMJ.* 2006;333(7575):942.
30. Rehman SU, Amoaku WM, Doran RM, et al. Randomized controlled clinical trial of beta irradiation as an adjunct to trabeculectomy in open-angle glaucoma. *Ophthalmology.* 2002;109(2):302-6.

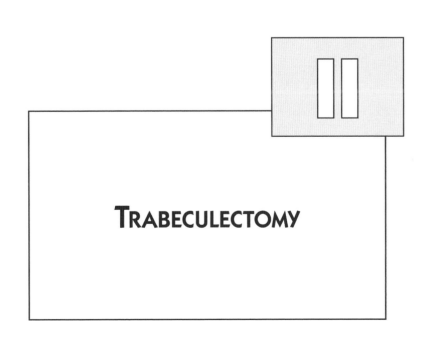

TRABECULECTOMY

4

Trabeculectomy Surgery
Decision Making and Technique

Marcos Reyes, MD; James A. Fox, MD;
and Mahmoud A. Khaimi, MD

The goal of glaucoma filtration surgery is to decrease the intraocular pressure (IOP) to a level that will arrest or retard the loss of the nerve fiber layer. The unifying feature of all glaucoma filtering surgery is to create a drainage system that flows into a newly created sub-Tenon's/conjunctival reservoir, the "bleb." The creation of a bleb allows the aqueous to bypass the nonfunctioning or, more commonly, poorly functioning trabecular meshwork and thereby lower the IOP.

Preoperative Assessment

Typically, the surgical option becomes a viable management alternative in the presence of advancing visual field defects and/or progressive loss of retinal nerve fiber layer, despite maximal tolerated medical therapy and laser trabeculoplasty (when appropriate).

Risk factors for surgical failure and the quality of postoperative care should be considered prior to filtration surgery. The risk factors for filtration failure[1,2] include young patients (except for young myopes <50 years old, who are at risk for overfiltration and hypotony maculopathy), diabetes, higher preoperative IOP, African American patients, iris/angle neovascularization, uveitis, and prior failed filtration surgery. The patient and/or caretakers must understand that the postoperative care is just as important as the surgery itself and that all postoperative instructions must be followed. Poor postoperative compliance can lead to prolonged uveitis, posterior synechia, cystoid macular edema, and bleb failure.

Kahook M.
Essentials of Glaucoma Surgery (pp 33-48).
© 2012 SLACK Incorporated.

Additional Perioperative Considerations

Hyperopic Eyes

1. Prone to shallow/flat anterior chambers postoperatively. Consider tighter scleral flap closure to avoid postoperative hypotony and shallow/flat anterior chamber.

2. When associated with chronic angle closure, there is an increased risk of malignant glaucoma.

Pseudophakic (Postoperative) Eyes

1. Check conjunctival mobility prior to choosing a filter site as prior cataract surgery might lead to conjunctival scarring if performed through a scleral tunnel.

2. Use caution when creating a scleral flap through an old cataract wound incision because there is a risk of scleral flap avulsion.

3. Perform anterior vitrectomy for vitreous in the anterior chamber.

PERIOPERATIVE SYSTEMIC MEDICATIONS

Oral steroids may be useful in patients with uveitic glaucoma but should only be used in selected cases and preferably after consultation with an internist or uveitis specialist. Intraocular inflammation at the time of surgery is highly associated with bleb failure.

If possible, both anticoagulants and antiplatelet agents should be stopped to decrease the risk of intraoperative, retrobulbar, or suprachorial hemorrhage. Cessation of blood thinners should be done only after consultation with the patient's internist or cardiologist.[3] Many surgeons choose not to discontinue these medications due to the elevated risk of vascular events. This issue should be discussed thoroughly with the patient.

BASIC SURGICAL TECHNIQUE

Glaucoma filtration surgery is performed in either the superonasal quadrant or directly superior, leaving the superotemporal quadrant available for a repeat filtration surgery or the use of a glaucoma drainage device. Anesthesia is typically accomplished effectively with a retrobulbar block consisting of a combination of lidocaine, bupivacaine, and hyaluronidase. Lid blocks and general anesthesia are rarely required.

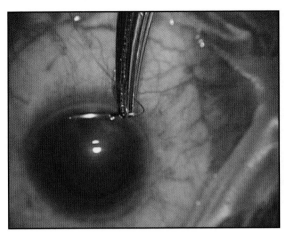

Figure 4-1. Superior corneal bridle suture.

Traction Sutures

A superior corneal bridle suture is the common approach used to rotate the eye inferiorly (Figure 4-1). This is performed with a 6-0 or 7-0 Vicryl or silk suture on a spatulated needle passed through clear, midstromal cornea approximately 1 mm from the superior limbus for approximately 2 to 2.5 mm. Gentle traction on the suture assures its integrity prior to taping or clamping the suture to the inferior drape or handing it over to an assistant to hold. An alternative approach is to place an inferior corneal bridle suture.

Avoid passing the needle into the anterior chamber, which produces a persistent aqueous leak at the suture site that could subsequently lead to intraoperative hypotony, a shallow anterior chamber, and possibly prevent the use of mitomycin C (MMC) due to the risk of intraocular tracking.

Creation of the Conjunctival Flap

The conjunctival flap may be either limbus- or fornix-based. Evidence suggests that both are successful.[4] However, debate continues regarding which is more efficacious. With either technique, the conjunctival tissue will ultimately function as a fluid flow resistor. It is therefore important to avoid excessive tissue manipulation, which can cause subconjunctival fibrosis, the most common cause of filtration failure. Only nontoothed forceps should be used on this tissue.

Limbus-Based Flap

Limbus-based conjunctival flaps are less likely to leak postoperatively, reducing their likelihood of flattening or scarring down.

Figure 4-2. Blunt dissection of the conjunctival–Tenon's flap.

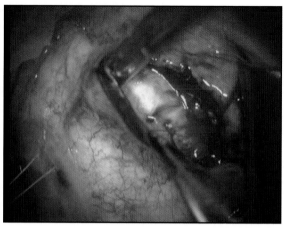

It is necessary to make the initial conjunctival incision parallel to the eyelid margin, a minimum of 8 mm posteriorly. The Tenon's fascia, in turn, is grasped and incised until the episclera is visualized. The conjunctival–Tenon's wound should be lengthened to approximately 2 clock hours. The conjunctiva and Tenon's tissue should only be incised when in the grasp of forceps and while they are raised over the episclera to avoid incorporating a rectus muscle with these tissues.

The conjunctival–Tenon's flap is bluntly dissected to the limbus through the insertion of Tenon's fascia (approximately 0.5 to 0.75 mm posterior to the limbus) to the insertion of the conjunctiva, which is approximately 0.5 mm onto clear cornea (Figure 4-2). Meticulous hemostasis using tapered tip cautery is then performed.

Fornix-Based Flap

Fornix-based conjunctival flaps have the advantage that they are easier to perform and can be used as an alternative to the limbal-based flap (Figure 4-3). These are initiated with a 1.5 to 2 clock-hour limbal peritomy and blunt dissection, which is carried posteriorly using blunt-tipped Westcott scissors through the insertion of Tenon's fascia. Blunt dissection is then carried posteriorly and laterally as far as the Westcott scissors can reach to obtain the most diffuse bleb possible.

Creating a Scleral Flap

The scleral flap, if adequately sutured, is a temporary resistor to the flow of aqueous through the sclerotomy site in the early postoperative period, reducing the incidence of hypotony. The shape of the scleral flap is of little consequence as long as the flap completely covers the sclerectomy. Our preference is to make a triangular flap 3.5 mm × 3.5 mm × 3.5 mm with

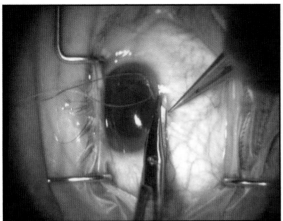

Figure 4-3. Limbal peritomy to create a fornix-based conjunctival flap.

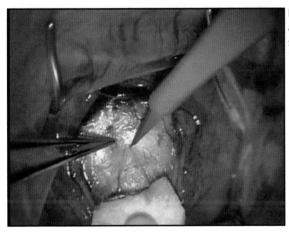

Figure 4-4. Creating a triangular-shaped scleral flap with a 15-degree blade.

a 15-degree blade, with a flap thickness of one-half to two-thirds sclera thickness (to avoid flap avulsion) (Figure 4-4). The flap is dissected anteriorly, beyond the gray line and into clear cornea anterior to the sclera spur and ciliary body, into clear cornea in a lamellar fashion with the same blade.

Mitomycin C

MMC is an antifibrotic agent used intraoperatively to reduce postoperative subconjunctival scarring, thus reducing the need for or eliminating multiple postoperative subconjunctival injections of 5-fluorouracil (5-FU), which historically was the antifibrotic agent used routinely prior to the widespread usage of MMC. When compared to 5-FU, MMC produces less corneal toxicity.[5] However, a dose-dependent complication associated with MMC

Figure 4-5. Anterior chamber paracentesis.

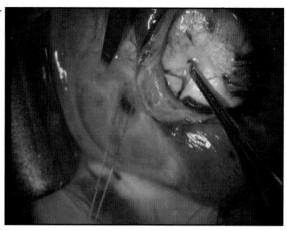

administration is long-term postoperative hypotony with associated maculopathy,[6] most commonly due to an avascular thin-walled bleb that over-filtrates. However, aqueous hypo-secretion secondary to ciliary body toxicity may play a role in some cases.[7]

The concentration of MMC (0.2 to 0.5 mg/mL) used and the duration (2 to 5 minutes) of application during glaucoma filtration surgery varies in the literature.[8-10] To reduce the risk of long-term hypotony with maculopathy, the duration of MMC exposure should be adjusted according to the risk factors of the individual patient.

Because MMC can be highly toxic to the corneal endothelium and tissues of the anterior segment,[11-12] it should be applied in a controlled manner to bare sclera prior to entering the eye. A cellulose or cut end of a Weck-Cel sponge saturated with MMC is applied to bare sclera. We recommend diffuse application of multiple MMC sponges, under all areas of Tenon's fascia, to decrease the incidence of high avascular localized blebs and to promote low diffuse filtering blebs. After the exposure period, the sponge is removed and the surgical site is thoroughly irrigated with a full container (15 mL) of balanced salt solution.

Paracentesis

Placement of a temporal-beveled, self-sealing paracentesis during filtration surgery before the sclerotomy but after application/rinsing of an antifibrotic agent is essential in allowing the surgeon access to the anterior chamber, similar to cataract surgery (Figure 4-5). A paracentesis enables the surgeon to allow for gradual pressure decline in patients in whom the IOP is high (reducing the risk of suprachoroidal hemorrhage), and to reform the anterior chamber to assess for adequate filtration at the flap margins after sclera flat closure.

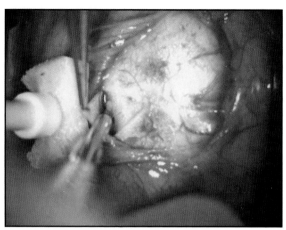

Figure 4-6. Creating a sclerotomy with a Kelly-Descemet punch.

Sclerectomy

There are 2 common methods for making the sclerotomy opening. For both methods, the anterior chamber is entered at the anterior most point of the scleral bed adjacent to the scleral flap with a 15-degree blade, or other such sharp knife. For the first method, 2 radial incisions centered under the scleral flap are made approximately 1.5 to 2 mm apart with Vannas scissors. The block is retracted posteriorly and excised with Vannas scissors. Alternatively, a sclerectomy can be made with a Kelly-Descemet punch (our preferred method). Two to 3 punches may be required to make a sclerectomy of adequate size (Figure 4-6). If the iris balloons forward through the surgical opening at any time during the construction of the sclerectomy, a small radial snip of the iris with Vannas scissors can deflate the ballooning.

Iridectomy

A peripheral iridectomy is performed to prevent obstruction/incarceration of the iris in the sclerectomy. The ideal iridectomy should be larger than the sclerectomy in all dimensions (wide at its base but short vertically to avoid iatrogenic polycoria and its associated monocular diplopia). With the scleral flap lifted, the iris is grasped 0.5 mm from the iris root and retracted through the sclerotomy. The scissors are opened enough to encompass the retracted iris, and then in one smooth cut, the iridectomy is made (Figure 4-7). The iris is reposited with a stream of balanced salt solution or by closing and gently massaging over the scleral flap. Upon completion of the iridectomy, the surgeon should have a view of the ciliary processes and occasionally the lens equator. If iris remnants or ciliary processes occlude the sclerectomy,

Figure 4-7. Surgical iridectomy.

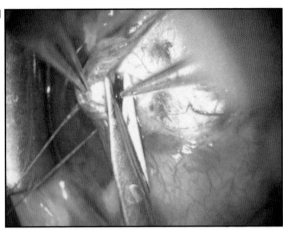

Figure 4-8. Scleral flap sutures.

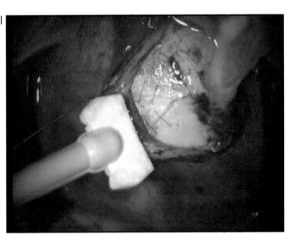

these should be excised only with great caution because it is exceedingly easy to damage the lens or hyaloid face.

Scleral Flap Closure

The scleral flap should be closed tightly enough to prevent postoperative hypotony. The flap is closed with interrupted 10-0 nylon sutures. A 3-1-1 knot buries well and secures the flap adequately. Usually 3 to 5 sutures are used to adequately close the flap (Figure 4-8). After the flap is secured, the anterior chamber is reformed through the paracentesis with balanced salt solution, and the filtration is checked at the flap margins with a Weck-Cel sponge. If the IOP and anterior chamber depth are

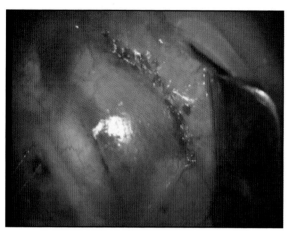

Figure 4-9. Limbal-based flap closure.

maintained with slow oozing of aqueous humor, then the scleral flap clo-sure is usually adequate. However, if aqueous humor flows freely and the anterior chamber shallows, additional sutures are required. Conversely, if aqueous humor does not flow, loosen, remove, or replace sutures. Also, it may be necessary to reopen the scleral flap and inspect the sclerectomy to ensure it is not obstructed.

Conjunctival Closure

Watertight conjunctival closure using nontoothed forceps is necessary to create an elevated filtering bleb. Tissues should be brought to apposi-tion only, as tight sutures "cheese-wire" postoperatively, creating a leaky, inflamed wound. Meticulous closure of the conjunctiva can save many postoperative hours dealing with the complications related to poorly closed wounds.

Limbus-Based Flap Closure

While the terminology is confusing, a limbus-based flap is performed with a conjunctival and Tenon's incision, typically performed in the superi-or fornix, approximately 8 to 10 mm posterior to the limbus. Most surgeons favor the use of running conjunctival closures with 8-0 or 9-0 absorbable suture (eg, Vicryl) on a BV needle, beginning on the side of the surgeon's dominant hand. The running suture closes the Tenon's fascia first, followed by the conjunctiva (Figure 4-9). Weck-Cel sponges are then used to assure the wound's watertight closure. It is useful to lock the running suture every second to third throw to provide watertight closure. Care should be taken not to take large bites of the anterior Tenon's fascia or conjunctiva, as this may cause the wound to migrate anteriorly, creating unwanted tension on the limbal conjunctiva.

Fornix-Based Flap Closure

While the terminology is confusing here as well, a fornix-based flap is created by incising the conjunctiva directly at the limbus, and dissecting posteriorly beneath Tenon's. Fornix-based flaps should be closed in a water-tight manner as well. Closure with winged sutures using nylon or Vicryl at either end of the conjunctival flap positions the leading edge of the flap over the limbus. Alternatively, if this closure is inadequate, 3 to 4 long mattress sutures are placed at the limbus using 10-0 nylon or 8-0 to 10-0 Vicryl on a spatulated needle. The suture should be placed through midstromal cornea. Exposed nonabsorbable sutures are removed after wound healing has occurred.

Seidel testing for bleb leaks with a saturated fluorescein strip should be performed at the conclusion of fornix-based surgery. If a bleb leak is detected, it should be closed with a single suture or a horizontal mattress suture and the wound rechecked with fluorescein.

INTRAOPERATIVE COMPLICATIONS

Buttonholes

Buttonholes can generally be avoided by meticulous handling of the conjunctiva with nontoothed forceps. If a large buttonhole overlying the filter site is found early in the surgery, the surgeon should consider relocating the filter to the adjacent quadrant. If the buttonhole is found or created late in the surgery, take care to not extend it while completing the surgery. Then make the repair with a tapered 9-0 or 10-0 Vicryl or nylon suture on a tapered needle in a mattress fashion, taking care to incorporate Tenon's tissue in your needle passes for stability, if possible.

Flap Dehiscence

A thin scleral flap is at risk for avulsion from the eye during the surgery. If done before making the sclerotomy, it is recommended to abandon that site and begin again in an adjacent area. If done after the sclerotomy, it is recommended that a scleral patch graft be placed over the sclerotomy and closed in watertight fashion, abandoning the filtration.

Bleeding

Bleeding from the sclerotomy edges and the iridectomy edges is not uncommon. Gentle cautery of small bleeders can be performed under direct visualization with taper tip cautery. To stop persistent bleeding, epinephrine 1:100,000 solution (sterile and unpreserved) can also be used. Take care to not inadvertently enlarge the sclerotomy site, as this can cause overfiltration. In addition, cautery of the iris should be performed with caution so as to not break the anterior hyaloid face and encounter vitreous or to violate the lens capsule in a phakic patient.

SUBCONJUNCTIVAL INJECTIONS

At the conclusion of filtering surgery, subconjunctival dexamethasone phosphate 5 mg is injected opposite the site of the filtering bleb. Injec anti-biotics can be used, but some surgeons feel it may increase postoperative inflammation. Cycloplegics (eg, atropine 1%, homatropine 5%, or scopol-amine 0.25%) may be given at the conclusion of the surgery if the patient is still phakic or has a shallow chamber to begin with. This is followed by a combination steroid/antibiotic ointment (eg, Tobradex or Maxitrol), which is then applied. The eye is then gently patched and an eye shield is applied.

POSTOPERATIVE MANAGEMENT

Topical steroids improve intermediate and long-term postoperative IOP control after filtering surgery by decreasing postoperative inflammation and scarring. Prednisolone acetate 1% is administered every 1 to 2 hours initially and tapered over 8 to 12 weeks, depending on the patient's response. No additional benefit has been demonstrated with the use of systemic pred-nisone.[13] Cycloplegics (eg, scopolamine 0.25%) can be used twice a day for 2 to 3 weeks after surgery to help maintain anterior chamber depth and prevent synechia. Antibiotics are given over a 2-week period. In addion, an antibiotic/steroid ointment is generally given at bedtime to aid in antibiotic and anti-inflammatory coverage while asleep.

It is important to understand that postoperatively there could be changes in the medical regimen that may affect the IOP in the fellow eye due to steroid response,[14] discontinuation of oral glaucoma medication, and confusion with medications. If the IOP reaches unsafe levels in the fellow eye, the surgeon must advance therapy accordingly.

Postoperative Scleral Flap Suture Release

If the IOP is not adequately lowered, laser suture lysis is a technique that allows the surgeon to modify scleral flap aqueous humor outflow resis-tance postoperatively.[15] With this available, the scleral flap can be closed more tightly intraoperatively, thus reducing the occurrence of postopera-tive hypotony and its attendant complications without as much concern for postoperative elevated IOP.

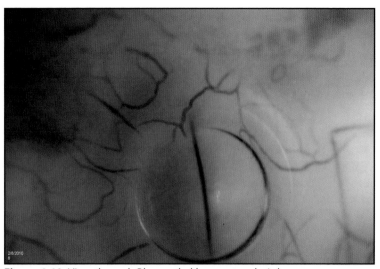

Figure 4-10. View through Blumenthal laser suture lysis lens.

Suture lysis is performed sequentially; that is, 1 suture at a time. The time interval between cutting sutures can be from hours to days, depending on the response. Suture lysis can be performed as early as 1 week after filtering surgery and as far out as 18 weeks after surgery.[16]

After application of topical anesthesia, a Zeiss, Hoskins, or Blumenthal lens is used to flatten the bleb overlying the scleral flap. The lens may need to be held in place for a short period of time (usually under a minute) to compress the bleb tissues and improve the view of the suture before laser application (Figure 4-10). An argon red or green wavelength is used with settings of 240 to 400 mW, 0.1 seconds, and a 50 μm spot size (see Appendix E for alternative laser settings). Argon red is useful if subconjunctival hemorrhage or pigmentation is present due to its reduced absorption by these substances. The suture should clearly separate when successfully cut. If there is no clear separation of the suture, it was not cut or it was not functionally closing the scleral flap. Additional sutures may need to be cut in the latter situation. Occasionally, a cut end stands vertically inside the bleb after lysis. This can be avoided if the suture is cut at its 2 ends. Releasable sutures, a method to remove scleral flap sutures at the slit lamp (beyond the scope of this chapter), can be used to circumvent the need for a laser.

After lysing or pulling a suture, it is important to judge the patency of the flap by using digital pressure (through the superior lid) or the Carlo Traverso maneuver (pressure using a cotton applicator adjacent to but outside the flap boundary)[17] to determine whether there is an elevation in the bleb after suture lysis.

THE FAILED FILTER

Unfortunately, even surgery performed and followed in the most meticulous manner may fail. Failure occurs when aqueous humor meets elevated resistance between the sclerectomy and the conjunctival epithelium.

Signs of bleb failure include the following:

1. Increased bleb vascularity.
2. Increased bleb wall thickness.
3. Decreased elevation of the bleb.
4. Reduction in conjunctival microcysts.
5. Increased IOP.

Causes of bleb failure include the following:

1. Subconjunctival (episcleral) fibrosis (most common cause).
2. Scleral flap fibrosis
3. "Tenon's cyst" formation (a fluid-filled cavity lined internally by fibrous tissue preventing filtration).
4. Obstruction of the sclerectomy by iris, vitreous or lens (as seen by gonioscopy).

Therapeutic options include the following:

1. Postoperative topical anti-inflammatory drop adherence, early digital massage, and 5-FU injections (for causes 1 and 2 prior to formation).
2. External bleb needle revision (for causes 1, 2, and 3).
3. Nd:YAG or argon laser reopening of the sclerectomy (for cause 4).

Digital Massage

Digital massage is used to push aqueous through the filter site in an attempt to prevent or slow the fibrosis that causes filtration surgery to ultimately fail.

While the patient is looking up and nasally, the index finger is used to identify the infraorbital rim. The patient should then place pressure on the globe through the lower lid with pressure directed inward and upward for 10 seconds with the soft fingerprint portion of the index finger. This is repeated 1 to 2 times per day until the patient is seen in clinic to reassess the filtering site. Risk is involved with this maneuver, and specific instructions and cautions must be given to ensure that the patient does not cause injury to him or herself. For this reason, many physicians choose not to use this manuever.

Bleb Needle Revision

In cases of bleb failure resulting from an elevated thick-walled encapsulated bleb (Tenon's cyst) or from advanced episcleral fibrosis causing a flat bleb, a needling procedure[18] may be used in an attempt to successfully revise the original filtering surgery. This is performed using a TB syringe to draw up 0.1 mL of sterile nonpreserved 1% lidocaine and 0.1 mL of 0.4 mg/mL MMC, yielding a final concentration of 0.2 mg/mL of MMC. Under sterile technique in the operating room or at the slit lamp, the diluted MMC is injected subconjunctivally in the superotemporal quadrant, far from the failed bleb (in the case of a superonasal bleb). If at the slit lamp, massage the MMC through the closed eyelid, toward the site of the initial surgery, until the area is flat. If in the operating room, you may use a cotton tip applicator on the conjunctiva to accomplish this flattening. A 25- or 27-gauge needle on a TB syringe or a 1.0 mm side-port blade is then inserted subconjuctivally, far from the bleb and away from the area of the MMC, and advanced until reaching the failed bleb. The sharp edges are then used to break up scar tissue, lift the flap, and enter the anterior chamber through the sclerotomy site to reinstate aqueous flow. Success is accomplished when the bleb reforms or becomes more diffuse after injecting balanced salt solution into the anterior chamber through a previously formed paracentesis. The conjunctival entry sites may be closed with suture or hand-held cautery.

CONCLUSION

Elevated IOP control via trabeculectomy is sometimes required to control glaucoma. Risk assessment, perioperative observation and management, and selection of the proper intraoperative technique are crucial to ensuring the success of the procedure. Gaining a comprehensive understanding of the theories underlying the various approaches and techniques of this classic filtration procedure will prepare the reader to learn glaucoma surgery. Additional pearls to more effective glaucoma surgery can be gleaned from Table 4-1.

TABLE 4-1. FILTRATION SURGERY KEY PEARLS	
Short conjunctival flap (limbus-based flap)	Reduces potential filtration area and increases likelihood of postoperative failure. Initiate conjunctival flap at least 8 mm from the limbus.
Toothed forceps for conjunctival manipulation	Use of nontoothed forceps and gentle handling of tissues reduces buttonholes and postoperative inflammation.
Thin or small scleral flap	The scleral flap should be at least half the total scleral thickness and large enough to functionally cover the sclerectomy site to prevent prolonged postoperative hypotony.
Paracentesis too small, cannot be found or cannot be cannulated	To cannulate easily, a paracentesis must have a large internal (endothelial) opening and known location and orientation (test paracentesis before continuing case).
Iridectomy imperforate or too small	The iridectomy must be patent and extend to the posterior sclerectomy margins (so one can see the red reflex or ciliary processes). Extreme caution must be used to enlarge a small iridectomy to avoid vitreous loss.
Sclerectomy site too far posteriorly	Excessive bleeding or occlusion of the sclerectomy by the ciliary body can be avoided by making the initial anterior chamber entry site as far anterior as possible (well into the limbal gray-blue zone).
Sclerectomy site too close to lateral scleral flap margin	The scleral flap must completely cover the sclerectomy, otherwise resistance to aqueous flow will be low and hypotony will result.
Occlusion of the sclerectomy by ciliary processes	Particularly seen in small hyperopic eyes. An anterior sclerectomy site is helpful. Ciliary processes can be gently cauterized, grasped with 0.12 forceps and excised with Vannas scissors if necessary.
Vitreous loss through sclerectomy site	Fortunately a rare complication. A meticulous Weck-Cel vitrectomy can salvage the bleb. Postoperative hypotony with a shallow anterior chamber must be avoided (to prevent posterior vitreous from entering the sclerectomy site).
Scleral flap closure (too tight or too loose)	With irrigation through the paracentesis, fluid should flow slowly with a maintained anterior chamber depth.
Conjunctival wound leak	Wound leaks can be reduced by meticulous wound closure and testing with fluorescein.

REFERENCES

1. AGIS Investigators. The Advanced Glaucoma Intervention Study (AGIS): 11. Risk factors for failure of trabeculectomy and argon laser trabeculoplasty. *Am J Ophthalmol.* 2002;134(4):481-498.
2. Phillips B, Krupin T. The risk profile of glaucoma filtration surgery. *Curr Opin Ophthalmol.* 1999;10(2):112-116.
3. Law SK, Song BJ, Yu F, Kurbanyan K, Yang TA, Caprioli J. Hemorrhagic complications from glaucoma surgery in patients on anticoagulation therapy or antiplatelet therapy. *Am J Ophthalmol.* 2008;145(4):736-746.
4. Kohl DA, Walton DS. Limbus-based versus fornix-based conjunctival flaps in trabeculectomy: 2005 update. *Int Ophthalmol Clin.* 2005;45(4):107-113.
5. Skuta GL, Beeson CC, Higginbotham EJ, et al. Intraoperative mitomycin versus postoperative 5-fluorouracil in high-risk glaucoma filtering surgery. *Ophthalmology.* 1992;99:438-444.
6. Shields MB, Scroggs MW, Sloop CM, et al. Clinical and histopathologic observations concerning hypotony after trabeculectomy with adjunctive mitomycin C. *Am J Ophthalmol.* 1993;116:673-683.
7. Rockwood EJ, Parrish RK II, Heuer DK, et al. Glaucoma filtering surgery with 5-fluorouracil. *Ophthalmology.* 1987;94:1071-1078.
8. Kitazawa Y, Suemori-Matsushita H, Yamamoto T, et al. Low-dose and high-dose mitomycin trabeculectomy as an initial surgery in primary open-angle glaucoma. *Ophthalmology.* 1993;100:1624-1628.
9. Neelakantan A, Rao BS, Vijaya L, et al. Effect of the concentration and duration of application of mitomycin C in trabeculectomy. *Ophthalmic Surg.* 1994;25:612-615.
10. Megevand GS, Salmon JF, Scholtz RP, Murray AD. The effect of reducing the exposure time of mitomycin C in glaucoma filtering surgery. *Ophthalmology.* 1995;102:84-90.
11. Derick RJ, Pasquale L, Quigley HA, Jampel H. Potential toxicity of mitomycin C. *Arch Ophthalmol.* 1991;109:1635.
12. Seah SK, Prata JA Jr, Minckler DS, et al. Mitomycin-C concentration in human aqueous humour following trabeculectomy. *Eye.* 1993;7:652-655.
13. Starita RJ, Fellman RL, Spaeth GL, et al. Short and long-term effects of postoperative corticosteroids on trabeculectomy. *Ophthalmology.* 1985;92:938-946.
14. Schwartz B. The response of ocular pressure to corticosteroids. *Int Ophthalmol Clin.* 1966;6(4):929-989.
15. Savage JA, Simmons RJ. Staged glaucoma filtration surgery with planned early conversion from scleral flap to full-thickness operation using the argon laser. *Ophthalmic Laser Therapy.* 1986;1:201.
16. Pappa KS, Derick RJ, Weber PA, et al. Late argon laser suture lysis after mitomycin C trabeculectomy. *Ophthalmology.* 1993;100(8):1268-1271.
17. Spaeth GL. *Ophthalmic Surgery: Principles and Practice.* Philadelphia, PA: Saunders; 2003.
18. Shetty RK, Wartluft L, Moster MR. Slit-lamp needle revision of failed filtering blebs using high-dose mitomycin C. *J Glaucoma.* 2005;14(1):52-56.

5

Trabeculectomy
Management of
Postoperative Complications

Jonathan A. Eisengart, MD

By its nature, trabeculectomy typically entails much more risk than cataract surgery. However, thoughtful and successful management of postoperative complications can significantly reduce the risk of long-term harm to the patient.

Hypotony

Assessment

Hypotony is one of the most dreaded complications of trabeculectomy and is one of the major causes of permanent reduction in visual acuity after glaucoma surgery. Hypotony itself, however, does not cause vision loss. Rather, the complications of hypotony, such as maculopathy, flat anterior chambers, and choroidal hemorrhages, can cause vision loss. The decision whether to intervene medically or surgically to reverse hypotony is dictated by the risk of vision loss. For example, a patient with an intraocular pressure (IOP) chronically in the range of 2 to 4 mm Hg can be safely observed if the anterior chamber is deep and the posterior segment examination is normal. Conversely, a flat anterior chamber with lens–cornea touch needs immediate intervention to prevent decompensation of the cornea. Hypotony maculopathy deserves definitive surgical treatment within several weeks to prevent permanent retinal damage (although significant recovery of vision can occur even after several years).[1]

Treatment for hypotony is directed at the underlying cause. In most cases, hypotony in the early postoperative period is due to overfiltration. Overfiltration is recognized by hypotony in the setting of a large and/or diffuse bleb and relatively quiet eye. A bleb leak can also contribute to

Kahook M.
Essentials of Glaucoma Surgery (pp 49-58).
© 2012 SLACK Incorporated.

Complications of Hypotony

- Shallowed anterior chamber
  - Mild to moderate shallowing
  - Iris–cornea touch
  - Lens–cornea touch
- Choroidal effusion/ciliary body detachment
- Choroidal hemorrhage
- Hypotony maculopathy
- Cystoid macular edema

---

hypotony, and needs to be ruled out with a Seidel test. More rarely, hypotony may be caused by aqueous hyposecretion, either from marked postoperative inflammation, uveitis, or ocular ischemia. Hyposecretion associated with inflammation is best treated with cycloplegia and frequent topical, and possibly systemic, steroids.

Medical Management

Most cases of postoperative hypotony, however, are due to overfiltration and typically respond to a reduction of topical steroids. This will allow for additional scarring and a natural rise in IOP over days to weeks. A cycloplegic is often added, which can be especially helpful in anterior chamber shallowing. In some patients, it might be prudent to temporarily discontinue topical beta-blockers in the contralateral eye. I also encourage behavior changes to help reduce aqueous egress, including strict instructions against eye rubbing, wearing an eye shield at night, and avoidance of Valsalva maneuver.

If hypotony is more profound, with marked shallowing of the anterior chamber and/or ciliary body detachment, viscoelastic can be injected into the anterior chamber.[2,3] Injection may be done with a cannula through a previously created paracentesis or through clear cornea with a 25-to 30-gauge needle. Injection should be performed in a sterile manner with a lid speculum after prepping with povidone-iodine and instilling a topical antibiotic. The viscoelastic will increase IOP for 24 to 48 hours, which may allow additional bleb scarring or reattachment of the ciliary body and increased aqueous secretion. Healon (sodium hyaluronate) is a common initial choice, whereas Healon GV (sodium hyaluronate 1.4%) and Healon 5 (sodium hyaluronate 2.3%) will allow progressively more retention and ability to raise IOP. Often, viscoelastic injections need to be repeated several times until IOP is maintained spontaneously. If viscoelastic injection is done, the IOP should be checked 1 to 2 hours later

---

Stepwise Treatment of Overfiltration

1. Medical and behavior management
   - Taper topical steroids
   - Cycloplegia
   - Avoid eye rubbing and Valsalva, wear eye shield
2. Minor procedures
   - Viscoelastic injection
   - Blood injection
3. Major procedures
   - Resuture the scleral flap ± excise avascular conjunctiva
   - Graft material to seal flap, ± additional drainage surgery

---

to monitor for an IOP rise. Especially with Healon GV and Healon 5, IOP can rise very high and remain there for days, therefore, marked care must be used when using these high-viscosity agents after a trabeculectomy.

One option to induce bleb scarring is an autologous blood injection.[4] Although I personally have found this to be rarely successful, it may be worthwhile in a few cases. After prepping the arm and eye with povidone-iodine, approximately 0.5 cc of blood is drawn from an antecubital or other convenient vein with an 18- to 20-gauge needle. The needle is changed to a 25-gauge, inserted subconjunctivally temporal to the bleb, and advanced to inject 0.1 to 0.5 cc of blood into and behind the bleb. The blood must be injected promptly following removal from the vein to avoid clotting in the syringe. Hyphema is a common but self-limited complication.

Surgical Management

It is necessary to intervene surgically for hypotony that is threatening vision, however, this is uncommon.

Transconjunctival Scleral Flap Resuturing

The easiest technique is to directly resuture the scleral flap. If the bleb is not avascular and the scleral flap is visible, the flap may be resutured directly through intact conjunctiva using 10-0 nylon.[5] The eye should be prepped sterilely, and a cotton-tip applicator can be used to push down and flatten the bleb overlying the scleral flap. The edges of the flap are then identified and sutured *tightly*. Over several days to a couple of weeks, the sutures will migrate into the bleb and become buried. As the bleb elevates again and tissue migrates out of the sutures, the sutures will loosen and the eye pressure will decrease.

Direct Scleral Flap Resuturing

More commonly, the scleral flap is resutured after opening conjunctiva. The conjunctival flap may be fornix- or limbus-based; it is often convenient to re-open the original conjunctival incision as long as the conjunctiva has not become avascular. Avascular tissue may not heal well and is prone to persistent leaks if incised. If avascular conjunctiva is believed to be playing a role in hypotony, it should be excised along with a narrow margin of healthy conjunctiva to ensure there is a bleeding, healthy, viable edge. The scleral flap is then identified, and if partially scarred down, may be sharply re-elevated and freshened. The flap should then be sutured tightly using 10-0 nylon to achieve a watertight (or nearly watertight) closure. The conjunctiva should then be closed in a watertight fashion, and suture lysis of the scleral flap sutures performed as needed. Achieving a controlled elevation of IOP in the early postoperative period may reverse some of the signs and symptoms of hypotony maculopathy and speed resolution of choroidal effusions.

Scleral Flap and Bleb Revision

Not infrequently, the scleral flap is found to be friable, partially "melted," or otherwise damaged from antimetabolite exposure and surgical manipulation, and it may be impossible to adequately restrict flow by resuturing the flap. These situations can be addressed by suturing graft material, typically sclera or pericardium, over the entire scleral flap site using 10-0 nylon. Although the graft should be sutured down tightly and securely, the closure may not need to be watertight because the new graft will typically scar down and permanently seal the old trabeculectomy site. Although some have tried to suture the new graft material in such a way to allow continued partial flow of aqueous posteriorly into the bleb, I have not found this technique to be successful.

As expected, covering the old trabeculectomy site frequently results in uncontrolled pressure. When sacrificing a bleb with graft material, I will frequently place a glaucoma tube shunt (typically a Baerveldt 350 mm^2 concomitantly to provide continuing control of IOP).

Choroidal Effusions

Although choroidal effusions are often approached as a distinct complication that requires directed treatment, I think it is better to consider them to be a complication of hypotony. I have found that drainage of choroidal effusions is rarely indicated. Rather, treatment of the underlying hypotony is typically curative.

Choroidal effusions themselves rarely cause permanent vision loss, although they are a risk factor for choroidal hemorrhage. Many effusions, even relatively large ones, can be carefully observed, while waiting for medical management, to allow spontaneous hypotony resolution. If effusions are "kissing," if there is lens–cornea touch, or if chronic ciliary body detachment is contributing to hypotony, drainage may be indicated as part of trabeculectomy revision.

AQUEOUS MISDIRECTION

Assessment

Glaucoma surgery is one of the most common reasons that eyes develop aqueous misdirection. Aqueous misdirection was previously called "malignant glaucoma," a moniker it earned due to the extremely high rate of blindness that occurred before ophthalmologists learned to treat this condition. Today, prompt recognition and appropriate treatment of this condition should prevent serious vision loss in most circumstances.

Aqueous misdirection is classically recognized by a shallow to flat anterior chamber and marked elevation of IOP. However, functioning outflow surgery can significantly blunt or prevent the elevation in IOP secondary to aqueous misdirection. For example, a markedly shallowed anterior chamber and an IOP of 16 mm Hg is highly suggestive of aqueous misdirection in the setting of recent trabeculectomy or tube shunt (by contrast, a shallowed chamber of overfiltration would typically be associated with IOP in the low single digits). Because pupillary block and choroidal hemorrhage can also present with a shallowed chamber and elevated IOP, a patent iridotomy and complete fundus exam are important before making the diagnosis of aqueous misdirection.

Medical Management

Initial treatment for aqueous misdirection is intense cycloplegia, augmented by topical aqueous suppressants and acetazolamide. Systemic hyperosmotics (intravenous mannitol, 0.5 to 1.5 gm/kg or oral glycerine 1 to 1.5 gm/kg) can be effective but must be used cautiously due to their systemic side effects. Often, medical management alone is not sufficient.

Laser Management

In pseudophakes, aqueous misdirection will often respond to nd:YAG capsulotomy and anterior hyaloidotomy to disrupt the anterior hyaloid face. After performing a typical nd:YAG capsulotomy, additional laser shots can be applied into the anterior vitreous. If successful, the anterior chamber will begin to deepen rather quickly, typically while the laser is still being performed. Retinal tears are a small risk when lasering the vitreous body.

Figure 5-1. Surgical management of aqueous misdirection. An iridozonulohyaloidectomy (IZH) is performed by passing the vitrector through the iris, zonules, and anterior hyaloid. This maneuver can be approached from the (a) anterior chamber via a clear cornea incision or (b) through the pars plana.

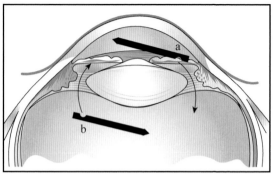

Alternatively, the YAG laser can be applied through a peripheral iridectomy to disrupt the zonules as well as the anterior vitreous face. Again, however, this is typically helpful only in pseudophakes.

Surgical Management

Complete removal of the vitreous body by a pars plana vitrectomy is currently the gold standard for curing aqueous misdirection. The vitreoretinal surgeon must be sure to break the anterior hyaloid face, which can be difficult to do in phakic patients without damaging the lens capsule.

Rarely, aqueous misdirection can persist despite a complete pars plana vitrectomy, presumably due in part to the presence of the retained vitreous skirt. In these cases, an iridozonulohyaloidectomy (IZH; this term was coined by Ike Ahmed, MD) should be performed (Figure 5-1). This can be done by passing an automated vitrector from the posterior segment, up through the zonules and iris, into the anterior chamber (or similarly from the anterior chamber down through iris and zonules into the anterior vitreous). A combined pars plana vitrectomy and IZH are highly curative but can be performed only in pseudophakes or aphakes. In phakic patients, the lens may need to be removed to allow resolution of aqueous misdirection.[6]

Some anterior segment surgeons have found that performing a limited anterior vitrectomy and IZH has allowed them to successfully treat aqueous misdirection without involving a vitreoretinal surgeon. I typically do not do this myself, but rarely I utilize this maneuver for "intraoperative aqueous/ infusion misdirection."

BLEB LEAK

Assessment

Although a bleb leak may lead to hypotony, the most serious complications are blebitis and endophthalmitis. It is for this reason that a frank bleb leak must always be treated.

A Seidel fluorescein test for leakage should be performed whenever a patient with a filtering bleb presents with epiphora, hypotony, or a low/flat bleb and hypotony. Additionally, it may be prudent to periodically check for leaks in high, thin avascular blebs.

Upon discovery of a leak, blebitis should be ruled out by ensuring there is no conjunctival injection, bleb infiltrate, or anterior chamber inflammatory cells. Initially, a simple bleb leak can be managed conservatively. The patient should be instructed to avoid touching the eye and practice good hygiene to avoid infection.

Medical Management

A majority of bleb leaks will resolve with conservative management, especially those leaks that occur in the early postoperative period. Shortly after a trabeculectomy, leaks will often respond to simply tapering topical steroids to allow scarring and healing.

Typically, when the leak is discovered, a topical antibiotic, such as a fourth-generation fluoroquinolone, is started to prevent the progression to blebitis. Although it is likely prudent to do so, it is not totally clear whether prophylactic antibiotics truly prevent blebitis or simply promote the emergence of a resistant organism.

Optimization of the ocular surface can help support healing of the leak. Erythromycin ointment or azithromycin gel, through their anti-inflammatory action and improvement in meibomian gland function, may help promote a healthy ocular surface and potential reepithelialization of the leak. Systemic doxycycline, up to 100 mg twice daily, can also improve ocular surface health in the same way. Additionally, its inhibition of matrix metalloproteinases may further promote closure of the leak.

The leak is likely kept open by continual aqueous flow through the conjunctival defect. Therefore, measures should be taken to reduce fluid egress through the leak. The patient should be instructed to avoid Valsalva, bending, and eye rubbing. Wearing an eye shield during sleep can be very helpful. To further reduce flow through the leak, aqueous suppressants can be tried.

Pressure-patching the eye for 24 hours may allow closure of the leak by temporally tamponading flow. Similarly, a bandage contact lens may be placed to completely cover the leak. Because infection and corneal decompensation are the main risks of a bandage contact lens, a topical third- or fourth-generation fluoroquinolone needs to be added, and the patient should be examined at least weekly. Typically, I replace the bandage lens every 1 to 2 weeks and will allow 2 to 4 weeks for healing before abandoning the bandage lens.

Surgical Management

If the leak occurs in a localized bleb (one surrounded by a ring of scar tissue), needling may be tried to allow aqueous to diffuse more broadly and lower the pressure within the bleb. In some cases, this may promote closure of the leak and prevent a return to the operating room.

The simplest repair is suturing the leak. Suturing is most likely to be helpful in the early postoperative period when the conjunctiva is actively healing and when the leak occurs in the previous conjunctival incision line. However, because every needle pass can create more leaks, resuturing is not helpful for thinned or avascular tissue.

If the leak does occur with thinned conjunctiva, most likely the leak will have to be repaired by conjunctival advancement, which provides an acceptable level of safety and success.[7] First, a peritomy is performed around the base of the bleb, taking care to keep the incision within bleeding, viable conjunctiva. Extensive undermining should then be performed to ensure fresh conjunctiva can be advanced to the limbus without tension. The avascular bleb tissue can then be deepithelialized with light cautery and the healthy conjunctiva advanced over the old bleb to the limbus. The closure should be as close to watertight as possible.

A few modifications to this technique may be helpful. The avascular, leaking bleb can be completely excised. Additional scleral flap sutures may be placed to reduce flow and promote healing of the newly advanced conjunctiva without leak; suture lysis may be performed a later date as necessary. If the conjunctiva cannot be closed without excessive tension, then a conjunctival autograft can be used or the bleb can be sacrificed by sealing it with donor graft material and placing a glaucoma tube shunt.

BLEBITIS

Assessment

Blebitis can rapidly progress to endophthalmitis and profound vision loss. Therefore, blebitis requires early recognition and aggressive management. The initial symptoms of blebitis are pain or discomfort, redness of the eye, and decreased vision. There may be antecedent epiphora from a bleb leak.

Signs on examination are injection of the bleb and/or surrounding conjunctiva, as well as a bleb infiltrate, giving the bleb a white or milky appearance. Occasionally, a hypopyon within the bleb can be seen. An anterior chamber reaction is common. If there are any vitreous inflammatory cells, retinal consultation should be obtained immediately to rule out endophthalmitis.

Management

If there is any question of blebitis, the patient should be started on a fourth-generation fluoroquinolone and rechecked in 24 hours or less. Alternatively, fortified antibiotics, typically vancomycin 25 to 50 mg/mL plus ceftazidime 50 mg/mL or tobramycin 14 mg/mL can be used for more assured microbial coverage (I tend to avoid the aminoglycosides, such as tobramycin, if there is any risk of intraocular penetration through a bleb leak due to their potential for extreme retinal toxicity). Typical dosing should begin with 1 drop every 15 minutes for the first hour, then 1 drop hourly thereafter. Subconjunctival injections of the same fortified antibiotics may be added if the patient's ability to fully adhere to the medical regimen is in doubt. Frequent follow-up is required to ensure the blebitis is resolving and not progressing to endophthalmitis.

If endophthalmitis is diagnosed, prompt treatment is essential. A pars plana vitrectomy is indicated earlier for a bleb-associated endophthalmitis than for a postcataract surgery endophthalmitis, although intravitreal antibiotic injections remain a viable alternative.

CHOROIDAL HEMORRHAGE

Assessment

Choroidal hemorrhages occur most commonly in the setting of hypotony. Other risk factors are glaucoma, systemic hypertension, vascular disease, and eyes that have had prior vitrectomies.[8,9] Systemic anticoagulation may not increase the risk of choroidal hemorrhage, but can make a small hemorrhage become one that is devastating.

Choroidal hemorrhages are recognized by pain and a dark choroidal mound on fundus examination. B-mode ultrasonography is confirmatory. Additional examination findings depend on the size of the hemorrhage and include shallowing or flattening of the anterior chamber, increased IOP, and variable loss of vision.

Management

Small, self-limited choroidal hemorrhages require observation only, along with instructing the patient to avoid Valsalva, eye rubbing, and, if possible, systemic anticoagulation. Larger hemorrhages may benefit from cycloplegia and topical or systemic steroids. If the anterior chamber is severely shallowed, if the choroidal hemorrhages are "kissing," or if IOP is uncontrolled, drainage is indicated. I typically refer patients to my vitreoretinal colleagues for drainage of choroidal hemorrhage, although some anterior segment surgeons prefer to perform the surgery themselves.

Key Points

1. Hypotony can often be observed but needs to be treated when it is causing (or likely will cause) vision-threatening complications.

2. Most early postoperative hypotony will resolve spontaneously if given enough time; supportive measures can help buy time for early bleb scarring to bring up the IOP.

3. All bleb leaks need to be addressed, and conjunctival advancement is often the best choice for late-onset leaks when more conservative measures fail.

4. Successful management of aqueous misdirection may respond to nd:YAG laser disruption of the anterior vitreous face but often requires a pars plana vitrectomy and/or an iridozonulohyaloidectomy.

References

1. Oyakhire JO, Moroi SE. Clinical and anatomical reversal of long-term hypotony maculopathy. *Am J Ophthalmol.* 2004;137(5):953-955.
2. Salvo EC Jr, Luntz MH, Medow NB. Use of viscoelastics post-trabeculectomy: a survey of members of the American Glaucoma Society. *Ophthalmic Surg Lasers.* 1999;30(4):271-275.
3. Hoffman RS, Fine IH, Packer M. Healon5 as a treatment option for recurrent flat anterior chamber after trabeculectomy. *J Cataract Refract Surg.* 2003;29(4):635.
4. Okada K, Tsukamoto H, Msumoto M, et al. Autologous blood injection for marked overfiltration early after trabeculectomy with mitomycin C. *Acta Ophthalmol Scand.* 2001;79(3):305-308.
5. Maruyama K, Shirato S. Efficacy and safety of transconjunctival scleral flap resuturing for hypotony after glaucoma filtering surgery. *Graefes Arch Clin Exp Ophthalmol.* 2008;246(12):175-176.
6. Tsai JC, Barton KA, Miller MH, Khaw PT, Hitchings RA. Surgical results in malignant glaucoma refractory to medical or laser therapy. *Eye (Lond).* 1997;11(Pt 5):677-681.
7. Burnsteil AL, WuDunn D, Knotts SL, Catoira Y, Cantor LB. Conjunctival advancement versus nonincisional treatment for late-onset glaucoma filtering bleb leaks. *Ophthalmology.* 2002;109(1):71-75.
8. Obushowska I, Mariak Z. Risk factors of massive suprachoroidal hemorrhage during extracapsular cataract extraction surgery. *Eur J Ophthalmol.* 2005;15(6):712-717.
9. Moshfeghi DM, Kim BY, Kaiser PK, Sears JE, Smith SD. Appositional suprachoroidal hemorrhage: a case-control study. *Am J Ophthalmol.* 2004;138(6):959-963.

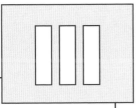

GLAUCOMA DRAINAGE DEVICE IMPLANTATION

6

Preoperative Evaluation for Glaucoma Drainage Device Surgery

Joshua D. Stein, MD, MS

The success of glaucoma drainage device (GDD) surgery depends not only on the technical skills necessary to perform the surgery but also on careful preoperative planning. During the preoperative evaluation, the surgeon must determine whether the patient is a good candidate for the surgery. Moreover, the surgeon must consider whether GDD surgery is the most appropriate option for lowering intraocular pressure (IOP) or whether other medical or surgical procedures would be better choices. The preoperative evaluation can affect the decisions regarding which type of GDD to use during the surgery, the best location to implant the GDD, and it may identify patients at increased risk for intraoperative or postoperative complications. This chapter discusses information that should be gathered and reviewed by the surgeon before performing GDD surgery.

Patient History

Ocular History

It is important to take a thorough ocular history to identify prior conditions and previously performed surgical procedures that may complicate GDD surgery. Specific conditions that one should inquire about include conditions that can result in scarring of the bulbar conjunctiva, including prior eye trauma and incisional surgical procedures, such as trabeculectomy surgery, intracapsular or extracapsular cataract surgery, or strabismus surgery. Previously placed implants, such as scleral buckles, need to be noted preoperatively, as their presence may affect the location of GDD implantation,

Kahook M.
Essentials of Glaucoma Surgery (pp 61-72).
© 2012 SLACK Incorporated.

or there may be extensive scar tissue around such devices, potentially preventing successful GDD implantation. If silicone oil or other substances that can obstruct the lumen of the GDD have previously been placed in the eye, these substances may need to be removed before a GDD can be successfully implanted. Other conditions, such as scleritis, ocular cicatricial pemphigoid, Stevens-Johnson syndrome, or chemical injuries can also cause thinning and scarring of the conjunctiva, which would make GDD surgery challenging, as would conditions that affect eyelid anatomy or the blink reflex. Whether a patient is phakic or pseudophakic and has undergone previous pars plana vitrectomy can also affect where the GDD can be inserted in the eye.

Medical History and Patient-Related Factors

The surgeon should inquire about acute and chronic medical conditions affecting the patient. For example, if a patient has an acute illness causing coughing, sneezing, nausea, or vomiting, it may be wise (when possible) to delay the GDD surgery, as these symptoms can cause sutures to break, wounds to dehisce, and can increase the risk for intraocular bleeding. Inquiring about chronic medical conditions such as obstructive pulmonary disease or back pain, which limit patients from lying flat on their back for the surgery, may affect the decision regarding the type of anesthesia to use for the surgery. Likewise, if a patient cannot lie still for prolonged periods of time due to Parkinson's or Alzheimer disease, this too can affect the type of anesthesia required. Patients who have a known history of poor adherence to glaucoma medication regimens need to be counseled about the importance of adhering to postoperative medication regimens to help reduce the risk for postoperative infection or inflammation.

Risk of Infection

Patients who are taking medications, such as corticosteroids or immunosuppressant agents, are at increased risk for infection during and after intraocular surgery. Persons who are immunocompromised are also predisposed to infection. Moreover, ocular conditions, such as blepharitis, can also lead to infection. In nonurgent surgeries, it is best to prophylactically treat conditions such as blepharitis to reduce the risk for serious infections (eg, endophthalmitis).

Risk of Hypotony

Patients with a history of chronic intraocular inflammation are at increased risk for ciliary body shutdown and postoperative hypotony after any intraocular surgery, including GDD implantation. Depending on the status of the patient's glaucoma, one may consider using a flow-restrictive glaucoma drainage implant, such as an Ahmed GDD (New World Medical, Inc), or a smaller-sized non–flow-restrictive device, such as a Baerveldt-250 (Abbott Medical Optics [AMO]), instead of a Baerveldt-350 (AMO) GDD.[1]

Risk of Bleeding

It is important to inquire about medical conditions and medications that can increase the risk for bleeding during surgery. Medical conditions associated with an increased risk for bleeding include liver disease, uremia, blood dyscrasias, and vitamin K deficiency. Medications that increase bleeding include aspirin, warfarin, and clopidogrel. Vitamins and supplements that can increase the risk for bleeding include vitamin E, ginkgo biloba, and garlic. Whenever possible, the patient should inquire with the medical provider who prescribed the medications about the possibility of discontinuing their use temporarily before surgery. If it is unsafe to discontinue use of these products, the surgery can still be performed, although the surgeon should be prepared to deal with any intra- and postoperative bleeding that may occur.

Risk of Suprachoroidal Hemorrhage

A serious, potentially sight-threatening complication of any intraocular procedure, including GDD surgery, is suprachoroidal hemorrhage. During the preoperative period, the surgeon should identify those patients who have multiple risk factors for this complication. Such risk factors include older age, arteriosclerosis, obesity, short axial length, high myopia, prior intraocular surgery (especially pars plana vitrectomy), use of blood-thinning agents, and a history of suprachoroidal hemorrhage.[2] In patients who have several of these risk factors, the surgeon should, whenever possible, try to prevent postoperative hypotony. Using flow-restrictive rather than non–flow-restrictive GDDs may be safer in these patients. Other techniques, such as injecting some viscoelastic into the anterior chamber at the end of the procedure or in clinic if profound hypotony occurs, can help reduce the risk for hypotony-related complications in these patients.

Patient Expectations

As part of the informed consent process before surgery, the patient needs to be made aware of the risks, benefits, and alternatives of performing the surgery. It is important to explain that it is not uncommon for patients to require one or more IOP-lowering medications, even if the surgery is successful and the GDD is functioning properly. Patients should also be informed that additional surgical interventions are necessary if the GDD becomes obstructed or does not sufficiently reduce the IOP. Discussing these points with the patient ahead of time and taking the time to answer questions about the surgery during the preoperative period can help prevent the patient from entering into the surgery with unrealistic expectations.

PREOPERATIVE OCULAR EXAMINATION

Best Corrected Visual Acuity

When evaluating a patient for GDD surgery, the surgeon must gauge the patient's visual potential by assessing his or her best corrected visual acuity (BCVA). In general, GDD surgery is offered to patients who have reasonable visual potential. In eyes known to have poor visual potential, a less invasive surgical procedure, such as cyclophotocoagulation, may be a more appropriate strategy to lower the IOP. Obtaining an accurate preoperative visual acuity is also useful for determining whether the vision has returned to baseline during the postoperative period after GDD surgery. If the GDD surgery is uncomplicated, the BCVA should quickly return to the preoperative level or better (if the patient had decreased vision as a result of microcystic corneal edema associated with elevated IOP), often within the first week. A decline in BCVA after GDD surgery may alert the clinician to a postoperative complication, such as cystoid macular edema or corneal edema.

Refractive Error

With any intraocular surgical procedure, including GDD surgery, obtaining a manifest refraction during the preoperative period can alert the surgeon to a patient's increased risk for intra- or postoperative complications. For example, patients who have high levels of myopia are at increased risk for a retinal tear or detachment in the postoperative period. These patients would benefit from a careful evaluation of the peripheral retina before proceeding with GDD surgery. Likewise, patients who have high levels of hypermetropia may have nanophthalmos. To reduce the risk for postoperative choroidal effusions in eyes with nanophthalmos, the surgeon may plan to perform prophylactic sclerostomies immediately before implanting the GDD.

Ocular Motility

One of the complications of GDD surgery is extraocular muscle restriction, which can result in binocular diplopia. Determining whether the ocular motility is normal in the preoperative examination can help the clinician identify whether self-report of diplopia after the surgery can be attributed to the surgery or to a pre-existing ocular or systemic condition.

Eyelids

When evaluating whether a patient is an appropriate candidate for GDD surgery, his eyelid function must be considered. Implanting a GDD in eyes with lagophthalmos or exophthalmos can be problematic because the ocular surface in these patients is often inadequately lubricated. Such patients have an increased likelihood of experiencing breakdown of the conjunctiva overlying the GDD. Before proceeding with GDD surgery, these patients may first require surgery to address their eyelid abnormalities. Alternatively, if a patient has significant eyelid abnormalities that are not easily correctable, endoscopic or transscleral diode cyclophotocoagulation may be more appropriate than GDD surgery. Because patients can develop ptosis as a result of GDD surgery, the clinician should document the presence of any pre-existing ptosis found in the preoperative evaluation.

Conjunctiva

One of the most important factors to consider when evaluating patients for GDD surgery is the health of the bulbar conjunctiva. Careful inspection is required to evaluate the viability of the bulbar conjunctiva in the quadrant where the surgeon is considering implanting the GDD. This is particularly critical in patients who have risk factors for scarring, such as those with a history of intraocular surgery, ocular trauma, or an acid or alkali burn. Extensive conjunctival scarring in the quadrant under consideration may make it technically challenging for the surgeon to adequately mobilize enough healthy conjunctival tissue to completely cover the implant and overlying patch graft. If conjunctival scarring is identified preoperatively, the surgeon may elect to implant the GDD in a different quadrant that has healthier bulbar conjunctival tissue. If considerable conjunctival scarring is present, the surgeon may need to perform a conjunctival autograft with tissue from an adjacent quadrant or from the contralateral eye. Alternatively, it may be preferable to consider performing a cyclodestructive procedure instead of attempting GDD surgery in these patients. In addition to visual inspection of the bulbar conjunctiva to identify scar tissue, one can instill a topical anesthetic in the eye and then gently manipulate the conjunctiva with a cotton tip applicator to get a sense of how adherent it is to the underlying sclera.

Sclera

Evaluating the quadrant where the GDD will be implanted for scleral thinning is necessary to avoid scleral perforation during the surgery. If the sclera is too thin, as a result of scleromalacia or other causes, it may be unsafe to attempt to implant a GDD in the affected quadrant. It is also useful during the preoperative period to check for evidence of previously created sclerostomies from prior glaucoma or retinal procedures. The surgeon would want to avoid prior trabeculectomy flaps and other sclerostomies during implantation of the GDD by rerouting the tube away from these locations. Inserting the tube through a previously created sclerostomy may lead to leakage of aqueous around the lumen of the tube, resulting in postoperative hypotony.

Cornea

During preoperative examination of the cornea, the surgeon should pay careful attention to the corneal endothelium. Corneal guttae on the surface of the endothelium may be a sign of Fuchs' endothelial dystrophy. Patients with Fuchs' endothelial corneal dystrophy are at increased risk for corneal decompensation after GDD surgery. In these patients, and with other patients who will likely undergo endothelial or penetrating keratoplasty in the future, the surgeon should plan to position the GDD as far away from the corneal endothelium as possible. If the patient is pseudophakic or aphakic, the surgeon should make every attempt to implant the GDD in the posterior chamber, and, if the patient had previous pars plana vitrectomy surgery, positioning the GDD in the vitreous cavity can reduce the risk for corneal decompensation after GDD surgery. It is also useful for the clinician to examine the cornea for scarring, as this may limit visualization of the tip of the tube both during the surgery and in the postoperative period. Often, patients with markedly elevated IOP before GDD surgery have microcystic corneal edema present. In these patients, temporarily lowering the IOP preoperatively with the use of aqueous suppressants and oral or intravenous carbonic anhydrase inhibitors may help clear up the edema and improve visualization of the tip of the tube during the surgery.

Anterior Chamber

When assessing the anterior chamber, one should take note of the anterior chamber depth and the presence of material in the anterior chamber that can get into and occlude the tube once it is inserted in the eye. There are several conditions that can result in the presence of a shallow anterior chamber. Individuals with high levels of hypermetropia often have short axial lengths and shallow anterior chambers. Persons who are phakic and who have large lenses that cause bulging forward of the iris can also exhibit shallowing of the anterior chamber. Scarring from previous intraocular surgery or trauma can result in iridocorneal touch, which can limit the depth of the anterior chamber. In all of these scenarios, it may be technically challenging to position the tip of the tube in the anterior chamber far enough away from the corneal endothelium. When possible, addressing the underlying condition (eg, by performing laser peripheral iridotomy or cataract extraction) may be necessary prior to or concurrent with GDD implantation. Materials that can occlude the lumen of the GDD include vitreous, fibrin, or blood. If these substances are known to be present during the preoperative examination, the surgeon may need to address them before implanting the GDD into the eye, by performing a vitrectomy to remove vitreous or an anterior chamber washout to remove extensive hemorrhage or fibrin. In patients with active uveitis, use of topical, subconjunctival, or sub-Tenon's corticosteroids during the preoperative period and at the time of surgery can limit postoperative inflammation.

Iris

If neovascularization of the iris is present in the preoperative evaluation, an injection of an anti-vascular endothelial growth factor (VEGF) agent should be considered. These agents can reduce the risk for intra- and postoperative bleeding during GDD surgery, and, occasionally, anti-VEGF agents can cause regression of neovascularization of the angle and resolution of the IOP elevation, thus negating the need for GDD surgery.[3] If anterior segment neovascularization is noted, the surgeon may consider indirect panretinal photocoagulation concurrent with GDD surgery. If the surgeon notes signs of iridocorneal endothelial (ICE) syndrome during the preoperative examination, he or she should try, whenever possible, to implant the GDD into the posterior chamber to reduce the chance that ICE material can proliferate into the lumen and obstruct the GDD.

Status of the Lens

When planning for GDD surgery, the surgeon should take note of whether the patient's eye is phakic, pseudophakic, or aphakic. Patients who are phakic should be informed that the surgery can hasten the development of cataracts. In addition, the surgeon should try to leave the tip of the tube short so that it will not get in the way during future cataract surgery. In patients who are phakic, it is necessary to implant the GDD in the anterior chamber. In patients with pseudophakia or aphakia, the surgeon may want to consider implanting the GDD into the posterior chamber, to reduce the risk for postoperative corneal decompensation in high-risk patients, such as those with Fuchs' endothelial dystrophy.

Intraocular Pressure

All patients who are being considered for GDD surgery have levels of IOP that are higher than desirable, which increases their risk for irreversible glaucomatous damage. During the preoperative evaluation, the surgeon should think about whether there is a need for short-term IOP control, long-term IOP control, or both. All patients who present with extensive glaucomatous damage will require long-term IOP control. However, there will be a subset of these patients who have such extensive damage to their optic nerve already or a high enough IOP that they are also at risk for vision loss in the short term if the surgeon implants a nonvalved GDD; it takes weeks before the GDD becomes functional. Other patients may present with a markedly elevated IOP, as a result of anterior segment neovascularization, uveitis, or exposure to corticosteroids, but the eye care provider has identified the problem before any glaucomatous damage has occurred. In this subset of patients, the goal of GDD surgery is to immediately lower the IOP to a safer level; yet, achieving a very low IOP over the long term may not be necessary because these patients have healthy nerves with little or no damage. In patients who present with markedly elevated IOP and require short-term IOP control, implanting a flow-restrictive GDD, such as an Ahmed FP7 (New World Medical, Inc), can be effective at immediately lowering the IOP. If the surgeon prefers to implant a nonvalved GDD, such as a Baerveldt GDD, because these devices are tied off for the first few weeks after implantation, venting slits must be created in the lumen of the GDD to help regulate the IOP in the short term until it is safe to open the tube. There is some evidence that GDDs with larger plates can achieve a lower IOP in the long term than can other devices with smaller plates. An ongoing randomized clinical trial is testing this theory.[4] Assuming this theory is correct, many surgeons prefer to implant GDDs that have larger-sized plates, such as the Baerveldt-350, in patients with advanced glaucoma who require a long-term low target IOP (in the low teens or lower), rather than devices with smaller-sized plates, such as an Ahmed GDD. Many of these patients can tolerate an IOP that is slightly above target for a few weeks after GDD implantation as they wait until it is safe for the tube to open and aqueous to flow through the GDD.

A small subset of patients have advanced glaucoma requiring long-term IOP control from a GDD with a larger plate size (eg, a Baerveldt-350), yet the preoperative IOP is also so high, or the damage to the optic nerve so advanced, that it would be too risky to implant a nonvalved GDD and simply wait a few weeks before the IOP can be lowered by opening the GDD. The surgeon has several options for managing these patients. One option is to implant a nonvalved Baerveldt-350 GDD and create venting slits in the lumen of the tube, with the hope that the venting slits will effectively lower the IOP in the short term until it is safe for fluid to flow through the GDD and collect around the plate. A second option is to combine the implantation of the Baerveldt-350 with an orphan trabeculectomy; one that is performed for the sole purpose of achieving an immediate lowering of IOP during the postoperative period until the GDD becomes functional. A third option is to perform a double-tube surgery, simultaneously implanting a Baerveldt-350 in the superotemporal quadrant to achieve long-term IOP control and an Ahmed S3 in the superonasal quadrant that, along with the use of aqueous suppressants, can achieve short-term IOP control until the Baerveldt-350 becomes functional. A fourth option is to implant a biplate Ahmed GDD. These devices contain a flow-restrictive element so that the IOP can be lowered immediately, but they also have 2 plates and thus a larger surface area for aqueous to accumulate, providing long-term IOP control.

Extent of Glaucomatous Damage

When evaluating a patient for GDD surgery, the surgeon must carefully consider the extent of glaucomatous damage present. Patients who have elevated IOPs with minimal or no damage to the optic nerve and retinal nerve fiber layer may not require a very low IOP during the postoperative period. In contrast, those who have extensive visual field loss and cupping of the optic nerve may require very low target pressures after the surgery. According to preliminary results of the Ahmed Baerveldt Comparison Trial, patients with extensive damage who require a very low IOP after GDD surgery may do better with a Baerveldt-350 than an Ahmed GDD.[5]

Retina

In patients who are undergoing GDD surgery for neovascular glaucoma, it is useful to inspect the retina to determine whether the patient would benefit from concomitant panretinal photocoagulation along with the GDD implantation.

Gonioscopy

Before proceeding with GDD surgery, it can be helpful to perform gonioscopy to identify the presence of peripheral anterior synechiae in the region of the drainage angle where the GDD will be implanted. In patients with pseudophakia, who have extensive peripheral anterior synechiae, the surgeon can avoid the synechiae and position the tube tip away from the corneal endothelium by implanting the GDD in the posterior chamber rather than the anterior chamber. Sulcus placement of the GDD can be ideal in this situation. In patients with neovascular glaucoma, preoperative gonioscopy can identify areas of active angle neovascularization, so these locations can be avoided during tube insertion. Patients with Fuchs' heterochromic iridocyclitis are also at increased risk for bleeding with GDD implantation, and gonioscopy can alert the surgeon to be prepared for this postoperative complication.

Hardware

During the preoperative assessment, the surgeon should check that there are no pieces of hardware, such as scleral buckle elements, present in the location where the plate of the GDD will be attached to the globe. If the patient has a scleral buckle present, the surgeon should consult with a retina specialist to determine whether it is safe, if necessary, to remove the element to free up space for the GDD. Some of the more modern scleral buckles may not require removal, as often the plate of the GDD can be positioned posterior to the buckle or sewn to the buckle element itself. If silicone oil is present in the eye, it will likely need to be removed before GDD implantation because it can obstruct the GDD or exit the eye via the GDD.

KEY POINTS

1. Decisions made during the preoperative evaluation can play an important role in the ultimate success of GDD surgery.

2. Factors affecting the decision about what type of GDD implant to use include the extent of glaucomatous damage present, the target IOP desired, the absolute level of IOP at the time of surgery and whether the eye can likely sustain this level of pressure for several weeks after implantation of a non–flow-restrictive device, and the type of glaucoma.

3. Important factors that affect the location of GDD placement in the eye include the presence of conjunctival scarring from prior surgery, whether the patient is phakic or pseudophakic, the depth of the anterior chamber, whether the eye has previously undergone pars plana vitrectomy, and the presence of previously placed hardware, such as scleral buckle elements.

4. Surgeons should plan ahead and, on occasion, modify their technique in patients at increased risk for infection, hypotony, bleeding, or suprachoroidal hemorrhage. Whenever possible, discontinuation of the use of medications that may predispose patients to intraoperative or postoperative bleeding should be considered.

5. Prior to proceeding with GDD surgery, it is essential to take the time to have a discussion of the risks, benefits, and alternatives of the surgery with the patient, to answer questions she may have, and to help set realistic expectations.

REFERENCES

1. Schwartz KS, Lee RK, Gedde SJ. Glaucoma drainage implants: a critical comparison of types. *Curr Opin Ophthalmol.* 2006;17(2):181-189.
2. Jeganathan VS, Ghosh S, Ruddle JB, et al. Risk factors for delayed suprachoroidal haemorrhage following glaucoma surgery. *Br J Ophthalmol.* 2008;92(10):1393-1396.
3. Duch S, Buchacra O, Milla E, et al. Intracameral bevacizumab (Avastin) for neovascular glaucoma: a pilot study in 6 patients. *J Glaucoma.* 2009;18(2):140-143.
4. Barton K, Gedde SJ, Budenz DL, Feuer WJ, Schiffman J; Ahmed Baerveldt Comparison Study Group. The Ahmed Baerveldt Comparison Study: methodology, baseline patient characteristics, and intraoperative complications. *Ophthalmology.* 2011;118(3):435-442.
5. Budenz DL, Barton K, Feuer WJ, et al. Treatment outcomes in the Ahmed Baerveldt Comparison Study after 1 year of follow-up. *Ophthalmology.* 2011;118(3):443-452.

7

TYPES OF GLAUCOMA
DRAINAGE IMPLANTS

Jeffrey M. Zink, MD

INTRODUCTION

Two basic types of glaucoma drainage implants are used in glaucoma surgery. One type that has no valve, and 1 type that has a valve mechanism to moderate against hypotony. Both types have a silicone tube that is attached to a plate with a 0.3mm-lumen.[1] The Baerveldt (Abbott Medical Optics, Abbott Laboratories Inc., Abbott Park, Illinois) and Molteno (Molteno Ophthalmic Limited, Dunedin, New Zealand) glaucoma drainage implants do not have a valve to restrict flow, and typically require a ligation suture to restrict flow in the early postoperative period to avoid hypotony. The first tube shunt equipped with a valve was the Krupin Valve (E. Benson Hood Laboratories, Inc., Pembroke, Massachusetts) in 1976, which is a tube attached to a plate with a unidirectional valve. Ahmed valve implants (New World Medical Inc., Rancho Cucamonga, California) are now the most commonly utilized glaucoma drainage implant equipped with a valve.

In both valved implants and nonvalved implants there exists a variety of sizes and, in some models, different implant material composition. Increasing the size of the glaucoma drainage implant plate is a strategy that has been used to try and achieve better intraocular pressure (IOP) lowering results. Heuer et al[2] showed lower postoperative IOPs in patients that received double-plate ($270mm^2$) compared to single-plate ($135 mm^2$) Molteno implants. Alternatively, Britt et al[3] found no additional IOP lowering benefit of the Baerveldt 500 mm^2 as compared to the 350 mm^2 in a randomized clinical trial. This suggests that there may be a benefit of lower IOP with increasing implant surface area to a certain degree, but this advantage is not necessarily consistent as implant size increases. Table 7-1 illustrates the characteristics of some of the most commonly used glaucoma drainage implants.[4]

Kahook M.
Essentials of Glaucoma Surgery (pp 73-80).
© 2012 SLACK Incorporated.

TABLE 7-1. CHARACTERISTICS OF MOST COMMON GLAUCOMA DRAINAGE IMPLANTS

Device	Ahmed		Molteno		Baerveldt	
Model	S2	FP7	DI	Molteno3	BG 103-250	BG 101-350
Device image						
Surface area	184 mm²	184 mm²	133 mm²	175 mm²	250 mm²	350 mm²
Side to side	13 mm	13 mm	13 mm	14.2 mm	22 mm	32 mm
Front to back	16 mm	16 mm	13 mm	13.6 mm	14 mm	15 mm
Implant profile	1.9 mm	0.9 mm	1.65 mm	1.5 mm	0.84 mm	0.84 mm
Single quadrant insertion	Yes	Yes	Yes	Yes	Yes	Yes
Plate material	Rigid polypropylene	Smooth silicone	Rigid polypropylene	Polypropylene	Smooth silicone	Smooth silicone
Drainage tube	Valved	Valved	Open	Open	Open	Open
Fixation suture holes	Yes	Yes	Yes	Yes	Yes	Yes
Manufacturer	New World Medical, Inc	New World Medical, Inc	Molteno Ophthalmic, Ltd	Molteno Ophthalmic, Ltd	Abbott Medical Optic	Abbott Medical Optic

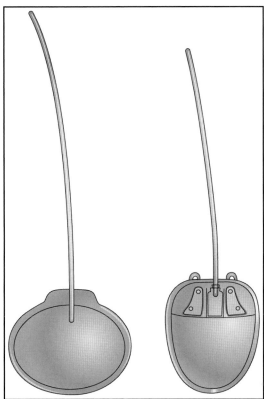

Figure 7-1. Krupin valve (left) and Ahmed valve (right). Both models contain a flow-restrictive valve designed to minimize the risk of hypotony.

Valved Implants

Valved implants were designed to lower the risk of hypotony by having a pressure valve that only lets fluid through the tube and into the subconjunctival space of the implant plate when the IOP exceeds around 8 to 11 mm Hg, depending on the type of the valved implant. They also provide the advantage of lowering pressure sooner, because there they are designed to establish filtration immediately upon insertion (Figure 7-1).

Ahmed Glaucoma Drainage Implant

Ahmed glaucoma drainage implants are made with either polypropylene or silicone for the plate body composition. The characteristics of the plate material are thought to have some effect on the capsule that forms over the plate. It has been shown that the polypropylene endplate of the Ahmed glaucoma valve induces greater amount of inflammation than the silicone end plate of the Baerveldt implant in the rabbit subconjunctival space.[5] The amount of inflammation generated by different biomaterials may influence capsular thickness and resistance characteristics, which can affect IOP. Clinically, it has been shown that the popular Ahmed model FP7 may provide better pressure control when compared to the Ahmed S2 polypropylene model.[6]

Because the valve mechanism is designed to reduce the chance of hypotony, valved implants are well suited for patients with compromised aqueous secretion. Patients with uveitis, ciliary body ischemia or fibrosis, and prior cyclodestructive procedures are good candidates for a valved implant, such as the Ahmed. Valved implants can also be ideal for patients that need immediate IOP lowering with a very high preoperative IOP (eg, neovascular glaucoma). The Ahmed silicone models include the FP7 (Flexible plate), FP8 (Flexible plate pediatric), FX1 (Flexible bi-plate), PC7 (FP 7 model with pars plana clip), and PC8 (FP 8 model with pars plana clip). The polypropylene models include the S2 (Ahmed glaucoma valve), S3 (Pediatric glaucoma valve), B1 (bi-plate), PS2 (S2 model with pars plana clip), and the PS3 (S3 model pediatric with pars plana clip).

Krupin Valve

Krupen et al[7] introduced the unidirectional, pressure-sensitive valve in 1976. The Krupin valve is designed to open at a pressure of 11 mm Hg and close at a pressure of 9 mm Hg.[8] This was the first valved implant to reduce the incidence of early postoperative hypotony following aqueous drainage implant surgery.[8] This valve has become less popular with the advent of the Ahmed glaucoma valve, which was introduced in 1993.

Nonvalved

Nonvalved implants do not contain a valve that restricts flow through the tube. As described previously, the nonvalved implants must be flow-restricted to allow time for adequate capsule formation and prevent immediate postoperative hypotony. Nonvalved implants can achieve immediate postoperative IOP control when tube fenestrations are performed. Tube fenestrations allow aqueous to drain from the tube, and into the subconjunctival space anterior to the suture ligation.[9] Although fenestrations are often helpful, they are not necessarily the most consistent way to lower pressure, as there is always some variability of the magnitude and the duration of their effect. Some surgeons prefer to combine a trabeculectomy with insertion of the nonvalved ligated implant to achieve immediate postoperative pressure control. This can be a very reliable way to titrate IOP when immediate pressure lowering is desired and the surgeon prefers the insertion of a nonvalved implant (Figure 7-2).

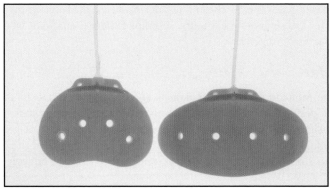

Figure 7-2. Baerveldt implant models 250 mm² (left) and 350 mm² (right) versions. These implants lack a flow-restrictive valve and require flow restriction in the early postoperative period to minimize the risk of hypotony. (Reprinted with permission from Allingham R, ed. *Shields Texbook of Glaucoma*. 6th ed. Philadelphia, PA: Lippincott Williams & Wilkins; 2011.)

Baerveldt

The Baerveldt glaucoma drainage implant has a large surface area plate attached to a tube for aqueous drainage. The Baerveldt implant is made of thin, durable, and flexible silicone material that is barium impregnated.[10] This implant is designed to maximize filtration surface area, while still allowing single quadrant insertion. There are 3 types of Baerveldt glaucoma drainage implants: The Baerveldt 101-350, the Baerveldt 103-250, and the 102-350 designed for pars plana insertion. The Baerveldt 101-350 has a 350 mm² surface area and is larger than the 103-250 that has a 250 mm² plate surface area. The Baerveldt 101-350 is a popular model, and the drainage implant plate is usually placed underneath the rectus muscles.

The Baerveldt 102-350 has a 350 mm² plate, as well as a smaller plate attached to the tube that is sutured to the sclera in the area of the pars plana. This smaller plate has a Hoffman elbow design that allows direct insertion of the tube into the pars plana, and is done through a 20-gauge pars plana sclerostomy incision.

All Baerveldt implants are designed with holes in the plate. The holes allow fibrous tissue to grow through and are designed to achieve a lower bleb profile and minimize extraocular muscle disturbances. The Baerveldt implant's lower profile enables it to be used in the inferior nasal or inferior temporal quadrant quite easily. A retrospective, noncomparative case series demonstrated the effectiveness of the Baerveldt glaucoma implant in the inferonasal quadrant.[11] I prefer the inferior nasal quadrant as my second choice for tube location next to the superior temporal quadrant when placing a Baerveldt implant.

Molteno

The Molteno glaucoma implant is another popular aqueous drainage implant design without a valve mechanism. Molteno implants come in multiple designs and have been studied for over 30 years in the management of glaucoma. In a rabbit model in 1969, Molteno first introduced the concept of a translimbal tube attached to an acrylic plate to facilitate aqueous drainage.[12]

Single-Plate Molteno

The Molteno single-plate design is ideal for single quadrant use and is relatively easy to insert with a relatively small conjunctival dissection. This is the original aqueous drainage implant design.

Double-Plate Molteno

The double-plate Molteno has a larger surface area, which is ideal when more IOP lowering effect is desired. This implant has the flexibility of additional postoperative control. The tube connecting the two plates, or the tube entering the eye, can be ligated with a temporary or permanent suture.[13] A ligature suture applied to the connecting tube can restrict excess flow to the second plate, which can give the surgeon more control over the amount of aqueous drainage depending on a patient's pressure lowering needs.

Molteno3

The newer Molteno3 has a more flexible, larger plate than the earlier designs, and has an oval subsidiary ridge designed to form a biological valve to reduce postoperative hypotony.[13] The biological valve works by limiting aqueous flow to the primary area of drainage until IOP increases to the point where the resistance of the overlying tissue is overcome, allowing aqueous drainage to expand over the whole plate.[13] The use of the biological valve on the Molteno3 is intended for glaucomas with very high preoperative IOPs, where acute pressure lowering is needed. It can be helpful in cases where a traditional valved shunt may become occluded by clot or fibrin, such as neovascular or inflammatory glaucomas. Hypotony can still be seen in the early postoperative period with this device if it is not ligated. Therefore, in most routine glaucoma cases, the Molteno3 is ligated similar to a nonvalved shunt and the biological valve mechanism is not utilized in the early postoperative period.

Schocket

The Schocket glaucoma implant, also known as the ACTSEB (anterior chamber tube shunt to encircling band), was described by Schocket et al[14] for the treatment of neovascular glaucoma. The Schocket implant technique utilizes a silastic tube used for nasolacrimal intubation (diameter 0.30 mm). One end is placed underneath and sutured into the groove of a #20 retinal encircling band that is placed underneath the rectus muscles. The other end is placed into the anterior chamber to allow aqueous outflow to the capsule that forms around the encircling band. Modifications of the Schocket technique have been reported using smaller buckle element segments.[15] This implant type has the advantage of being relatively inexpensive and can be used in places where glaucoma drainage implants are difficult to obtain, such as in developing countries. However, this implant is currently rarely used due to the existence of more modern implant designs.

OTHER IMPLANTS

Ahmed implants also have 2 commercially available models of non-valved implants: a silicone nonvalved flexible plate implant (the FX4), and a polypropylene nonvalved model (the B4).

KEY POINTS

1. Nonvalved implants require a ligature suture, sometimes combined with a stent suture, to restrict flow in the early postoperative period.

2. Valved implants establish flow immediately and do not require a ligation suture.

3. IOP control may be influenced by the size of the glaucoma drainage implant plate, up to a certain point.

4. The type of material of the glaucoma drainage implant plate (silicone versus polypropylene) may influence the capsule characteristics and affect IOP control.

5. Smaller implants are available for pediatric glaucoma cases.

6. Pars plana models are available in the Baerveldt and Ahmed implants.

REFERENCES

1. Sidoti P. Glaucoma drainage implants. In: Morrison JC, Pollack IC, eds. *Glaucoma: Science and Practice.* New York, NY: Thieme; 2002:481.

2. Heuer DK, Lloyd MA, Abrams DA, et al. Which is better? One or two? A randomized clinical trial of single-plate versus double-plate Molteno implantation for glaucomas in aphakia and pseudophakia. *Ophthalmology.* 1992;99(10):1512-1519.

3. Britt MT, LaBree LD, Lloyd MA, et al. Randomized clinical trial of the 350-mm² versus the 500-mm² Baerveldt implant: long term results. Is bigger better? *Ophthalmology.* 1999;106(12):2312-2318.

4. Kahook, MY, Noecker RJ, Pantcheva MB, Schuman JS. Location of glaucoma drainage devices relative to the optic nerve. *Br J Ophthalmol.* 2006;90(8):1010-1013.

5. Ayyala RS, Harman LE, Michelini-Norris, et al. Comparison of different biomaterials for glaucoma drainage devices. *Arch Ophthalmol.* 1999;117(2):233-236.

6. Ishida K, Netland, PA, Costa VP, Shrioma L, Khan B, Ahmed II. Comparison of polypropylene and silicone Ahmed Glaucoma Valves. *Ophthalmology.* 2006;113(8):1320-1326.

7. Krupin T, Podos SM, Becker B, et al. Valve implants in filtering surgery. *Am J Ophthalmol.* 1976;81(2):232-235.

8. Hong C, Arosememena A, Zurakowski D, Ayyala S. Glaucoma drainage devices: a systematic literature review and current controversies. *Surv Ophthalmol.* 2005;50(1):48-60.

9. Emerick GT, Gedde SJ, Budenz DL. Tube fenestrations in the Baerveldt glaucoma implant surgery: 1-year results compared with standard implant surgery. *J Glaucoma.* 2002;11(4):340-346.

10. Baerveldt glaucoma implant [package insert]. Kalamazoo, MI: Abbott Medical Optics & Upjohn, Inc; 2000.

11. Harbick KH, Sidoti PA, Budenz DL, et al. Outcomes of inferonasal Baerveldt glaucoma drainage implant surgery. *J Glaucoma.* 2006;15(1):7-12.

12. Molteno ACB. New implant for draining in glaucoma. *Br J Ophthalmol.* 1969;53(3):161-168.

13. Molteno Ophthalmic Web site. http://www.molteno.com/.

14. Schocket SS, Nirankari VS, Lakhanpal V, et al. Anterior chamber tube shunt to an encircling band in the treatment of neovascular glaucoma. *Ophthalmology.* 1982;89:1188-1194.

15. Omi CA, Almeida GV, Cohen R, Mandia C, Kwitko S. Modified Schocket implant for refractory glaucoma. *Ophthalmology.* 1991;98(2):211-214.

8

STANDARD TECHNIQUE FOR IMPLANTING GLAUCOMA DRAINAGE DEVICES

Joshua D. Stein, MD, MS

This chapter will review a basic step-by-step technique for implantation of non–flow-restrictive (eg, Baerveldt) and flow-restrictive (eg, Ahmed) glaucoma drainage devices (GDDs). The chapter will cover suggested instruments used to perform each step of the procedure, a description of how to perform each step of the surgery, the rationale for why each step of the procedure is performed, and a description of some pearls and pitfalls associated with each step of the procedure. The focus of this chapter is the description of the basic technique for GDD implantation. Please see subsequent chapters for a description of modifications of the techniques described below to address more complicated situations that one may encounter when performing GDD surgery.

OBTAINING ADEQUATE EXPOSURE

Adequate exposure is essential when performing GDD surgery. Two options are available for improving exposure. One option is to place a traction suture through the superior cornea. A 7-0 polyglactin suture is passed through the peripheral cornea at the 12 o'clock position. For inferior tube placement, an inferior corneal traction suture can be placed in a similar fashion at the 6 o'clock position. Care should be taken not to take too deep a pass and penetrate into the anterior chamber. If the patient has had a prior penetrating keratoplasty or other incisional corneal surgery, the corneal traction suture should be placed in a manner to avoid these sites. An alternative option to a corneal traction suture is to place the suture around the superior rectus muscle. After the traction suture is placed, the eye is rotated inferonasally to maximize exposure to the superotemporal bulbar

Kahook M.
Essentials of Glaucoma Surgery (pp 81–94).
© 2012 SLACK Incorporated.

conjunctiva. The traction suture is secured to the operative drape with a hemostat. A corneal protector is then placed over the cornea to protect it during the procedure and reduce retinal exposure to bright light from the operating microscope. Placement of viscoelastic beneath the corneal shield in patients with severe surface disease or corneal pathology can help to reduce the chance of a corneal epithelial defect developing during surgery.

CONJUNCTIVAL INCISION

The technique I prefer is to create a conjunctival peritomy 5 mm posterior to the limbus. A caliper is used to measure 5 mm posterior to the limbus in the superotemporal quadrant. Using nontoothed forceps, such as Pierce-Hoskins forceps (Katena Eye Instruments, Denville, New Jersey) or Max Fine forceps (Altomed, Boldon, United Kingdom), the bulbar conjunctiva is gently tented up, and an incision is made through the conjunctiva with Westcott scissors. Using the Pierce-Hoskins forceps to hold up the conjunctiva adjacent to the incision, use Westcott scissors though the conjunctival incision to perform blunt dissection of the surrounding bulbar conjunctiva. Extend the initial conjunctival incision temporally and superiorly for 2 clock hours. The incision should follow the curve of the limbus. When extending the incision laterally and superiorly, the surgeon should be careful not to cut the superior or lateral recti muscles. Next, grasp Tenon's capsule with the Pierce-Hoskins forceps and cut through it with Westcott scissors down to bare sclera. After Tenon's tissue has been cut, it is best (whenever possible) to avoid grasping the conjunctiva until the time of closure so this tissue does not become damaged. Instead of grasping conjunctival tissue, grasp Tenon's tissue with the Pierce-Hoskins forceps and use the Westcott scissors to perform blunt dissection to create a pocket in the superotemporal quadrant for the implant to be placed (Figure 8-1). Enter with the curved Stevens scissors (Katena Eye Instruments) and continue with blunt dissection. Adequate blunt dissection is achieved when one can insert closed curved Stevens scissors into the superotemporal quadrant and open them wide with little resistance. If bleeding is encountered during the blunt dissection, use cautery to achieve hemostasis. Instead of performing the conjunctival perimetry 5 mm posterior to the limbus as described above, an alternative technique is to create the conjunctival peritomy directly at the limbus.

ANESTHESIA

My preference for anesthesia is to provide a sub-Tenon's injection of 3 to 4 cc of a 50/50 mixture of 2% lidocaine and 0.5% bupivicaine in the superotemporal quadrant around the superior and lateral rectus muscles. This should be done with a curved blunt-tip cannula (an olive tip works well). When injecting the anesthesia using the dominant hand,

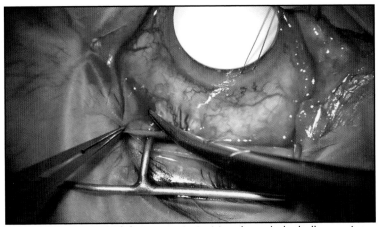

Figure 8-1. Conjunctival dissection. An incision through the bulbar conjunctiva was made 5 mm posterior to the limbus in the superotemporal quadrant. Pierce-Hoskins forceps are used to grasp Tenon's tissue, and Westcott scissors are used to perform blunt dissection separating the bulbar conjunctiva and Tenon's tissue from the underlying sclera.

simultaneously use a Pierce-Hoskins forceps with the nondominant hand to press down on the conjunctiva, which helps trap the anesthetic in the desired location. An alternative means of anesthetizing the eye for the GDD surgery would be to perform a peribulbar or retrobulbar block prior to beginning the surgery.

PREPARING THE GLAUCOMA DRAINAGE DEVICE FOR IMPLANTATION

Ahmed Glaucoma Drainage Device

Ahmed glaucoma drainage devices (models S2, FP7, and S3) contain a built-in element that acts like a one-way valve to restrict the flow of aqueous through the implant. Before an Ahmed glaucoma drainage device can be implanted into the eye, it is necessary to first prime the tube. Priming involves injecting balanced salt solution through the tube to assure tube patency. A 27- or 30-gauge cannula is attached to the tip of the tube. Balanced salt solution is injected through the tube. As one presses down on the plunger to flush the tube with balanced salt solution, one should encounter moderate resistance. If there is little or no resistance (ie, balanced salt solution exits through the tube with little or no force exerted on the plunger of the cannula), the implant may be defective. If it is inserted into the eye and the flow restrictive element is not properly restricting flow, the patient is at risk for postoperative hypotony. If extensive resistance is encountered during flushing with balanced salt solution, this may also indicate a defective flow-restrictive element, and if the tube is implanted, it may be nonfunctional. In either case, if the tube does not flush properly, ask for a new GDD and send the defective one back to the manufacturer.

Baerveldt Glaucoma Drainage Device

Baerveldt glaucoma drainage devices (models BG 103-250 and BG 101-350) do not contain a flow-restrictive element. However, they still need to be primed with balanced salt solution to verify the patency of the tube. A 27-gauge cannula is attached to the tip of the tube. There should be no resistance when balanced salt solution is passed through the tube.

Next, a piece of 6-0 Prolene (Ethicon, Somerville, New Jersey) or 5-0 nylon suture is passed through the lumen of the Baerveldt implant.[1] This piece of suture will serve as a ripcord that will allow the surgeon a means of opening the implant at the slit lamp during the postoperative period, thus making it functional. Although some surgeons elect not to use a ripcord with this procedure, I routinely use ripcords because it allows me to control the precise timing of the opening of the tube. Without a ripcord, if the 7-0 polyglactin ligature obstructing the GDD is not easily accessible to be able to apply laser to dissolve the suture in the clinic during the postoperative period (because it is covered by a scleral patch graft), the tube will open spontaneously and the surgeon will be unaware if the intraocular pressure becomes too low, putting the patient at increased risk for complications associated with hypotony.

The final step in preparing a Baerveldt GDD is to tightly tie off the tube using a piece of 7-0 absorbable polyglactin suture so that no aqueous can exit through the tube until a capsule has formed around the plate. Because Baerveldt implants have no mechanism to restrict the flow of aqueous, if a capsule of tissue has yet to form around the plate, the patient will experience hypotony during the immediate postoperative period if the tube is not tied off completely. To help assure that the tube is completely tied off and will remain so until a capsule has formed, the tube is tied off with the 7-0 polyglactin suture by using at least 3 knots. I routinely use 6 knots to tie off the tube to be absolutely sure it will not open prematurely. Next, the cannula containing balanced salt solution is reattached to the tip of the tube. An attempt is made to forcefully pass balanced salt solution through the occluded tube. With forceful irrigation, if the surgeon is able to pass balanced salt solution through the occluded tube, this indicates that it is not completely occluded. Additional 7-0 polyglactin sutures should be placed adjacent to the first suture and tied off in the same manner described above.

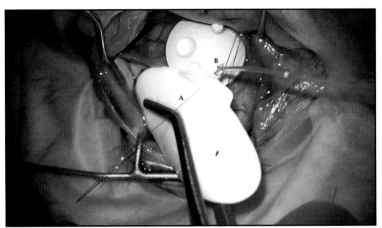

Figure 8-2. Preparing a Baerveldt 350 glaucoma drainage device for implantation. In preparation for implanting a Baerveldt 350 glaucoma drainage device, after flushing the tube with balanced salt solution, a 6-0 Prolene suture has been inserted through the lumen of the tube (A) and the tube is tied off with 7-0 polygalactin suture (B). The surgeon grasps the implant with Nugent forceps and is about to position it under an extraocular muscle.

Repeated testing with balanced salt solution should be performed until the surgeon is unable to forcefully pass any balanced salt solution through the tube, indicating it is completely occluded (Figure 8-2).

SECURING THE PLATE OF THE IMPLANT TO THE SCLERA

Ahmed Glaucoma Drainage Device

Ahmed GDDs are small enough that the plate can fit in between the superior and lateral rectus muscles. When grasping the Ahmed GDD to position it in the superotemporal quadrant, care should be taken to avoid touching the valvular element because it can easily get damaged. With the nondominant hand, the surgeon should use Pierce-Hoskins forceps to grasp and retract back the Tenon's tissue, exposing the underlying bare sclera in the superotemporal quadrant. Using Nugent forceps, the surgeon should grasp the plate of the Ahmed implant behind the valvular element and place it in the superotemporal quadrant between Tenon's tissue and bare sclera. When positioning the plate in the superotemporal quadrant, if resistance is encountered, one may need to perform additional blunt dissection using the Westcott or curved Stevens scissors. Next, the surgeon should use a caliper to mark the sclera 8 mm posterior to the limbus in the superotemporal quadrant. It is important that the plate is secured at least 8 mm posterior to the limbus, as a more anterior placement of the plate can increase the risk of developing dellen during the postoperative period. Next, the surgeon should pass a 9-0 nylon suture through the sclera, at least 8 mm posterior to the limbus. Although it is important to take an adequate bite of sclera with the suture pass so that the suture does not cheese-wire through the sclera when it is tied off, one needs to be careful not to take too deep of a pass through the sclera so that the suture penetrates the choroid or retina. After taking the scleral bite, the suture should then be passed through the eyelet of the implant and tied off. A second 9-0 nylon suture should be passed through the sclera and then through the other eyelet and tied off. Tying forceps are then used to bury the knots within the eyelets to reduce the risk of them eroding through the conjunctiva during the postoperative period. After the plate is secured to the underlying sclera, calipers should be used to verify that the plate is situated at least 8 mm posterior to the limbus. If the implant is more anterior than 8 mm, one or both of the nylon sutures may need to be cut and resecured further back from the limbus.

Baerveldt Glaucoma Drainage Device

Baerveldt glaucoma drainage devices have a larger surface area relative to Ahmed glaucoma drainage implants and must be positioned under the insertions of the superior and lateral rectus muscles. The Baerveldt 250 implant can be positioned with 1 wing under either the lateral or superior rectus muscle, whereas the Baerveldt 350 model is larger and needs to be positioned with both wings under the recti muscles. In general, this implant is designed to be placed underneath the extraocular muscles, but it can also be placed on top of the muscles in special circumstances, such as with prior strabismus surgery or traumatic globe injuries. In these cases, the normal extraocular muscle anatomy can be significantly disrupted, making standard placement underneath the muscles difficult or impossible.

Before attempting to place the implant in the superotemporal quadrant, the surgeon should use a muscle hook to identify and isolate the superior and lateral rectus muscles. It is important to clean and check ligaments beneath the muscles to ensure that the wing of the implant passes freely underneath the muscle. Next, with the nondominant hand, the surgeon should use Pierce-Hoskins forceps to grasp and retract back the Tenon's tissue, exposing the underlying bare sclera in the superotemporal quadrant. With the dominant hand, the surgeon should next isolate and hook either the superior or lateral rectus muscles. After the muscle is hooked, the surgeon should hold the hooked muscle with the nondominant hand, freeing the dominant hand to be able to position the plate of the implant under the muscle. Using Nugent forceps, the surgeon should grasp the plate of the Baerveldt implant and place 1 wing of the plate behind the hooked rectus muscle. After the wing is situated behind the rectus muscle, the surgeon can release the hooked muscle and slide the muscle hook out from between the rectus muscle and wing of the plate. When removing the muscle hook, care should be taken to ensure that the wing of the Baerveldt remains properly positioned posterior to the rectus muscle.

When implanting the Baerveldt 350 model implant, the surgeon must next isolate and hook the second rectus muscle with the muscle hook. After this muscle is hooked, the plate of the implant is manipulated so that the second wing is positioned posterior to the hooked rectus muscle. When the wing is visualized behind the insertion of the rectus muscle, the hooked rectus muscle can be released and the muscle hook can be slid out from between the rectus muscle and the wing of the plate. Before securing the plate to the underlying sclera, the surgeon can check to verify that both wings of the implant are posterior to the recti muscles by grasping one of the eyelets with 0.12 forceps and tugging the plate toward the limbus. If both wings of the plate are posterior to the muscle insertions, resistance will be met when attempting to tug the plate more anterior toward the limbus. If there is little or no resistance with this maneuver, it may indicate that one or both of the wings may not be posterior to the rectus muscles, and the plate will need to be repositioned before it can be secured to the sclera.

Next, the surgeon should use calipers to mark the sclera 8 mm posterior to the limbus in the superotemporal quadrant. It is important that the plate is secured at least 8 mm posterior to the limbus, as a more anterior placement of the plate can increase the risk of developing dellen or plate erosions during the postoperative period. The surgeon should then pass a 9-0 nylon suture through the sclera, at least 8 mm posterior to the limbus. Although it is important to take an adequate bite of sclera with the suture pass so that the suture does not cheese-wire through the sclera when it is tied off, one needs to be careful not to take too deep of a pass through the sclera so that the suture penetrates the choroid or retina. After taking the sclera bite, the suture should then be passed through the eyelet of the implant and tied off. A second 9-0 nylon suture should be passed through the sclera and then through the other eyelet and tied off. Tying forceps are then used to bury the knots within the eyelets to reduce the risk of them eroding through the conjunctiva during the postoperative period. After the plate is secured to the underlying sclera, the calipers should be used to verify that the plate is situated at least 8 mm posterior to the limbus. If the implant is more anterior than 8 mm, one or both of the nylon sutures may need to be cut and resecured further back from the limbus. For placement of Baerveldt GDDs in the inferonasal and inferotemporal quadrants, a similar technique is followed except that the wings of the implant are placed beneath the inferior rectus and corresponding medial or lateral rectus muscles.

ADDITIONAL CONJUNCTIVAL DISSECTION

The bulbar conjunctiva adjacent to the limbus can be thin and friable, and after it is dissected away from the underlying sclera it can lose its viability if it dries out. For this reason, I find it useful to hold off performing blunt dissection of this tissue away from the underlying sclera until after the plate is secured to the sclera. Using Westcott scissors, blunt dissection of the conjunctiva and Tenon's tissue is performed all the way anterior up to the limbus. Additional blunt dissection can be performed by using Weck-Cel spears (Medtronic, Jacksonville, Florida) to gently lyse any additional adhesions that are present at the limbus. It is important to exert care when manipulating this tissue so it does not tear. If bleeding is encountered, cautery should be applied, when necessary, to achieve hemostasis. If there is scar tissue at the superotemporal limbus from prior intraocular surgery, the tube may need to be rerouted to adjacent tissue, which may be more viable. Likewise, if there is a prior trabeculectomy flap present in the superotemporal quadrant, care should be taken to avoid routing the tube through the flap of the trabeculectomy. Note, this step is not necessary if the initial conjunctival incision was performed at the limbus rather than 5 mm posterior to the limbus.

TRIMMING THE TUBE

Corneal traction is released so that the eye can return to its normal position and the surgeon can determine the optimal location to trim the tube. Release of corneal traction is important because if the surgeon trims the tube while the eye is torqued inferonasally without accounting for this, the tip of the tube may end up too long in the anterior chamber after traction is released. If the tube needs to be rerouted around scar tissue, this should be taken into consideration when deciding the location to trim the tube, as it may need to be longer to account for such rerouting. With the nondominant hand, the tube is grasped with tying forceps and Westcott or Vannas scissors are used with the dominant hand to trim the tube in a manner so that a sharp bevel is created (Figure 8-3). It is important not to forcefully tug the tube toward the center of the cornea when grasping it with the nondominant hand prior to trimming it, as this can cause the surgeon to inadvertently trim the tube so that it is too short. When trimming the tube, one should err on the side of too long rather than too short. If it is too long, it can always be trimmed shorter, whereas if the tube is trimmed too short, a tube extender may be required to lengthen it.

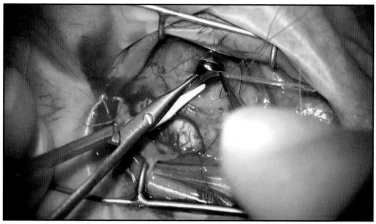

Figure 8-3. Trimming the tube. Westcott scissors are used to trim the tube to the proper length. When trimming the tube, by positioning the Westcott scissors in a plane that is nearly parallel to that of the tube, the surgeon is able to create a sharp bevel, which can facilitate insertion of the tube through the sclerostomy.

If the plan is to insert the tube into the anterior chamber, one should trim the tube so that it will extend 2 to 3 mm into the anterior chamber with its bevel directed upward. If the tube is trimmed too short, there is a possibility it may retract posteriorly during the postoperative period and out of the anterior chamber. If the tube is trimmed too long, it increases the risk of the tip contacting the corneal endothelium, which would lead to corneal decompensation. If the plan is to insert the tube into the posterior chamber, the surgeon should create a downward rather than an upward bevel and should trim the tube so that it is longer. If the tube is cut short, it will be completely hidden behind the iris after it is inserted into the posterior chamber. By trimming the tube longer, it will be easier to visualize the tip of the tube during the postoperative period. If the plan is to insert the tube into the vitreous cavity to facilitate visualization of the tube tip, the surgeon should trim it so that it will extend at least 6 mm within the vitreous cavity. In eyes with prior vitrectomy, a longer tube in the vitreous cavity will also reduce the risk of tube occlusion from retained vitreous. This can happen in the setting of an incomplete vitrectomy where the vitreous skirt may not have been adequately trimmed prior to the tube insertion.

PARACENTESIS

A 75/15 blade or microvitreoretinal blade is used to create a paracentesis through temporal clear cornea. The purpose of creating a paracentesis is so that the surgeon can easily access the anterior chamber to reinflate the anterior chamber with balanced salt solution if it gets too shallow or to insert a cyclodiaylsis spatula in the event that the tip of the tube happens to get stuck in the iris during insertion. The paracentesis also gives the surgeon access to the anterior chamber in the early postoperative period to acutely lower or raise the intraocular pressure (IOP) by "burping" aqueous from the paracentesis or injecting viscoelastic through the paracentesis in the setting of profound hypotony.

SCLEROSTOMY

Arguably, the most important step of the surgery is the creation of the sclerostomy, as this will determine where the tube will be positioned within the eye. The sclerostomy is created with a 22- or 23-gauge needle. An advantage of using a 22-gauge needle to create the sclerostomy is that it creates a larger sclerostomy so that it is easier to insert the tube into the anterior chamber. A disadvantage of a larger-size sclerostomy is that aqueous can exit through the sclerostomy around the lumen of the tube, increasing the risk of postoperative hypotony. For this reason, I prefer using a 23-gauge needle to create the sclerostomy. Although it creates a sclerostomy with a tighter fit, there is less room for aqueous to exit through the sclerostomy around the tube and thus a reduced risk of postoperative hypotony.

For implantation of the tube into the anterior chamber, I choose an entry site as anterior to the limbus as possible approximately at the 10:30 or 11 o'clock position whenoperating on a right eye; I use 1 o'clock for left eyes. If a buttonhole is present in the overlying conjunctiva at the planned site of the sclerostomy, I will create the sclerostomy at a different location to avoid the conjunctival buttonhole. If the plan is to place the tube into the posterior chamber, I create the sclerostomy 2 mm posterior to the limbus, whereas if the plan is to implant the tube into the vitreous cavity, the sclerostomy should be created 3.5 mm posterior to the limbus. When creating the sclerostomy, the 23-gauge needle should be grasped with its bevel upward. To assure proper positioning of the tube in the anterior chamber, it is helpful to enter with the needle into the anterior chamber following a pathway that is parallel to the plane of the iris (Figure 8-4). If the needle does not enter parallel to the iris plane, the tip of the tube may end up positioned against the corneal endothelium, which can increase the risk of corneal decompensation, or with the tube tip embedded into the iris stroma so that aqueous is unable to exit through the tube. If the patient is phakic, care should be taken when creating the sclerostomy not to enter too deep into the anterior chamber with the needle so as to risk damaging the lens or lens capsule. When placing the tube into the vitreous cavity, the needle should be oriented so the tube will be positioned just anterior to the center of the vitreous cavity.

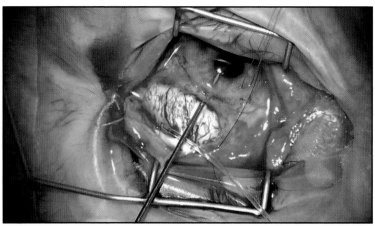

Figure 8-4. Creating the sclerostomy. A 23-gauge needle is used to create a sclerostomy. The angle of entry of the needle into the anterior chamber should be parallel to the plane of the iris with the bevel of the needle positioned upward.

Tube Insertion Through the Sclerostomy

Once the sclerostomy is created, the next step is to insert the tube through the sclerostomy. Gently retract the bulbar conjunctiva adjacent to the sclerostomy toward the limbus so it is not in the way during the tube insertion. Grasp the tube at its bevel with a tube introducer or angled Kelman forceps (Katena Eye Instruments) and insert the bevel completely into the sclerostomy. To facilitate the insertion, hold the bevel of the tube in the sclerostomy for 20 to 30 seconds before regrasping the tube slightly posteriorly and continue pushing the tube into the sclerostomy. Continue passing the tube through the sclerostomy until it can be visualized in the anterior chamber. Watch the tip of the tube as it enters into the anterior chamber to be sure that it is properly positioned in the anterior chamber. If the tip of the tube gets embedded in the iris, it can often be repositioned by inserting a cyclodialysis spatula through the paracentesis and sweeping the tip away from the iris. If the tube tip is visualized abutting the peripheral cornea, the tube will need to be pulled back out through the sclerostomy, the sclerostomy sutured shut, and a new sclerostomy created. If the tube tip is visualized to be too long, it should be pulled back out of the sclerostomy, trimmed to the proper length, and reinserted.

Securing the Tube to Sclera

To aid in the remaining steps of the surgery, the eye should again be rotated inferonasally and held in this position using the traction suture.

Once the tube is visualized to be properly positioned within the eye, the exposed portion of the tube is secured to the underlying sclera using a 9-0 nylon suture by creating a figure-of-eight knot. Care should be taken not to penetrate the lumen of the tube when passing this suture.

VENTING SLITS

Because Baerveldt implants are completely tied off, until the ripcord is pulled and the tube is opened or the tube opens spontaneously, the IOP will continue to remain elevated during the immediate postoperative period. Some surgeons elect to make 1 to 5 small punctures into the lumen of the tube between the sclerostomy and the plate that serve as venting slits to help lower the IOP during the immediate postoperative period.[2] The venting slits are created by using a spatulated needle. A TG-140 needle works well.

COVERING THE TUBE WITH A PATCH GRAFT

To prevent the tube from eroding through the overlying bulbar conjunctiva, it is strongly recommended to cover the exposed tube from the plate to the sclerostomy with a patch graft.[3] Different materials including donor sclera, donor cornea, or Tutoplast (New World Medical, Inc) can be used as a patch graft to cover the exposed tube. The most important portion of the tube requiring coverage with the patch graft is the site where the tube enters into the sclerostomy. The patch graft can be tacked down to the underlying sclera by using 2 to 4 7-0 polyglactin sutures (Figure 8-5). When securing the patch graft to the underlying sclera, care should be taken not to penetrate the lumen of the tube.

CONJUNCTIVAL CLOSURE

Prior to reapproximation of the conjunctival wound during Baerveldt implant surgery, one will need to trim the ripcord and tuck it under the bulbar conjunctiva before closing the conjunctival wound if the ripcord technique was used. The ripcord should be tucked under the conjunctiva in a location where it is easy to get to at the slit lamp, such as under the temporal bulbar conjunctiva, close to the limbus.

To reapproximate the conjunctiva, the posterior edge of the bulbar conjunctival wound is grasped with 2 Pierce-Hoskins forceps and gently shimmied forward so it can be sutured to the anterior edge of the bulbar conjunctival wound. Two to 3 evenly spaced interrupted 8-0 polyglactin sutures on a vascular needle are used to secure the 2 edges of the conjunctival wound. Next, the conjunctival wound is reapproximated by using a running locked 8-0 polyglactin suture on a vascular needle. During wound

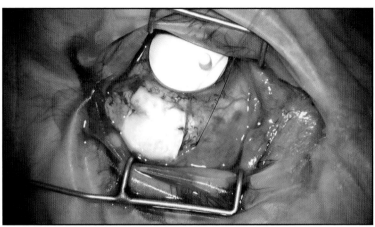

Figure 8-5. Covering the tube with a scleral patch graft. A scleral patch graft covers the tube its entire length from the plate to the sclerostomy. The patch graft has been secured in place by using two 7-0 polygalactin sutures. The 6-0 Prolene ripcord can be seen to the right of the scleral patch graft.

closure, it is very important to be sure that one is reapproximating bulbar conjunctiva to bulbar conjunctiva and not conjunctiva to Tenon's tissue.

COMPLETION OF THE SURGERY

At the conclusion of the surgery, one should inspect the depth of the anterior chamber and evaluate whether the IOP is physiologic. The traction suture is removed. A fluorescein strip is used to check the conjunctival wound and paracentesis site for leaks. A subconjunctival injection of steroids and antibiotics is given inferiorly. In cases of uveitic or neovascular glaucoma, a drop of atropine 1% can be helpful to help maximize the anterior chamber depth and stabilize the blood-ocular barrier. The eyelid speculum is removed. The eye is dressed with bacitracin or erythromycin ointment and closed. A patch and metal shield are placed over the eye for protection.

KEY POINTS

1. When preparing a non–flow-restrictive implant such as a Baerveldt GDD or Molteno GDD, is it essential that the tube is completely tied off before such devices are implanted into the eye. Without complete ligature of these devices, all of the aqueous can escape through the GDD, resulting in hypotony with a shallow or flat anterior chamber. These patients are at significantly increased risk for experiencing serious sight-threatening complications such as suprachoroidal hemorrhage.

2. One of the most important steps of GDD surgery is the creation of the sclerostomy though which the GDD will course into the eye. The entry should be parallel to the plane of the iris. An entry that is too anterior can result in the tip of the tube adjacent to the cornea, increasing the risk of corneal decompensation. If the entry is too posterior, the tube tip may become embedded in the iris.

3. When trimming the GDD to the proper length, one should err on the side of leaving the tube tip too long, as it is much easier to trim the tube further than to risk creating a tube that is too short.

4. When covering the tube with a patch graft, it is important to attain complete coverage of the exposed tube from the sclerostomy site to the site where the tube attaches to the plate.

REFERENCES

1. Lerner SF, Parrish RK. Glaucoma aqueous humor drainage devices. In: Chen TC, ed. *Glaucoma Surgery*. Philadelphia, PA: Lippincott Williams & Wilkins; 2003:111-125.
2. Fechter HP, Lee PP, Walsh MM. Non-valved single-plate tube shunt procedures: Baerveldt and Molteno implants. In: Chen TC, ed. *Glaucoma Surgery*. Philadelphia, PA: Elsevier Inc.; 2008:87-121.
3. Raviv T, Greenfield DS, Liebmann JM, Sidoti PA, Ishikawa H, Ritch R. Pericardial patch grafts in glaucoma implant surgery. *J Glaucoma*. 1998;7(1):27-32.

9

LOCATION OF GLAUCOMA DRAINAGE IMPLANTS AND TUBES

Gabriel T. Chong, MD and Richard K. Lee, MD, PhD

Glaucoma drainage implants (GDIs) are an important treatment modality for glaucoma, especially for refractory types, such as neovascular and uveitic glaucomas. Organic materials (eg, horse hair and silk) or inert materials (eg, gold and platinum) were used as conduits to shunt aqueous from the anterior chamber to the subconjunctival space at the limbus as early GDIs prior to the 1900s.[1] The nonvalved Molteno implant was the first widely used GDI device of the modern era.[2] Shortly thereafter, Krupin developed a valved glaucoma implant to reduce the risk of early hypotony.[1] The Ahmed and Baerveldt GDIs were introduced in the 1990s and are now also widely used.[1]

REASONS FOR GLAUCOMA DRAINAGE IMPLANTS

Although trabeculectomy with antifibrotic agents remains a common IOP-lowering glaucoma surgery worldwide, glaucoma patients with high risk for surgical failure (eg, uveitic and neovascular glaucoma) can achieve long-term intraocular pressure (IOP) control with GDI surgery. The Tube Versus Trabeculectomy (TVT) study's 1-year results indicated comparable IOPs with GDIs compared with trabeculectomies, with a trend toward fewer reoperations in the GDI group.[3] The TVT study also suggested that GDIs are less likely to cause hypotony-related issues and are more likely to achieve IOP control compared with trabeculectomies.[3] GDIs also offer good IOP control in refractory glaucomas, such as those associated with uveitis, trauma, epithelial and fibrous downgrowth, aniridia, and iridocorneal endothelial syndromes, whereas trabeculectomy is frequently less successful.[4]

Kahook M.
Essentials of Glaucoma Surgery (pp 95-104).
© 2012 SLACK Incorporated.

TYPES OF GLAUCOMA DRAINAGE IMPLANTS

GDIs in popular use include the nonvalved single- and double-plate Molteno, the nonvalved Baerveldt, the valved Ahmed, and the valved Krupin glaucoma drainage implants.[1] The first widely used GDI was the Molteno implant, which has a round polypropylene end plate with a surface area of 134 mm^2 for the single plate and 268 mm^2 for the double plate GDI. The rounded plates of the double-plate Molteno implant are connected by a 10-mm silicone tube.[4] The Ahmed valved implant is made from either polypropylene (models S2, S3, and B1) or silicone (models FP7, FP8, and FX1).[4] Different plate sizes are available with surface areas ranging from 96 mm^2 (S3 and FP8) to 184 mm^2 (S2 and FP7) to 364 mm^2 (B1 and FX1).[4] The Ahmed valve mechanism consists of 2 thin membrane-like elastomer sheets, which, in principle, restrict flow until a pressure of greater than 8 to 12 mm Hg is experienced intraocularly.[4] The Krupin slit valve consists of an oval silastic disc (13×18 mm)[5] with an area of 183 mm^{2,4} The pressure is regulated by horizontal and vertical slit valves. As an alternative, the tube end may be connected to a #220 silastic band. The Baerveldt nonvalved GDI plate is a barium-impregnated X-ray–visible smooth and flexible silicone plate that comes in 2 sizes—plate areas of 250 mm^2 or 350 mm^2 (the larger 500 mm^2 model was discontinued).[6] The plate has fenestrations to allow bridging superior and inferior plate surface fibrous strands to develop, thereby reducing the vertical profile of the resultant bleb from 10.6 mm to 4.9 mm.[7]

Several GDIs offer multiple plate options, such as for the Molteno and the Ahmed. Various studies have shown that the larger the end plate size, the larger the surface area of encapsulation around the plate and thus the greater the degree of IOP reduction with a greater surface area of filtration.[8] Although larger surface area may be better for IOP lowering, an upper limit beyond which a larger size plate may not lead to lower IOP exists, and larger plates may lead to more surgical complications.[7]

The profile of each type of GDI ranges from a flatter 0.84 mm for the 2 Baerveldt plate sizes and 0.9 mm for the silicone FP7 Ahmed, to a higher profile for the Ahmed S2 (which is 1.9 mm high) and the Krupin (which is 1.75 mm high).[5,6] Capsule profile height is an important consideration because patient comfort and ocular motility may be decreased by greater plate height. Depending on the quadrant of GDI implantation, cosmesis may also be affected.

The composition of the plate affects capsule formation. A prospective, comparative study in which polypropylene Ahmed and silicone GDIs were compared showed a greater incidence of Tenon cysts formation in the polypropylene group, and better IOP lowering was observed with the silicone plate group.[9] The more rigid polypropylene Ahmed plate is also believed to cause more movement of the plate against the globe, which can stimulate a more aggressive inflammatory reaction and thicker capsule wall formation associated with higher IOP outcomes. The more flexible silicone plate is suggested to reduce formation of thick filtering capsules. Also, valved GDIs have immediate fluid drainage to the plate, which may induce thicker capsule formation compared with nonvalved GDIs, with which aqueous flow is occluded until after capsule formation.[10] Cosmetically, this information is useful when choosing the quadrant of insertion for a GDI because thicker, higher capsules may be less desirable in the inferior quadrants. A lower-profile Baerveldt implant may be a better choice than an Ahmed for inferior quadrant placement.

OCULAR ANATOMY AND ORBITAL CONSIDERATIONS FOR GLAUCOMA DRAINAGE IMPLANT PLACEMENT

Of the 4 orbital quadrants available for GDI placement, the most common and recommended site is the superotemporal quadrant. Key reasons for this recommendation include ease of plate implantation access in this quadrant for the surgeon, avoidance of the oblique extraocular muscles, and available conjunctival tissue for plate and tube coverage. The various GDI plate placement locations in the 4 orbital quadrants in relation to the limbus and the optic nerve were studied in human cadaver eyes. The Ahmed (S2 and FP7), Molteno (single-plate), and Baerveldt (250 and 350 mm^2) GDIs were implanted onto cadaveric eyes with axial lengths ranging from 22.5 mm to 26.0 mm.[6] The measured variable was the maximum distance that a GDI could be placed posterior to the limbus in the various quadrants without encroaching within 2 mm of the optic nerve. The location of the GDI relative to the various muscles was also examined. The average maximum distance from the limbus to the anterior plate edge ranged between 9.0 and 15.0 mm in the superotemporal (ST) quadrant for all GDI types tested.[6]

For the other 3 quadrants, the distances spanned 8.0 to 14.0 mm, 9.0 to 14.0 mm, and 11.0 to 17.0 mm for the superonasal (SN), inferonasal (IN), and inferotemporal (IT) quadrants, respectively.[6] The "safe zone" from the plate to the optic nerve head was defined as 2 mm based on optic nerve changes found in rabbits after plates were implanted either abutting the optic nerve or within 1 mm of the nerve sheath.[11] Changes included microglial cell loss and localized astrocyte clustering.[11] Based on this study, the SN quadrant may offer the least amount of distance from the optic nerve for a GDI plate. This may be especially important for Ahmed GDIs, which have an anterior-posterior length of 16 mm compared with Molteno, Baerveldt 250 mm^2, and Baerveldt 350 mm^2 GDIs, having lengths of 13, 14, and 15 mm, respectively.[6] The width of the plate is also an important factor to consider. The Baervelt 250 mm^2 GDI has a width of 22 mm, whereas the Baerveldt 350 mm^2 GDI has a width of 32 mm. The Ahmed, Molteno, and Krupin GDIs are 13 mm in width. The Baerveldt GDI plates, due to their wider plate widths, may be more likely to impinge on surrounding muscles, such as the rectus and oblique muscles. Such plate–muscle impingement may lead to patient discomfort and diplopia.

The IT quadrant is prone to more ocular muscle problems secondary to the close proximity of the inferior rectus and inferior oblique muscles. All GDIs, except for the Molteno, consistently contact the insertion site of the inferior oblique.[6] If a ST quadrant placement is not ideal, the next best quadrant for GDI placement is the inferonasal quadrant. Despite a potentially more difficult insertion due to exposure issues, an IN plate insertion is less likely to interfere with the adjacent inferior oblique muscle, as suggested by comparison of inferonasal to IT placement of Baerveldt 350 mm² GDIs.[12] The variability of each patient's eye means that surgeons should be aware of the differences in the "safe" range for GDI placement from eye to eye and quadrant to quadrant. This is especially important in nanophthalmos and in small eyes in hyperopes and children.[6]

ADVANTAGES AND DISADVANTAGES OF TUBE AND PLATE LOCATIONS

Previous ocular surgery is an important factor when considering GDI placement. Quadrants that have had previous ocular surgery, especially trabeculectomy with antifibrotic therapy, may have thin, friable conjunctiva, which may make conjunctival closure over the plate difficult. If a superior trabeculectomy is present, a GDI placed inferonasally may be a good option. In cases of a previous scleral buckling procedure, the GDI plate can be placed above the fibrotic band of tissue without the need for dissecting away fibrous tissue to access extraocular muscles. A fibrous capsule forms around the plate without difficulty, and some glaucoma surgeons routinely place Baerveldt GDI plates over the muscle. Although the capsule profile may be slightly higher, patients typically have good cosmetic results, IOP control, and minimal risk of diplopia.

Our recommended site for placement of Molteno, Ahmed, or Baerveldt GDIs is the ST quadrant to avoid motility problems and for easier surgical access.[1] In cases of certain previous ocular surgery, such as trabeculectomy with antifibrotic agents or superior extracapsular cataract extraction (ECCE), the conjunctiva in the ST quadrant may be too scarred, thinned, or friable for placement of a superior GDI. In such cases, a GDI placed inferonasally may be appropriate (Figure 9-1). The IT quadrant is avoided for cosmetic reasons, as well as for the risk of diplopia or other motility problems associated with inferior oblique muscle dysfunction. Also, IN GDI placement may be preferable to a superior placement to avoid obstruction of

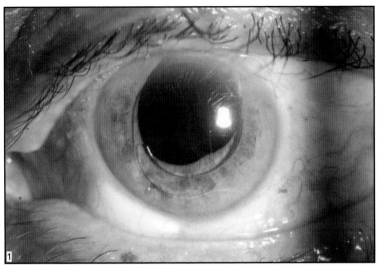

Figure 9-1. Inferonasal tube placement. This patient had a large superior extracapsular limbal wound from placement of an anterior chamber IOL. Note the 1 o'clock X-stitch that was part of the scleral wound closure which left the superior region with scarred conjunctiva. An inferonasal Baerveldt GDI was placed with a patch graft. The Baerveldt tube tip was placed right over the IOL haptic aimed away from the cornea.

the tube by silicone oil or egress of silicone oil into the subconjunctival space via the GDI, leading to significant inflammation.[1] The risk of hyphema (eg, in neovascular glaucoma) may preclude placing an inferior tube, as inferiorly layered blood may obstruct the filtering GDI tube tip, or the tube should be placed strategically longer for the tube tip to be higher within the anterior chamber.

The Ahmed S2 GDI has the highest profile at 1.9 mm and Baerveldt GDIs (both sizes) have the lowest profile at 0.84 mm.[6] The size of the plate for the various GDIs is important not only for IOP-lowering considerations but also in terms of where the implant can and should be placed. Molteno introduced the idea of draining aqueous to a posterior plate away from the limbus in 1969.[13,14] Although this led to decreased rates of exposure of the plate due to its posterior location, the risk of interference with extraocular muscles and even optic neuropathy from compression of the optic nerve increased. Similar to the Molteno GDI, the Ahmed GDI can be presumed to have similar plate characteristics in the various quadrants due to a similar plate profile and size ($1.75 \times 13 \times 18$ mm).[5]

The ST quadrant is the ideal plate location due to its combination of space, avoidance of the oblique muscles, and ease of exposure at the time of surgery. If the ST quadrant is not accessible, the IN quadrant is the next best site based upon our clinical experience. The IT quadrant is not an ideal location due to the potential for inferior oblique impingement leading to ocular motility disturbance. Also, large bleb formation inferotemporally can lead to an undesired cosmetic result. Although superior and inferior Ahmed GDI placements have similar results in terms of IOP reduction and preservation of vision, Pakravan et al[15] reported that inferiorly placed Ahmeds (which included a significant number placed inferotemporally) had more complications, including higher rates of wound dehiscence, tube or implant exposure, disfiguring encapsulation, lower lid bulge, exposure of the sclera patch graft, and endophthalmitis.

Anterior Chamber Tube Placement

Besides type of plate and plate placement location, the location of the GDI tube is also important. The GDI tube can be placed in different quadrants and different anterior-posterior chamber locations, such as anterior chamber (AC), sulcus, or pars plana (PP). AC tube placement is typically the most common location due to direct visualization and ease of placement during surgery. Postoperatively, the tube tip can be readily visualized to verify its placement and patency. Occlusion of the tube by iris, blood, fibrin, vitreous, and other ocular contents can be directly visualized for diagnosis and treatment of tube occlusion. An AC tube is also amenable for ripcord suture removal for early tube opening in the clinic. Also, if tube retraction is a concern, gonioscopy can be performed to verify the tube is in the AC. Some disadvantages to AC tube placement include corneal damage if the tube is in contact with the corneal endothelium, which can result in endothelial cell loss, corneal edema, and possible need for keratoplasty.[16] Eye rubbing can also cause areas of focal corneal edema due to intermittent tube–cornea contact. Another disadvantage is the difficulty of placing a tube in the AC in a quadrant where pre-existing high peripheral anterior synechia (PAS) is present.

The ST quadrant is ideal for AC placement of the tube, partly because it is the most spacious quadrant for plate placement and surgical site access during surgery. The tube is also easy to visualize with inferior gaze for laser suture lysis (LSL) through a corneal patch graft if early tube opening is necessary. For issues regarding patency of the tube or whether the GDI is filtering properly, the ST quadrant is relatively simple for ultrasound to visualize fluid over the plate and, at the slit lamp, a view of plate edge for the presence of a filtering bleb is relatively simple compared with other quadrants. A disadvantage of the ST location is that eye rubbing can more easily cause extrusion of the tube or erosion of the conjunctiva overlying the tube, especially in the early postoperative course. The risk of tube erosion can be minimized by routing the tube to enter the AC more superiorly toward the 12 o'clock meridian, which places the tube and patch graft entirely underneath the upper lid.[16]

If the ST quadrant is unavailable for GDI placement secondary to previous trabeculectomy, superior ECCE wound, or other reason for scarred or friable superior conjunctiva, the IN quadrant is our preferred next option for AC tube insertion. Adequate space exists inferonasally for most GDI plates and oblique muscles are avoided for a lower risk of diplopia. Tube erosion or extrusion is also less likely in the IN quadrant. If silicone oil is in the eye or may be needed in the future, the IN quadrant location of the tube minimizes the risk of silicone oil obstructing the tube. Some disadvantages of an IN tube include poorer cosmesis (the upper lid usually helps hide the tube in the ST AC), and hyphema can occlude an inferior tube tip if not above the level of the hyphema. For IN tubes, we typically use a transparent corneal patch graft to minimize cosmesis issues.

Placement of a tube in the AC in the SN and IT quadrants is often not ideal because of more difficult surgical site access for plate implantation, risk of diplopia, and cosmesis. Even implanting the plate in the ST or IN quadrants and routing the tube to the SN and IT quadrants is not ideal and may require use of a tube extender for optimal tube placement. The IT quadrant location is difficult due to possible interference with inferior oblique muscle function, hyphema obstructing the tube, and poorer cosmetic results with increased patch graft show.

Posterior Chamber Tube Placement

In eyes with a disorganized anterior segment, current or future need for keratoplasty, neovascularization of the angle, significant and/or high peripheral anterior synechiae, a shallow anterior chamber, history of PP vitrectomy, or future need for vitrectomy, a posterior chamber placement of a tube may be ideal.[17] A tube placed in the PP probably has a lower risk of erosion by virtue of the tube location being more posterior from the limbus and covered by Tenon's and other soft tissue.[16] If a tube is placed in the PP, a complete vitrectomy to the vitreous skirt or base needs to be performed to prevent tube tip blockage by residual vitreous.[18] If blocked by vitreous, PP tube placement makes visualization of the tube tip difficult, and lasering the tube tip or needling the tube tip to remove the obstruction is typically not an option. A PP tube is also associated with a risk of retinal detachment, especially if significant inflammation occurs upon opening of a nonvalved tube with ligature release. Other contraindications of a PP tube include abnormalities of the sclera and lens status of the eye.[18] A higher postoperative hypotony risk was observed when a GDI tube was placed through a sclerostomy as opposed to AC placement.[18] When placing a tube in the PP

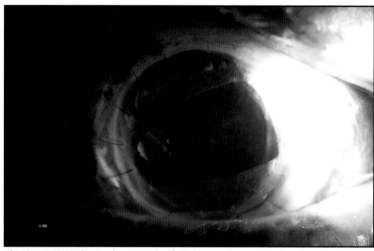

Figure 9-2. Sulcus placement of superotemporal GDI tube. This pseudophakic patient with a history of a penetrating keratoplasty had a superotemporal GDI placed for chronic angle-closure glaucoma. Secondary to high PAS associated with the history of corneal transplantation, the tube was placed in the sulcus, which kept it away from the cornea and above the IOL, minimizing the risk of vitreous tube occlusion and allowing for easy insertion of the tube.

(unless employing the Hoffman elbow for tube insertion), use of a 20-gauge microvitreoretinal blade creates a larger opening compared with a 23-gauge needle, and the resulting leakage around the sclerostomy site can lead to postoperative hypotony.

Sulcus placement of a tube may be an ideal compromise between an AC and a PP tube location in pseudophakic eyes. When a tube is placed in the sulcus, the tube is posterior to the iris, which keeps the tip below the iris plane and prevents tube contact with the cornea. This should prevent any direct corneal endothelial loss associated with tube corneal contact. A sulcus placement is also away from the vitreous and above the IOL, which typically prevents vitreous obstruction of the tube, especially with the tip bevel turned toward the IOL to minimize iris incarceration. Placing a tube in the sulcus may be more technically challenging. Ideal eyes for a sulcus tube placement are nonvitrectomy pseudophakic eyes with high PAS, such as neovascular or chronic angle-closure eyes (Figure 9-2).

Tube Entry Location

In certain cases, the length of the tube in a GDI may be inadequate after placement and may need to be relocated to a different position. This may occur in pediatric patients, in whom axial growth can lead to tube retraction from the globe.[19] Acute trauma, malposition of the tube, tube tip occlusion, accidently shortened tubes (eg, cutting in the operating room), and eye-rubbing–associated tube extrusion may require that the tube location be changed.[20] Various methods for relocating a tube exist, including using a connecting segment of 22-gauge angiocatheter tubing,[21] a silastic sleeve,[22] a small-diameter silastic tube connected to the original tube,[23] or a commercially available tube extender, such as the Model TE (New World Medical, Inc).[20] A tube extender allows the surgeon to reroute a tube away from areas of high PAS or reoperated or scarred conjunctiva without having to explant an existing GDI and place a new GDI in a separate location for IOP control. Relocating an extruded tube is a relatively straightforward method to preserve a filtering GDI.

KEY POINTS

1. Our preference for GDI placement location is in the superotemporal quadrant, and in the inferonasal quadrant as the second choice for reasons including ease of surgical access, improved cosmesis, decreased risk of diplopia, access for laser suture lysis in nonvalved GDIs, and decreased risk of optic nerve damage.

2. A larger glaucoma drainage plate size improves IOP control, but only to a certain point (ie, bigger is not always better and may increase the risks of complications such as diplopia).

3. Anterior chamber GDI tube placement is preferred because visualization of the tube tip can aid in the diagnosis of poor or blocked filtration secondary to iris incarceration, fibrin, and other occlusions that are amenable to manipulation, such as laser treatment.

4. Posterior chamber GDI tube placement is preferred in cases of a shallow anterior chamber, other corneal problems (eg, Fuchs' dystrophy, penetrating keratoplasty, or iridocorneal endothelial syndromes), or anterior segment problems that are planned for a vitrectomy. Sulcus GDI tube placement is often ideal for pseudophakic eyes with high PAS.

REFERENCES

1. Dietlein TS, Jordan J, Lueke C, Krieglstein GK. Modern concepts in antiglaucomatous implant surgery. *Graefes Arch Clin Exp Ophthalmol.* 2008;246(12):1653-1664.
2. Minckler DS, Vedula SS, Li TJ, et al. Aqueous shunts for glaucoma. *Cochrane Database Syst Rev.* 2006(2):CD004918.
3. Gedde SJ, Schiffman JC, Feuer WJ, et al. Treatment outcomes in the tube versus trabeculectomy study after one year of follow-up. *Am J Ophthalmol.* 2007;143(1):9-22.
4. Schwartz KS, Lee RK, Gedde SJ. Glaucoma drainage implants: a critical comparison of types. *Curr Opin Ophthalmol.* 2006;17(2):181-189.

5. Krupin eye valve with disk for filtration surgery. The Krupin Eye Valve Filtering Surgery Study Group. *Ophthalmology.* 1994;101(4):651-658.

6. Kahook MY, Noecker RJ, Pantcheva MB, Schuman JS. Location of glaucoma drainage devices relative to the optic nerve. *Br J Ophthalmol.* 2006;90(8):1010-1013.

7. Lloyd MA, Baerveldt G, Fellenbaum PS, et al. Intermediate-term results of a randomized clinical trial of the 350- versus the 500-mm^2 Baerveldt implant. *Ophthalmology.* 1994;101(8):1456-1463.

8. Heuer DK, Lloyd MA, Abrams DA, et al. Which is better? One or two? A randomized clinical trial of single-plate versus double-plate Molteno implantation for glaucomas in aphakia and pseudophakia. *Ophthalmology.* 1992;99(10):1512-1519.

9. Ishida K, Netland PA, Costa VP, et al. Comparison of polypropylene and silicone Ahmed Glaucoma valves. *Ophthalmology.* 2006;113(8):1320-1326.

10. Nouri-Mahdavi K, Caprioli J. Evaluation of the hypertensive phase after insertion of the Ahmed Glaucoma Valve. *Am J Ophthalmol.* 2003;136(6):1001-1008.

11. Ayyala RS, Parma SE, Karcioglu ZA. Optic nerve changes following posterior insertion of glaucoma drainage device in rabbit model. *J Glaucoma.* 2004;13(2):145-148.

12. Sidoti PA. Inferonasal placement of aqueous shunts. *J Glaucoma.* 2004;13(6):520-523.

13. Molteno AC. New implant for drainage in glaucoma. Clinical trial. *Br J Ophthalmol.* 1969;53(9):606-615.

14. Molteno AC. New implant for drainage in glaucoma. Animal trial. *Br J Ophthalmol.* 1969;53(3):161-168.

15. Pakravan M, Yazdani S, Shahabi C, Yaseri M. Superior versus inferior Ahmed glaucoma valve implantation. *Ophthalmology.* 2009;116(2):208-213.

16. Heuer DK, Budenz D, Coleman A. Aqueous shunt tube erosion. *J Glaucoma.* 2001;10(6):493-496.

17. de Guzman MH, Valencia A, Farinelli AC. Pars plana insertion of glaucoma drainage devices for refractory glaucoma. *Clin Experiment Ophthalmol.* 2006;34(2):102-107.

18. Scott IU, Alexandrakis G, Flynn HW Jr, et al. Combined pars plana vitrectomy and glaucoma drainage implant placement for refractory glaucoma. *Am J Ophthalmol.* 2000;129(3):334-341.

19. Dawodu O, Levin AV. Spontaneous disconnection of glaucoma tube shunt extenders. *J AAPOS.* 2010;14(4):361-363.

20. Sarkisian SR, Netland PA. Tube extender for revision of glaucoma drainage implants. *J Glaucoma.* 2007;16(7):637-639.

21. Smith MF, Doyle JW. Results of another modality for extending glaucoma drainage tubes. *J Glaucoma.* 1999;8(5):310-314.

22. Kooner KS. Repair of Molteno implant during surgery. *Am J Ophthalmol.* 1994;117(5):673.

23. Minckler D. Pathophysiology, indications, and surgical technique: glaucoma drainage devices. In: Weinreb RN, Mills RP, eds. *Glaucoma Surgery: Principles and Techniques.* San Francisco, CA: American Academy of Ophthalmology; 1998.

USE OF ANTIMETABOLITES
WITH TUBE SHUNT SURGERY

Anup K. Khatana, MD

Glaucoma surgeons struggle with the adverse effects of scarring on a daily basis. Tube shunts were able to increase the success rate of filtration surgery in certain complex glaucomas and eyes that had either failed or were unable to undergo a trabeculectomy. However, they were still limited to varying degrees by the nature of the fibrotic capsule that formed over the distal plate of the shunt. The ability of 5-fluorouracil (5-FU) and mitomycin C (MMC) to increase the success rate of trabeculectomy stirred interest among glaucoma surgeons to investigate their effects with tube shunts.

TUBE VERSUS TRABECULECTOMY

Before we assess the potential role for antimetabolite use in glaucoma implant surgery, it is helpful to look at how implants without antimetabolites compare with standard trabeculectomy with mitomycin C. In 2009, the 3-year follow-up results were published for the Tube Versus Trabeculectomy (TVT) Study. This study was a multicenter US trial that included open-angle glaucoma patients with previous trabeculectomy or cataract extraction with intraocular lens (IOL) implantation, or both, and uncontrolled glaucoma with intraocular pressure (IOP) between 18 and 40 mm Hg, inclusive. Patients were randomized to undergo either a 350-mm^2 Baerveldt glaucoma implant or trabeculectomy with MMC. Of the 212 patients enrolled, the mean IOP at 3 years was 13.0 ± 4.9 mm Hg on 1.3 ± 1.3 glaucoma medications in the tube group, and 13.3 ± 6.8 mm Hg on 1.0 ± 1.5 glaucoma medications in the trabeculectomy group. Interestingly, the cumulative probability of failure was 15.1% in the tube group and 30.7% in the trabeculectomy group during this 3-year follow-up. It was also interesting to note that 39% of patients in the tube group and 60% in the trabeculectomy group developed some postoperative complication, although most were transient and self-limited.[1] As we discuss

Kahook M.
Essentials of Glaucoma Surgery **(pp 105-110).**
© 2012 SLACK Incorporated.

the role for antimetabolites in tube shunt surgery, the results of the TVT trial demonstrate the effectiveness of the Baerveldt glaucoma implant in controlling pressure without the use of antimetabolites. The question remains as to whether we can safely augment the IOP reduction from tube shunt surgery with antimetabolites in a manner similar to that seen with trabeculectomy.

EARLY ANIMAL STUDIES

The first published report of the use of MMC with a tube shunt was in 1993 by Choi and colleagues, using an anterior chamber silicone tube to an expanded polytetrafluoroethylene membrane in rabbit eyes. Histologically, the capsules that formed over the membrane in the MMC group were less cellular and less dense, with less proliferating fibrous connective tissue and more microcystic spaces, suggesting higher permeability to aqueous humor.[2] Another rabbit study done by Prata, Minckler and colleagues investigated the use of 0.5 mg/mL MMC for 5 minutes with Baerveldt glaucoma implants followed for 24 weeks postoperatively. No postoperative steroids were used. The MMC eyes had thinner and less cellular capsules with less dense collagen layers over the implant compared to the controls. The IOP was lower in the MMC-treated eyes at all time points, but the difference was only statistically significant up to 8 weeks postoperatively. The control eyes demonstrated a "hypertensive phase" that peaked at 4 weeks, but a gradual rise in IOP until 6 weeks followed by a gradual decline through the 11th week. The MMC-treated group demonstrated a minimal "hypertensive phase" with only a small rise in IOP by 6 weeks. Resistance to flow was lower in the MMC-treated group at all time points, but this difference was only statistically significant through 6 weeks postoperatively. Flow rates through the implant bleb were also higher at all time points in the MMC-treated group, and were statistically significant at 2, 4, 6, and 24 weeks postoperatively. The complication rate was also higher, with wound dehiscence, bleb leaks, and extraocular muscle hemorrhagic necrosis observed only in some of the MMC-treated eyes, but none of the controls.[3] It is important to keep in mind that the extraocular muscle capsule has been noted to be thinner in rabbits than humans. This may help explain the higher rate of related complications in the MMC group.

HUMAN CLINICAL STUDIES

There have been a number of publications on the use of MMC with tube shunts in humans. Some have been prospective and randomized, while others have been observational retrospective case series. These studies vary in the type of implant used, MMC application, length of follow-up, definitions of success, etc. Two early studies by Susanna et al[4] and Perkins et al[5] compared MMC in the implantation of Molteno implants to historical controls where no MMC was used. These studies suggested a beneficial effect of MMC. Cantor et al[6] prospectively randomized patients undergoing double-plate Molteno implantation to either MMC 0.4 mg/mL for 2 minutes or a balanced salt solution control. Costa et al[7] prospectively randomized patients undergoing Ahmed glaucoma valve implantation to an intraoperative application of either MMC 0.5 mg/mL for 5 minutes or balanced salt solution. Neither of these studies found a statistically significant difference between the MMC and control groups in IOP, number of antiglaucoma medications, or complications. Three retrospective studies that used a historical control group also found no evidence of higher surgical success with adjunctive MMC in single-plate Molteno, Baerveldt 350 mm², and Ahmed valve tube shunts, respectively.[8-10]

In another retrospective comparative series in a pediatric population, Al-Mobarak and Khan[11] found a shorter survival at 2 years' follow-up with Ahmed valves implanted with intraoperative MMC than those without MMC in children during the first 2 years of life (mean age at implantation: 11.1 months). Pakravan et al[12] found comparable outcomes between trabeculectomy with MMC versus Ahmed valve with MMC for the treatment of aphakic glaucoma in children under the age of 16.

The classic hypertensive phase after tube shunt surgery is a period of IOP elevation that begins typically approximately 5 weeks postoperatively from the formation of a bleb capsule over the plate of the shunt and can last up to 6 months postoperatively. It is presumed to be due to the lower permeability of the initial capsule that forms over the plate of the shunt. Through wound remodeling, the permeability of the capsule slowly increases, resulting in a gradual decline in IOP. Ellingham et al[13] showed that MMC (0.3 mg/mL for 3 minutes) applied to Tenon's capsule over the secondary plate of double-plate Molteno implants was able to blunt the hypertensive phase. However, no significant difference was seen with the use of MMC on the hypertensive phase in the Cantor study.[6] Part of the rise in IOP that occurs approximately 3 to 4 weeks postoperatively in nonvalved shunts that are ligated and receive venting slits is due to fibrosis around the tube in the area of the venting slits. Trible and Brown[14] investigated the effect of 5-FU and MMC applied locally only to the sclera in the area of a standardized venting slit (but not directly to the area over the plate where the bleb would form) after the plate was secured to the sclera. There was no statistically significant difference between the 5-FU and MMC groups. Susanna[15] studied the effect of adjunctive MMC in Ahmed glaucoma valve surgery with or without partial Tenon's capsule resection. They found no benefit or no increase in complications from partial Tenon's capsule resection.

MMC has also been studied and used with tube shunt revisions. Zarei and Shahhosseini[16] found limited benefit to needling bleb revision with

MMC for failed Molteno tubes. The success rate was 87.5% at 3 months, 37.5% at 6 months, and 12.5% at 24-months follow-up. The reader is also referred to an excellent Cochrane review analyzing all of the published literature on aqueous shunts in glaucoma by Minckler et al[17] in 2006.

LABORATORY STUDIES

Freedman and Goddard[18] studied aqueous humor samples obtained from eyes that underwent Molteno implants, trabeculectomy, and cataract surgery. They found that transforming growth factor beta (TGF-β) and prostaglandin E2 (PGE2) levels were higher in the Molteno and trabeculectomy eyes than in cataract surgery eyes. There was also a trend toward higher levels of PGE2 and TGF-β in patients with a higher IOP. They postulated that a sustained IOP rise, such as that seen with encapsulated blebs and during the hypertensive phase, stimulates production of PGE2 and TGF-β. These factors mediate ongoing inflammation, progressive fibrosis, and a sustained rise in IOP.

Occleston et al[19] showed that one 5-minute in vitro exposure of 5-FU or MMC significantly inhibited cultured human Tenon's capsule fibroblast migration and decreased growth factor production, growth factor receptor expression, and extracellular matrix production initially. The effects were greater with MMC than 5-FU as expected. However, these values gradually returned to control levels starting approximately 1 week after the exposure and reached control levels approximately 5 weeks after the exposure. In addition, even the growth-arrested cells appeared to be capable of producing growth factors, expressing growth factor receptors, and producing extracellular matrix. This may perhaps explain the inability of antimetabolites to completely prevent failure from fibrosis in all glaucoma surgeries.

PERSONAL EXPERIENCE

I first began to use MMC with tube shunts in 2002, based on the goal of trying to achieve lower IOPs and reduce the need for adjunctive medical therapy. Minimizing topical therapy is particularly important when managing glaucoma in eyes with complex ocular surface disease, such as those that have undergone limbal stem cell transplantation. It was felt that the potential inflammatory effects of IOP-lowering eye drops could adversely affect the limbal stem cell transplants.

I have not observed any higher incidence of complications since beginning to use MMC, nor do my complication rates seem higher than published reports. Although I have not performed a comparative trial, it is my impression that MMC does help achieve lower IOPs and may also reduce the dependence on medications to achieve IOP control. It is also my clinical impression that MMC helps to blunt the hypertensive phase.

When one begins to use an agent like MMC, it is advised to use the standard concentration that one is already familiar with when performing trabeculectomies. I recommend starting with a relatively short duration of 30 to 60 seconds. Observe the clinical course of these patients and then gradually adjust the exposure as needed. MMC has been accepted to increase the success rate of trabeculectomies and has been widely adopted in that setting. Animal studies with MMC and tube shunts have also suggested a (mostly) beneficial effect on the exposed tissue. However, it is curious that the majority of the clinical studies have not shown any significant long-term benefit from adjunctive MMC with tube shunts. The answer may well be multifactorial. The Occleston study,[19] showing that growth-arrested cells still produce growth factors, may shed light on at least part of the cause. It is also possible that an inadequate dose of MMC has been used.

KEY POINTS

1. The 3-year results of the TVT study showed comparable results between Baerveldt 350 tube shunts without MMC and trabeculectomy with MMC.

2. Adjunctive use of MMC during tube shunt implantation in rabbit eyes created less dense and less cellular fibrous capsules over the implant plate, and less resistance to outflow compared to controls.

3. Human clinical studies have shown mixed results, but the majority of them have not shown any long-term benefit from MMC. One study did show a positive effect on the hypertensive phase from MMC use.

4. Some evidence suggests a correlation between elevated levels of TGF-β and PGE2 in eyes that have an elevated IOP after tube shunt surgery.

5. In vitro evidence indicates incomplete inhibition of fibroblasts from a single exposure of 5-FU or MMC and a gradual loss of the physiologic effects on the fibroblasts over 1 to 5 weeks after the exposure.

REFERENCES

1. Gedde SJ, Schiffman JC, Feuer WJ, Herndon LW, Brandt JD, Budenz DL. Three-year follow-up of the tube versus trabeculectomy study. *Am J Ophthalmol.* 2009;148(5):670-684.

2. Choi WS, Park SJ, Kim DM. Mitomycin C in anterior chamber tube shunt to a surgical membrane. *Korean J Ophthalmol.* 1993;7(2):48-54.

3. Prata JA, Minckler DS, Mermoud A, Baerveldt G. Effects of intraoperative mitomycin-C on the function of Baerveldt glaucoma drainage implants in rabbits. *J Glaucoma.* 1996;5(1):29-38.

4. Susanna R Jr, Nicolela MT, Takahashi WY. Mitomycin C as adjunctive therapy with glaucoma implant surgery. *Ophthalmic Surg.* 1994;25(7):458-462.

5. Perkins TW, Cardakli UF, Eisele JR, Kaufman PL, Heatley GA. Adjunctive mitomycin C in Molteno implant surgery. *Ophthalmology*. 1995;102(1):91-97.
6. Cantor L, Burgoyne J, Sanders S, Bhavnani V, Hoop J, Brizendine E. The effect of mitomycin C on Molteno implant surgery: a 1-year randomized, masked, prospective study. *J Glaucoma*. 1998;7(4):240-246.
7. Costa VP, Azuara-Blanco A, Netland PA, Lesk MR, Arcieri ES. Efficacy and safety of adjunctive mitomycin C during Ahmed Glaucoma Valve implantation: a prospective randomized clinical trial. *Ophthalmology*. 2004;111(6):1071-1076.
8. Lee D, Shin DH, Birt CM, et al. The effect of adjunctive mitomycin C in Molteno implant surgery. *Ophthalmology*. 1997;104(12):2126-2135.
9. Irak I, Moster MR, Fontanarosa J. Intermediate-term results of Baerveldt tube shunt surgery with mitomycin C use. *Ophthalmic Surg Lasers Imaging*. 2004;35(3):189-196.
10. Kurnaz E, Kubaloglu A, Yilmaz Y, Koytak A, Ozerturk Y. The effect of adjunctive Mitomycin C in Ahmed glaucoma valve implantation. *Eur J Ophthalmol*. 2005;15(1):27-31.
11. Al-Mobarak F, Khan AO. Two-year survival of Ahmed valve implantation in the first 2 years of life with and without intraoperative mitomycin-C. *Ophthalmology*. 2009;116(10):1862-1865.
12. Pakravan M, Homayoon N, Shahin Y, Ali Reza BR. Trabeculectomy with mitomycin C versus Ahmed glaucoma implant with mitomycin C for treatment of pediatric aphakic glaucoma. *J Glaucoma*. 2007;16(7):631-636.
13. Ellingham RB, Morgan WH, Westlake W, House PH. Mitomycin C eliminates the short-term intraocular pressure rise found following Molteno tube implantation. *Clin Experiment Ophthalmol*. 2003;31(3):191-198.
14. Trible JR, Brown DB. Occlusive ligature and standardized fenestration of a Baerveldt tube with and without antimetabolites for early postoperative intraocular pressure control. *Ophthalmology*. 1998;105(12):2243-2250.
15. Susanna R Jr; Latin American Glaucoma Society Investigators. Partial Tenon's capsule resection with adjunctive mitomycin C in Ahmed glaucoma valve implant surgery. *Br J Ophthalmol*. 2003;87(8):994-998.
16. Zarei R, Shahhosseini S. Needling revision with mitomycin C for failed Molteno tube shunt implant. *Asian J Ophthalmol*. 2007;9:27-29.
17. Minckler DS, Vedula SS, Li TJ, Mathew MC, Ayyala RS, Francis BA. Aqueous shunts for glaucoma. *Cochrane Database Syst Rev*. 2006;19(2):CD004918.
18. Freedman J, Goddard D. Elevated levels of transforming growth factor beta and prostaglandin E2 in aqueous humor from patients undergoing filtration surgery for glaucoma. *Can J Ophthalmol*. 2008;43(3):370.
19. Occleston NL, Daniels JT, Tarnuzzer RW, et al. Single exposures to antiproliferatives. Long-term effects on ocular fibroblast Wound-healing behavior. *Invest Ophthalmol Vis Sci*. 1997;38:1998-2007.

Considerations on Day of Glaucoma Drainage Implant Surgery

Jeffrey M. Zink, MD

On the day of aqueous drainage implant surgery, there are some important things to consider to help achieve desired results. Although it is necessary to plan in advance prior to surgery, there are some important considerations on the actual day of surgery as well. Attention to detail regarding preparations in the holding area, preoperative equipment check, anesthesia type, operative positioning for surgeon and patient, last-minute implant considerations, and intraoperative tissue and anatomical assessments can help to achieve more optimal results.

Holding Area

The holding area is where you want to make sure that the patient understands the surgery and that you answer any last-minute questions or concerns. The surgeon must make sure the patient has signed the consent form for the appropriate tube shunt surgery and that the correct eye is scheduled. Mark the patient's operative eye in the holding area and confirm the correct eye with the patient. Review the surgical consent form and ensure that placement of a tissue patch graft is included in the surgical consent form. Ensure that the patient is willing to accept donor tissue, as most patients do not consider glaucoma surgery as involving transplanted tissue. Some patients will not accept transplanted tissue for religious reasons, and it is important to have this conversation and make them aware that transplanted patch graft material is part of this type of glaucoma surgery. If the patient is on warfarin, I like to check an international normalized ratio blood test on the day of surgery. If the patient is taking clopidogrel or other blood thinners, ask when these medications were discontinued. If blood thinners were

Kahook M.
Essentials of Glaucoma Surgery (pp 111–114).
© 2012 SLACK Incorporated.

not stopped, you may want to consider topical or intraoperative sub-Tenon's anesthesia.

PREOPERATIVE CHECK

It is important to make sure you have the correct implant available prior to the surgery. I like to have a second implant of similar type available in case one is defective or if the device is damaged during surgery. I also recommend having a tube extender available, especially in training programs. If the tube is inadvertently cut too short, a tube extender will allow the tube to be extended and placed at the desired length in the anterior chamber. Make sure that the donor patch graft material is present and stored appropriately. If there is the possibility of placing an inferior tube, I prefer to have corneal patch graft available for cosmetic reasons. Corneal patch material is clear and does not show up on the sclera as conspicuously as scleral patch grafts when placed inferiorly. For cosmesis, processed pericardium is preferable to sclera but less preferable than cornea. If patch graft tissue is ordered from an eye bank, make sure to check the eye bank paperwork to ensure that all proper serologic testing has been done and the appropriate titers are negative.

ANESTHESIA

Anesthesia for glaucoma drainage implant surgery can vary from topical with subconjunctival supplementation, peribulbar block, or retrobulbar block. The type of anesthesia that is needed should be tailored to the level of complexity of the case in terms of tissue manipulation and the patient's ability to cooperate during the surgical procedure. I prefer intraoperative sub-Tenon's anesthesia or a peribulbar block in the holding area. I use a long block consisting of a 50:50 mixture of 0.5% marcaine and 2% lidocaine. In complex cases that require extensive tissue dissection and manipulation, a standard retrobulbar block may be required.

POSITIONING

The importance of proper patient and surgeon positioning in the operating room cannot be overstated. Make sure your patient is comfortable and you have adjusted the head positioning so that it minimizes neck and back discomfort during the surgery. If your patient is not comfortable, they are more likely to move suddenly. Consider taping the patient's head to minimize the risk of sudden movement. Some surgeons prefer to use a wrist rest to stabilize their hands during surgery. I like to sit superiorly during aqueous drainage implant surgery. Some surgeons prefer to sit slightly offset from 12 o'clock to the side of implant placement location to give them better access to the superior temporal quadrant.

IMPLANT CONSIDERATIONS

Intraoperative examination is important when determining implant location. If patients have a very tight orbital space, you may favor implanting a smaller plate tube shunt. Sometimes, you may not be able to determine the appropriate size of the implant until you have started the dissection and better evaluate orbital anatomy in the operating room. In patients with a prior scleral buckling procedure, I prefer a lower profile tube shunt, such as a Baerveldt 250 mm^2 implant, which can be sewn to the buckle itself or just posterior to the buckle, depending on the buckle location.

Normally, the preferred location of implant placement is the superior temporal quadrant. Intraoperatively, you may notice extensive conjunctival scarring superiorly in some cases. The conjunctiva may also be very thin and friable from previous trabeculectomy surgery and mitomycin C (MMC) exposure. In these cases, the inferior nasal quadrant can be a great alternative location for implant placement. If you think that inferior tube shunt placement may be necessary, it is a good idea to have corneal tissue available for patch material, as previously mentioned, to provide a less conspicuous patch graft. A scleral patch graft can be quiet visible when placed inferiorly. In addition, I prefer a tube that achieves a lower profile, such as the Baerveldt 250 mm^2 or 350 mm^2 for inferior tube placement. Although Ahmed implants can be placed in the inferior nasal quadrant, I have found that an implant with a lower profile is a better alternative cosmetically.

CONJUNCTIVAL CLOSURE CONSIDERATIONS

In general, with healthy conjunctival tissue, I prefer closure with an 8-0 braided Vicryl suture on a TG-140 needle. For very friable tissue, or tissue with previous MMC exposure, a 9-0 monofilament Vicryl suture on a VAS-100 needle works well. Monofilament Vicryl can be used in routine cases, but it costs more than braided Vicryl and is usually not necessary.

KEY POINTS

1. Attention to detail and being prepared on the day of surgery is important to be able to provide optimal patient care.
2. If considering inferior glaucoma drainage implant placement, consider having corneal patch tissue and a lower-profile implant, such as a Baerveldt, available to achieve more desirable cosmetic results.

SUGGESTED READINGS

Minckler DS, Vedula SS, Li TJ, Mathew MC, Ayyala RS, Francis BA. Aqueous shunts for glaucoma. *Cochrane Database Syst Rev.* 2006;(2):CD004918.

Patel S, Pasquale LR. Glaucoma drainage devices: a review of the past, present, and future. *Semin Ophthalmol.* 2010;25(5-6):265-270.

Sidoti PA, Baerveldt G. Glaucoma drainage implants. *Curr Opin Ophthalmol.* 1994;5(2): 85-98.

12

POSTOPERATIVE MANAGEMENT OF GLAUCOMA DRAINAGE IMPLANTS

Jeffrey M. Zink, MD

The postoperative management of glaucoma drainage implants is important in determining the success of the surgery. Patient education, medications, and in-office procedures are important things to consider when managing the postoperative glaucoma drainage implant patient.

PATIENT EDUCATION

The first part of successful glaucoma surgery is patient education. It is important to spend time educating your patients about what to expect, proper eye drop usage and compliance following surgery. Proper eye drop use is critical for postoperative intraocular pressure (IOP) control, inflammation treatment, and infection prophylaxis. Many glaucoma drainage implant patients may have medical conditions that make drop instillation difficult, such as dementia, arthritis, tremor, or coordination issues. In these patients, I find it helpful to elicit the aid of a reliable family member of the patient to assist with postoperative drop instillation. I like to provide a detailed sheet with drop instructions for the patient to take home following surgery. It is important to include bottle top colors and use large font to facilitate the reading and understanding of drop instructions. Giving patients a written schedule to follow, in a form they can understand and read, will improve compliance with complicated postoperative drop schedules.

As with any other intraocular surgery, it is important to tell patients to call if they notice worsening redness, pain, sudden loss of vision, discharge, or swelling. Most patients are very concerned about the appearance and comfort of their eye following tube shunt surgery. Foreign body sensation from sutures, moderate conjunctival injection, and subconjunctival hemorrhages are commonly seen following surgery. It is important to have patients look at their eye on the first postoperative day, so they know if the appearance of the

Kahook M.
Essentials of Glaucoma Surgery (pp 115-120).
© 2012 SLACK Incorporated.

eye changes for the worse. Educating patients on what to be concerned about and when to call their surgeon is an important first step in managing and avoiding problems following glaucoma drainage implant surgery.

MEDICATIONS

A typical postoperative drop regimen for tube shunt surgery includes prednisolone acetate 1% 4 times a day and an antibiotic drop 4 times a day for the first week after surgery. If a patient is a known steroid responder, one can substitute loteprednol etabonate instead of prednisolone acetate. I prefer a flouroquinolone antibiotic for 1 week following surgery. I prefer a longer antibiotic course for some conditions, such as wound leaks, surface disease requiring contact lens use, or moderate to severe blepharitis. Higher doses of steroids may be necessary in patients with known uveitis or a predisposition to intraocular inflammation. Cycloplegics should be used when hypotony, shallow chamber, and choroidal effusions are present to facilitate anterior chamber deepening. Steroids and cycloplegics will help reduce the risk of peripheral anterior synechiae formation in the setting of hypotony.

VALVED IMPLANTS

Typically, the steroids can be slowly tapered in the case of valved implants over the course of the first month or 2. They may need to be continued longer if a hypertensive phase develops. For further details on the hypertensive phase, please see Chapter 13.

When a valved glaucoma drainage implant is placed, flow is immediately established between the anterior chamber and the subconjunctival space over the implant, assuming that the valve is functioning and has been primed appropriately. This creates a higher likelihood of a low IOP in the immediate postoperative period for valved implants. These patients may need to be followed more closely during the early postoperative period for shallow chambers, hypotony, and choroidal effusions. Rarely, it may be necessary to reform the anterior chamber with viscoelastic if there is profound hypotony with a flat chamber in the early postoperative period (the reader is referred to the next section for further details on viscoelastic injections). In most cases, the early hypotony seen on valved implants can be managed with cycloplegics, steroids, and close monitoring. When hypotony is present, it is important to tell patients to avoid lifting, bending, or straining. I prefer to have them keep their head elevated on a pillow when sleeping and wear a protective shield at night. Typically, when there is hypotony following the implantation of a valved implant, it resolves in the first week or 2 with conservative treatment. Some surgeons advocate performing suture ligature of valved implants, such as the Ahmed, to avoid the risk of early postoperative hypotony.

NONVALVED IMPLANTS

Management Prior to Tube Opening

In a typical nonvalved implant, such as a Baervedlt or Molteno, there is a higher likelihood that you may be dealing with higher pressures in the immediate postoperative period due to the tube ligature and stent suture. These patients often need to restart their glaucoma drops and sometimes require oral carbonic anhydrase inhibitors following surgery until the tube opens. Initially, I like to start with aqueous suppressants. In general, I avoid prostaglandin analogues unless absolutely necessary out of concern for augmenting postoperative inflammation.

Because the nonvalved aqueous drainage implant is ligated in most cases in the early postoperative period, sometimes there is a need to lower IOP beyond what medicines can provide. In the very early postoperative period, one can use a TG-140 needle to fenestrate the tube proximal to the tube ligature site to allow egress of fluid through the fenestration. This can be done as a simple in-office procedure at the slit lamp. A betadine drop, antibiotic, and 2% lidocaine gel are placed in the eye. A temporal lid speculum is placed and a locking needle driver with a TG-140 needle is used to enter to subconjunctival space adjacent to the tube. The tube is then visualized anterior to the ligature suture and the needle is used to put a fenestration in the tube. The surgeon needs to take great care during this procedure to avoid violating the sclera and avoid globe perforation. The needle is then removed from the subconjunctival space after a fluid wave is observed. A cotton tip applicator is used to apply direct pressure to the needle entry site until no leak of aqueous is confirmed. This procedure can be accomplished when the ligature suture is visible posterior to the tissue patch graft. When placing the tube initially, I leave a little space between the tissue patch graft and the Vicryl ligature to allow for this type of in-office fenestration, if necessary. This technique can temporarily allow aqueous to be released until the tube opens.[1-3]

In addition to slit-lamp fenestrations, the tube can be opened early before the Vicryl suture dissolves. It is important to place the suture behind the tissue patch graft during the original surgery to allow access to the Vicryl ligature. Argon laser suture lysis of a Vicryl suture can be performed to open the tube prematurely using a 50-μm spot size, 500 mW, and 500 ms settings (Figure 12-1). I prefer not to open the tube prior to 4 weeks postoperatively to allow the capsule to mature and decrease the risk of hypotony. If forced to open the tube earlier in the setting of a very high pressure in a very advanced glaucoma patient, it is important to have viscoelastic (Healon or Healon GV, Abbott Medical Optics Inc, Abbott Park, Illinois) available to reform the anterior chamber if profound hypotony ensues.

Figure 12-1. Hoskins lens placed over a Vicryl ligature suture to allow good visualization for laser suture lysis. The argon laser can be used to weaken the Vicryl suture and open the tube. The ligation suture was placed posterior to the tissue patch graft to allow access for laser suture lysis.

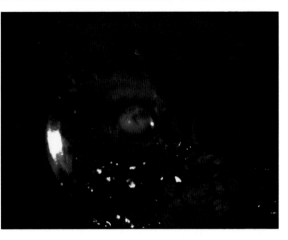

If the surgeon uses a ripcord suture technique, pulling the ripcord can be a great way to increase the flow of aqueous to the bleb space over the implant if forced to do so by an unacceptable pressure. Again, it is better to wait as long as possible to pull the ripcord suture to allow adequate capsular maturation and lower the risk of hypotony. For very rare cases of unacceptable high IOP before the Vicryl dissolves, the ripcord suture can be removed. This can be done in the office by making a small incision in the conjunctiva overlying the suture with Vannas scissors, and gently removing the suture from the tube lumen with Jeweler's forceps. It is especially useful for those eyes with orbital and lid anatomy that preclude visualization of the posterior tube, making laser suture lysis of the Vicryl ligature suture difficult. See Chapter 8 for more details about the ripcord suture technique.

Management Following Tube Opening

In tubes that are ligated, the type of suture used for ligature will determine when the tube will open. An 8-0 Vicryl suture ligature typically opens at approximately 4 weeks and with a 7-0 Vicryl ligation suture it typically occurs 5 to 7 weeks postoperatively. When the tube opens, the ridge that is seen over the glaucoma drainage implant plate lessens, and a nice bleb is seen over the glaucoma drainage implant plate (Figures 12-2 and 12-3). It is important to see the patient more frequently around the time that the tube is likely to open. I often tell patients this is the second phase of the surgery and much akin to having a "second operation" in terms of frequency of follow-up. It is important to warn patients with ligated, nonvalved implants about the signs and symptoms of tube opening and need for immediate follow-up. Patients should call their surgeon if they notice a change in vision, increased

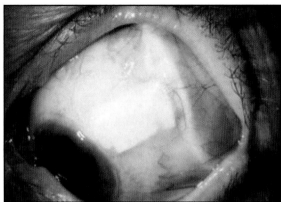

Figure 12-2. Baerveldt glaucoma drainage implant is seen beneath the superior temporal conjunctiva prior to tube opening. The ridge of the glaucoma drainage implant plate is prominent beneath the conjunctiva. (Reprinted with permission from Steve Gedde, MD.)

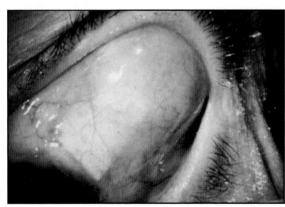

Figure 12-3. Baerveldt glaucoma drainage implant is seen beneath the superior temporal conjunctiva after tube opening. A nice diffuse bleb is seen overlying the glaucoma drainage implant plate. (Reprinted with permission from Steve Gedde, MD.)

redness, or pain. Some surgeons prefer to open the tube in the office at 5 to 6 weeks following tube placement, by lasering the Vicryl ligature or pulling the ripcord suture. It is often necessary to increase the frequency of steroid drops at the time of tube opening due to increased inflammation and sometimes fibrin formation. Some patients may exhibit profound inflammation following the tube opening with significant fibrin formation in the anterior chamber. In these cases, I have found it helpful to use 2 to 4 mg of subconjunctival dexamethasone, which can aid in controlling the inflammation. At times, a longer-acting steroid is needed and sub-Tenon's triamcinolone acetate injection can be very effective.

Rarely, following tube opening, the presence of profound hypotony, with a flat chamber, may require injection of viscoelastic to maintain the chamber. I prefer to use regular Healon for the initial injection and move to a more viscous viscoelastic, such as Healon GV, if the patient fails initially with Healon. It is important to titrate the amount of viscoelastic used to reform the chamber to avoid a very high pressure. It is better, initially, to use only the amount necessary to deepen the chamber and assess for a response. A viscoelastic overfill can lead to very high pressures, which can require urgent viscoelastic removal. The injection of viscoelastic in the setting of profound hypotony and flat chamber will decrease the risk of a choroidal effusion or hemorrhage, chronic iridocorneal adhesions, or corneal decompensation. This technique should be used with caution in very advanced patients with visual field loss involving fixation, as there is a small risk of very high pressure following viscoelastic injections. It is important to warn patients to call immediately with increased eye pain or brow pain following a viscoelastic injection, which may indicate a high IOP. For management of patients in whom conservative measures fail to address the hypotony, the reader is referred to Chapter 13.

KEY POINTS

1. Valved implants tend to have lower IOP in the early postoperative period.

2. Nonvalved implants, because of ligature and stent sutures, tend to have higher pressures in the immediate postoperative period. Patients and often need to be started back on glaucoma medicines until the tube opens.

3. Fenestrations can provide immediate pressure lowering in a ligated, nonvalved glaucoma drainage implant until the tube has opened.

4. Nonvalved implant patients need to be followed very closely around the time of tube opening because they can exhibit low IOP and increased inflammation.

5. Treat inflammation aggressively to avoid inflammatory complications such as posterior or anterior synechiae, fibrin plug formation causing tube blockage, or pupillary membrane formation.

REFERENCES

1. Trible JR, Brown DB. Occlusive ligature and standardized fenestration of a Baerveldt tube with and without antimetabolites for early postoperative intraocular pressure control. *Ophthalmology*. 1998;105(12):2243-2250.
2. Emerick GT, Gedde SJ, Budenz DL. Tube fenestrations in Baerveldt Glaucoma Implant surgery: 1-year results compared with standard implant surgery. *J Glaucoma*. 2002;11(4):340-346.
3. Kansal S, Moster MR, Kim D, Schmidt CM Jr, Wilson RP, Katz LJ. Effectiveness of nonocclusive ligature and fenestration used in Baerveldt aqueous shunts for early postoperative intraocular pressure control. *J Glaucoma*. 2002;11(1):65-70.

13

GLAUCOMA DRAINAGE DEVICES
MANAGEMENT OF INTRAOPERATIVE
AND POSTOPERATIVE COMPLICATIONS

Jonathan A. Eisengart, MD

INTRAOPERATIVE COMPLICATIONS

Tube Transection

Transection of a tube is more common during a revision than during initial insertion. If transaction happens at the time of initial insertion, it may be prudent to simply replace the device. However, the techniques described below can be used as well.

If transection occurs during revision or inadvertently during other ocular surgery, it may not be feasible to replace the device. Once transection has occurred, the eye will be very hypotonous, so consider placing viscoelastic into the anterior chamber. The transection itself can be repaired with a commercially available tube extender, the Model TE (New World Medical, Inc. Rancho Cucamonga, California). Although this is easy, the extender is somewhat bulky, needs to be covered with graft material, and may not be immediately available.

An alternative to an extender is to splice in a segment of 22-gauge angiocatheter (Figure 13-1). A short segment can easily slip over each cut end of the transected tube as a sleeve. A 9-0 Prolene suture can then be placed directly through the angiocatheter sleeve and cut tube segment end at each end to secure the sleeve.

Tube Trimmed Too Short

If the tube is placed in the anterior chamber and is 1 to 2 mm too short, the plate can usually be moved forward on the eye. Simply cut 1 or both

Kahook M.
Essentials of Glaucoma Surgery (pp 121-132).
© 2012 SLACK Incorporated.

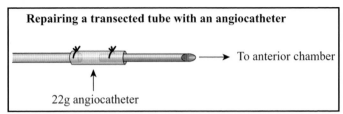

Repairing a transected tube with an angiocatheter

To anterior chamber

22g angiocatheter

Figure 13-1. A 22-gauge angiocatheter placed over the cut tube ends and secured with 9-0 Prolene can be used to lengthen a tube or repair a transection.

plate anchoring sutures, and resecure the plate a little more anteriorly. It is important, however, to make sure the plate is still at least 8 mm or more posterior to the limbus.

If the plate cannot be moved forward enough, then the device can be replaced or the tube can be extended using one of 2 techniques described above.

Scleral Perforation

Scleral perforation is most likely to occur when the plate is being anchored to the sclera, but can occur during any scleral suture pass. Perforation may be recognized by vitreous presenting through the suture tract, pigment egress, and less commonly by hemorrhage or hypotony. Once recognized, the suture should be removed. If the needle may have passed through the retina, then cryotherapy should be applied over and surrounding the needle tract (typically 1 to 3 spots). The temperature is allowed to reach −40 degrees Celsius and remain there for approximately 5 to 10 seconds.

After applying cryotherapy, the surgery is resumed and the plate can be anchored in the same area (it may, in fact, provide a small scleral buckle effect if part of the plate is overlying the perforation). A cycloplegic should be instilled at the end of surgery, and a careful fundus examination performed as soon as possible. A vitreoretinal consultation may be prudent.

Leakage Through Sclerostomy Around the Tube

If there is not a good seal around the tube, then profound hypotony can result.[1] Minimal ooze will typically stop on its own in a few days. If you recognize more then slow ooze around the tube, the tube should be removed, the sclerostomy sutured tight with an 8-0 Vicryl suture, and a new sclerostomy made. Occasionally it may work to tighten the existing sclerostomy with an 8-0 Vicryl suture, but serious hypotony can result if a good seal is not achieved.

Postoperative Complications

Although glaucoma tube shunts are subject to some unique complications, many are similar to those found in trabeculectomy. The reader is encouraged to review Chapter 4.

Hypotony

Assessment

Final intraocular pressure (IOP) after tube shunt placement is determined by the rate of aqueous production and the rate of aqueous egress through the tube and capsule. Egress is controlled by the thickness/permeability of the capsule surrounding the plate and the surface area of the plate. Hypotony is caused by an imbalance in which aqueous egress is relatively too high for the level of aqueous production.

In the early postoperative period, overfiltration is the most common cause of hypotony after tube implant surgery. In a valved device, overfiltration is usually due to a failure of the valve mechanism. In a nonvalved tube shunt, very early postoperative overfiltration may be due to inadequate occlusion of the tube, over-zealous fenestration of the tube, or leakage through the sclerostomy around the tube. Overfiltration occurring later than 5 to 6 weeks postoperatively is likely due to lack of adequate encapsulation of the plate.

Aqueous hyposecretion from active iridocyclitis, ischemia, cyclitic membranes, or other forms of ciliary atrophy can also lead to hypotony. Often, a combination of the above factors is at play (eg, an elderly white woman with poor healing and subnormal aqueous secretion develops intractable hypotony after implantation of a large, nonvalved plate).

As is the case after trabeculectomy, the decision of whether to intervene for hypotony must be made based on the present risk to vision. Uncomplicated hypotony can often be observed, wheras a flat anterior chamber needs immediate intervention.

Medical Management

Similar to trabeculectomy overfiltration, tube-shunt overfiltration will often respond to a reduction in steroid dose and, if necessary, cycloplegia. Tapering the steroids will facilitate plate encapsulation, a process than can take several weeks. Having the patient wear a shield at night and avoid eye rubbing can help prevent intermittent tube-corneal endothelial touch. Avoidance of the Valsalva maneuver should be recommended to reduce the risk of choroidal hemorrhage.

If hypotony is not resolving or if the anterior chamber is extremely shallow or flattened, viscoelastic can be injected into the anterior chamber to temporarily restrict flow through the tube. This can allow some time for the plate to encapsulate. In the setting of ciliary body detachment, which characteristically causes aqueous hyposecretion, the temporary rise in IOP provided the viscoelastic can allow reattachment of the ciliary body and improvement in aqueous secretion. Viscoelastic should be injected through a 27-gauge needle after sterilely prepping the eye and administering a topical antibiotic. Healon is a typical standard choice, and may be retained in the anterior chamber less than 24 hours. Healon GV and Healon 5 allow progressively longer retention and higher achievable IOP.

Surgical Management

If hypotony is not resolving spontaneously or if it is profound, surgical intervention is indicated. The easiest approach is to re-occlude the tube to give the plate more time to encapsulate. This may be done by making a small conjunctival cut-down just anterior to the plate and tightly occluding with a 7-0 Vicryl or 8-0 Prolene suture (the latter option should be wound twice around the tube). Alternatively, the tip of the tube can be delivered from the eye, occluded with an 8-0 Prolene suture wrapped twice, and replaced into the anterior chamber. (The occluding suture will be within the anterior chamber, allowing for easy laser access later.) Prolene sutures can then be "warmed" and loosened at a later date with an argon laser, 500 mW for 500 msec. A red laser may work better than a green laser for Prolene sutures.

If there is recalcitrant or late hypotony, the plate may simply be too large for the eye's ability to produce aqueous and encapsulate the plate. The most assured "cure" of the hypotony is to remove the device (or cut off and remove the tube), although uncontrolled IOP elevation will often result. If the original device was a large, nonvalved plate, it may be replaced with a valved device. A perhaps less successful alternative is to replace it with a smaller version of the same device (eg, changing a Baerveldt 350 mm^2 to a 250 mm^2 or a Molteno3) or trimming the existing plate to a smaller size. Silicone or flexible plates can be easily cut to a smaller size with Stevens scissors.

Removing a tube shunt begins by making a conjunctival incision 2 to 3 mm anterior to the plate, parallel to the plate, and at least as wide. The incision is then carried down through Tenon's capsule to sclera and posteriorly to expose the anterior edge of the plate capsule. To help mobilize conjunctiva and eventual wound closure, blunt dissection is then used to separate conjunctiva from underlying capsule. A paracentesis is made so that the anterior chamber can be reformed as needed. The tube is then grasped near the plate (Figure 13-2) and pulled from the anterior chamber. Given the long tract under the conjunctiva and patch graft, there should not be much leakage, but the sclerostomy can be sutured as necessary by making a small peritomy at the limbus to elevate the patch graft. The capsule

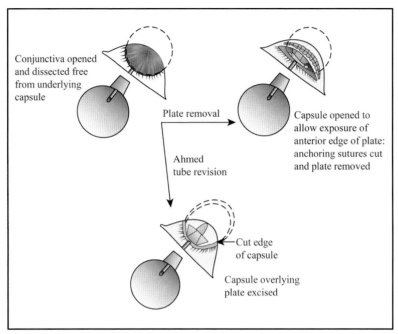

Figure 13-2. Accessing the plate for removal or revision.

surrounding the plate should then be sharply entered near the anterior edge of the plate and the incision extended widely to expose the entire anterior edge of the plate. Next, cut the sutures anchoring the plate to the sclera. To find and cut the fibrous "stalks" that have grown through a Baerveldt's plate fenestrations, place blunt-tipped scissors on top of the plate and "strum" the stalks to locate them. Most plates can now be easily pulled out, although large Baerveldt plates may be more easily removed if one wing is cut off first. If necessary, a smaller tube shunt can then be placed in the existing Tenon's "pocket" or placed in a new quadrant.

Hypertensive Phase

Any type of glaucoma drainage device can go through a hypertensive phase, but it is more common, or at least more easily noticed, in valved devices that are not tied off initially. The hypertensive phase is typically seen at 4 to 5 weeks[2] postoperatively, when the IOP begins to rise. Often, a moderate to high encapsulated bleb is noted.

First-line treatment is to taper steroids if possible, because steroid-responsive IOP rise is definitely possible despite a functioning tube. Early use of aqueous suppressants can also be helpful, not only to lower the IOP but also to potentially "soften" the capsule by lessening internal pressure and stretching of the capsule. Typically, I will avoid early use outflow agents (ie, prostaglandin analogs) because they can be somewhat inflammatory in the early postoperative period and because there is already some functional outflow from the tube shunt.

Tube Exposure

Assessment

Erosion of the tissues overlying the tube usually occurs months to years after tube placement, although occasionally it can occur earlier. It is typically seen approximately 2 to 4 mm posterior to the limbus, presumably due to pressure and rubbing from the upper lid tarsus. Tube exposure needs to be repaired because it can lead to endophthalmitis and even orbital cellulitis. Although a patient may be temporized with topical antibiotics, management of tube exposures is purely surgical.

If signs of infection are seen, such as anterior chamber reaction or purulence, intense antibiotic treatment should be instituted and consideration given to tube removal. Clearly, any hint of endophthalmitis should be referred to a vitreoretinal specialist.

Surgical Management

In my experience, most cases of tube exposure have occurred in tubes originally covered by pericardium. If that is the case, I will try once to re-cover the tube with donor sclera or rarely split-thickness cornea, both of which are more durable in the eye than pericardium (if the tube erodes through sclera, I will often reposition the tube as described below). I typically make my incision at the limbus, anterior to the plate, or along the area of erosion depending on the location and amount of scarring. Careful, gentle dissection is then used to elevate conjunctiva off the tube and surrounding sclera to make a pocket large enough to accommodate a new graft. The new graft material is slipped into place and sutured with 8-0 Vicryl. Often, there is extensive scarring, and mobilizing adequate conjunctiva is difficult. Additionally, the original erosion leaves a hole in the conjunctiva that may overlie the new patch graft. Exposed scleral patch grafts will typically epithelialize and then vascularize in a few weeks. If a large area of patch graft remains exposed at the end of the surgery, amniotic membrane or a free conjunctival graft can be sutured to fill in the conjunctival defect.

If the tube erosion is recurrent or there is not enough mobile conjunctiva to allow re-covering of the tube, then the tube needs to be repositioned to change the way it interacts with the eyelid. One option is to remove the device (or just cut off and remove the tube) and place a new device in another quadrant. However, I have had excellent success by repositioning the tube into the pars plana. If the patient has not already had a complete pars plana vitrectomy with trimming of the vitreous skirt, I will perform the surgery in conjunction with one of my vitreoretinal colleagues. Once the vitreous has been cleared, I begin repositioning the tube by making a 2 to 3 clock-hour limbal peritomy with short radial relaxing incisions in the quadrant with the tube. Conjunctiva is elevated, the tube tip is removed from the eye, and the sclerostomy is sutured with 8-0 Vicryl. The tube is then placed into the pars plana through a fresh 23-gauge needle tract. For further details on pars plana placement of the tube, please see Chapter 38.

Plate Erosion

Late erosion of the plate is uncommon but cannot be repaired. Direct suturing of the conjunctiva or covering the plate with graft material almost always fails. In these cases, the exposed device should be removed. If necessary, another tube can be placed in a different quadrant, or ciliary body ablation can be performed.

Early postoperative wound dehiscence can be successfully resutured if there is healthy conjunctiva and minimal wound tension. Friable conjunctiva or excessive wound tension should be approached by replacing the device into another quadrant.

Tube Occlusion

Occlusion in the Anterior Chamber

Tube occlusion can occur at the tip of the tube in the anterior chamber. Occlusion is easily recognized in the anterior chamber if iris, fibrin/blood clot, silicone oil, or other substance is seen at the end of the tube in association with an elevated IOP.

Frequently, these occlusions may be cleared with the YAG laser. Rarely, pilocarpine helps pull iris out of the tube, but the iris may come back up into the tube at a later date. Fibrin or blood clot may be treated with tissue plasminogen activator (tPA), 3 to 25 µg injected into the anterior chamber through a 30-gauge needle. (An inpatient hospital pharmacy or compounding pharmacy can dilute the intravenous tPA solution to 100 to 250 microgram/mL, and 0.1 cc is injected at the slit lamp.[3]) Of course, intracameral tPA can lead to a total hyphema if fresh wounds or fragile vessels remain.

Occlusion of the Valve Mechanism

A valved device, in particular Ahmed tubes, can also become obstructed at the level of the valve mechanism. Obstruction can be due to material lodged in the valve mechanism or from fibrous bands growing retrograde from the plate up the tube. Valve obstruction is often difficult to differentiate from simple plate encapsulation. However, when the IOP is elevated, careful inspection of the bleb can be revealing. When the valve is obstructed, the bleb will be absent, the conjunctiva will be closely adherent to the plate, and detailed structures of the plate will frequently be visible through the conjunctiva. With plate encapsulation, the bleb may be low but not flat, and detailed structures of the plate are not visible. B-scan ultrasonography also may be helpful to look for fluid surrounding the plate.

If valve obstruction is confirmed, firm ocular massage may force aqueous through the valve and occasionally relieve the obstruction. This technique tends to work best in the first few days after surgery.

If massage fails, the tube may be considered to have failed. Options for managing tube failure are discussed below in the section on cyclodestruction.

However, I have had success in surgically clearing a valve obstruction with a planned 2-step approach. In the operating room, begin by getting a careful baseline examination of the flat bleb because you will be looking for it to elevate when the obstruction is relieved. The first attempt to clear the obstruction is made by passing a 3-0 Prolene suture up the tube through the valve. The Prolene can be placed into the tube by delivering the tip of the tube from the eye, or by making a paracentesis 180 degrees away from the tube and running the tube across the anterior chamber. As the suture is advanced, you may feel resistance and then a "give" as the suture passes through the valve. Once the suture is inserted as far as it can go, it is important to ensure it has passed the valve (Figure 13-3), especially if it cannot be directly seen through the conjunctiva. With tying forceps, grasp the Prolene right at the tip of the tube (or at the paracentesis if the suture was passed through the cornea) and *without letting go*, pull the Prolene out. Your forceps now mark the maximum point where the suture was inserted, so you can lay the Prolene on the eye, lining up your forceps with the tube tip/paracentesis, to make sure adequate suture length was inserted to pass through the valve. Next, deepen the anterior chamber and raise the IOP substantially. Check to make sure that the bleb forms and that the IOP comes down over several minutes. Many times this maneuver will be successful.

If there is still no evidence of tube function, the obstruction is more likely due to fibrous growth into the valve or tight encapsulation overlying the valve outlet. I have found success in these situations by cutting away the capsule overlying the plate (only in valved devices, otherwise profound hypotony will

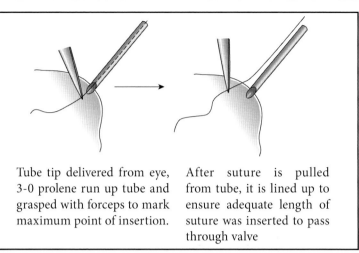

Tube tip delivered from eye, 3-0 prolene run up tube and grasped with forceps to mark maximum point of insertion.	After suture is pulled from tube, it is lined up to ensure adequate length of suture was inserted to pass through valve

Figure 13-3. Passing suture up Ahmed tube and ensuring adequate length was inserted to clear valve.

result). Begin by making a conjunctival incision 2 to 3 mm anterior to, and parallel to, the plate and at least as wide as the plate. Carry it deep to the sclera, taking care to avoid cutting the tube. Identify the anterior edge of plate, and bluntly and broadly dissect conjunctiva and Tenon's off of the capsule surrounding the plate. Next, sharply enter the capsule at the anterior edge of the plate and excise as much capsule tissue as possible. Often, as the thick encapsulation is pulled up off the plate, a fibrous extension can be seen extending into the valve. Once the valve is cleared, aqueous should flow immediately (if it does not, the plate should be replaced or the valve mechanism disassembled). Close the conjunctiva–Tenon's complex with a running 8-0 Vicryl suture. To prevent the incision from overlying the plate where it can leak, take anterior anchoring bites of Tenon's, scar, and/or sclera as the suture is run.

Tube Failure

For the purpose of this discussion, tube failure is considered to occur when the IOP remains too high despite a bleb over the plate and maximum tolerated hypotensive therapy.

This situation can be difficult to manage, and there are essentially 3 options: revision of the existing tube, placement of a second tube, or cyclodestruction.

Revision of the Existing Tube

This involves cutting away the thick capsule overlying the plate as described above. This can be successful in some cases, but the capsule may reform. In a valved device, this technique has the advantage of relatively rapid patient recovery and low operative risk. I will often try a revision of an Ahmed tube before placing a second device.

If a nonvalved device is revised, then it must be temporarily reoccluded to prevent profound hypotony. For that reason, I do not attempt to revise nonvalved devices.

Placement of a Second Tube Shunt

A second tube shunt is often quite successful, as long as there is an available quadrant to place it in. In most cases, I will implant a Baerveldt 250 mm^2 or 350 mm^2 as a second tube because it is low profile and highly effective. An Ahmed may be a reasonable second choice, but its higher profile can lead to proptosis or inferior globe displacement when another drainage device is already in place. However, if the first implant provided very minimal benefit, then a second device may not work much better.

Cyclodestruction

Transscleral or endoscopic cyclophotocoagulation can be highly effective in the setting of some functional outflow (eg, the tube shunt). Treatment parameters are the same as for an eye without a tube shunt in place. For a transscleral approach, however, I will typically avoid treating the quadrant with the tube shunt because the graft and tube itself will make treatment of the underlying ciliary body less predictable. Cyclodestruction may be a less desirable in phakic patients, however, due to the rapid formation of advanced cataract.

Corneal Edema and Decompensation

The presence of any foreign object within the anterior chamber can lead to progressive loss of corneal endothelial cells and eventual corneal edema. The rate of endothelial cell loss has been reported at 18.6% at 24 months and even higher in the quadrant with the tube.[4]

Prevention

Progressive corneal endothelial cell loss is thought to be due to intermittent tube–corneal touch. A long tube or an anteriorly directed tube are risk factors for progressive corneal edema. Additionally, corneal endothelial cells may be lost at the site of the sclerostomy. Ideally, the sclerostomy should be made so that the tube enters *posterior* to Schwalbe's line, which will ensure no portion of the tube is in contact with the corneal endothelium.

Surgical Management

If a tube is too long, the tip can be delivered from the anterior segment and trimmed. Alternatively, it can be trimmed directly within the anterior chamber.[5] If the tube is anteriorly directed, the tip should be removed, the sclerostomy sutured closed, and the tube reinserted in an appropriate direction.

When corneal edema related to a tube is noted, the tube should ideally be removed or repositioned into the posterior segment (please see Chapter 38). If visually significant corneal edema has already developed, a corneal endothelial graft or penetrating keratoplasty may be required. The success of a corneal graft in this situation may be improved if the tube is removed or repositioned posteriorly.

KEY POINTS

1. A piece of 22-gauge angiocatheter can be spliced in to extend or repair a tube.

2. Leakage around the tube can result in intractable hypotony, and anything more than a minimal ooze needs to be addressed before leaving the operating room.

3. Early postoperative hypotony is likely due to failure of the valve mechanism is valved devices, poor occlusion or over-fenestration in nonvalved devices, or leakage around the tube in either type of device.

4. Late postoperative hypotony is due to poor encapsulation of the plate and/or reduced aqueous production.

5. A "hypertensive" phase is common, but typically IOP can be controlled by tapering steroids and adding ocular hypotensive medications.

6. When the IOP is too high after implantation of a valved device, look for a flat bleb to rule out valve obstruction.

7. Failed drainage devices can be addressed by revision (for valved devices), placing a second device, or cyclodestruction.

REFERENCES

1. García-Feijoó J, Cuiña-Sardiña R, Méndez-Fernández C, Castillo-Gómez A, García-Sánchez J. Peritubular filtration as a cause of severe hypotony after Ahmed valve implantation for glaucoma. *Am J Ophthalmol.* 2001;132(4):571-572.

2. Nouri-Mahdavi K, Caprioli J. Evaluation of the hypertensive phase after insertion of the Ahmed Glaucoma Valve. *Am J Ophthalmol.* 2003;136(6):1001-1008.

3. Zalta AH, Sweeney CP, Zalta AK, Kaufman AH. Intracameral tissue plasminogen activator use in a large series of eyes with valved glaucoma drainage implants. *Arch Ophthalmol.* 2002;120(11):1487-1493.

4. Lee EK, Yun YJ, Lee JE, Yim JH, Kim CS. Changes in corneal endothelial cells after Ahmed glaucoma valve implantation: 2-year follow-up. *Am J Ophthalmol.* 2009;148(3):361-367.

5. Asrani S, Herndon L, Allingham RR. A newer technique for glaucoma tube trimming. *Arch Ophthalmol.* 2003;121(9):1324-1326.

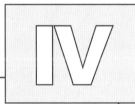

GLAUCOMA SURGERY COMBINED WITH CATARACT EXTRACTION

14

CATARACT SURGERY AND INTRAOCULAR PRESSURE

John P. Berdahl, MD and Thomas W. Samuelson, MD

Cataracts and glaucoma are the first and second leading causes of blindness worldwide.[1,2] Because both diseases usually occur after the fifth decade of life, it is not surprising that these 2 diseases occur simultaneously in many patients. Intraocular pressure (IOP) reduction after cataract surgery has been shown in many studies, and the most recent data indicates that IOP reduction after cataract surgery is more significant and sustained than previously thought.[3,4]

Lowering IOP is the mainstay of glaucoma treatment. Traditional glaucoma surgeries such a trabeculectomy and tube shunts work well to lower IOP and decrease progression of glaucoma; however, these procedures carry significant morbidity. Many patients with glaucoma have concurrent cataracts, and some studies have suggested that glaucoma itself is a risk factor for cataract development. Certainly glaucoma-filtering procedures, peripheral iridotomy, and some glaucoma medications increase the risk of cataract formation. Historically, patients with moderate to advanced glaucoma with concurrent cataracts would have either a combined procedure or a 2-stage surgery. Surgeons have traditionally felt that cataract surgery lowers IOP in open-angle glaucoma (OAG) only slightly and temporarily, despite a paucity of robust data. In contrast, current data demonstrate a greater and more sustained IOP reduction.[4,5] As such, cataract surgery may be a safe alternative to glaucoma surgery in some patients and could shift the surgeon's approach in treating concurrent cataract and glaucoma, especially in the early or moderate stages of glaucoma.

SUMMARY OF VARIOUS STUDIES

The earliest studies of IOP after cataract surgery showed little if any reduction of IOP. However, these results probably do not apply today

Kahook M.
Essentials of Glaucoma Surgery (pp 135-138).
© 2012 SLACK Incorporated.

because of advances in surgical technique and intraocular lens (IOL) technology. As phacoemulsification became the standard, studies began to demonstrate more sustained IOP lowering following cataract surgery.[5] The conventional wisdom that cataract surgery lowers IOP by 2 to 4 mm Hg for a couple of years was partially confirmed by the only meta-analysis of the topic;[6] however, nearly all of the studies showed only mean IOP change and did not stratify patients based on preoperative IOP, which has critical significance in data interpretation because only a subset of patients had an elevated and, therefore, modifiable IOP. Those studies that did stratify patients based on preoperative IOP clearly demonstrated that patients with higher preoperative IOP enjoy the greatest reduction of IOP after cataract surgery.[4,7,8] IOP reduction is maintained in 75% to 85% of patients at 5 years, and IOP can be controlled in 20% of patients with OAG without drops after cataract surgery.[9]

The method of cataract extraction may influence the reduction of IOP. Phacoemulsification (particularly clear corneal phacoemulsification) seems to lower IOP more than manual extracapsular cataract extraction. The type of OAG may also influence IOP reduction. Pseudoexfoliation patients may have an even greater long-term decrease in IOP than primary OAG patients although IOP often rises on postoperative day 1. However, the early IOP variability following cataract surgery rarely has clinical consequence. Many other factors, such as pressurization at the time of surgery, immediate postoperative medications (especially corticosteroid), and viscoelastic type, contribute to short-term IOP fluctuations following cataract surgery.

PATHOPHYSIOLOGY OF REDUCED INTRAOCULAR PRESSURE AFTER CATARACT SURGERY

Although the physiological reasons for decreased IOP after cataract surgery remain speculative, the facility of outflow is known to increase after cataract surgery.[10] Angle width changes less than one would expect following cataract surgery, suggesting improved function of the trabecular meshwork itself rather than improved aqueous access to the trabecular meshwork. Three or more different mechanisms may contribute to the observed reduction in IOP after cataract surgery.

Lens-Induced Changes to Outflow Pathway

As the eye ages, the crystalline lens increases significantly in volume. This may initiate a series of anatomical changes that ultimately leads to the increase in IOP observed with aging. As the lens grows, the anterior lens capsule is displaced forward causing the zonules to place anteriorly directed traction on the ciliary body and uveal tract, which in turn compresses the canal of Schlemm and the trabecular meshwork. Because the anterior tendons of the ciliary muscles contribute to the architecture of the trabecular meshwork, as the ciliary body is displaced forward by the enlarging lens, the tendons relax and the space between trabecular plates becomes narrowed.

Inflammation Induced by Cataract Surgery

Phacoemulsification typically induces a low-grade inflammation in the immediate postoperative period. It is plausible that the induced inflammation lowers IOP by either decreasing aqueous production of the ciliary body, as seen in uveitis, or it could increase outflow similar to the mechanism of selective laser trabeculoplasty or prostaglandin analogues. Although these options seem plausible, little experimental data exist currently to support these hypotheses.

Fluidics of Phacoemulsification

Another possible for lower IOP after cataract surgery is that high flow of fluid and high IOP (up to 90 mm Hg) experienced during cataract surgery forces fluid through the trabecular meshwork into the canal of Schlemm and the episcleral veins. Forcing this large amount of fluid through the drainage system may increase patency and promote flow. Again, little evidence exists to support or refute this hypothesis.

IS CATARACT SURGERY A GLAUCOMA SURGERY?

Cataract surgery is a very common, successful, highly refined surgery with a favorable risk–benefit profile including improved visual acuity and visual field. The widespread general belief that cataract extraction alone lowers IOP 2 to 4 mm Hg is slowly evolving toward an understanding of a larger and more sustained IOP reduction, especially in patients with higher preoperative IOP.[4,6,11] Although cataract surgery alone lowers IOP, combined glaucoma/cataract surgery lowers IOP more with fewer postoperative pressure spikes. Surgeons should carefully monitor IOP after cataract surgery to prevent a postoperative pressure spike that could "snuff" the nerve, especially in patients with pseudoexfoliation syndrome. Moreover, the influence of corticosteroid on IOP must be monitored. It often takes weeks or months following surgery to achieve the new postoperative baseline. During this period, IOP should be managed with the knowledge that temporary factors, such as typical postsurgical inflammation and topical steroid, may cause IOP to be elevated. The clinician should not interpret the early postoperative IOP as the new postsurgical baseline until all inflammation has subsided and steroids discontinued. Nonetheless, cataract surgery seems to be emerging as a safe way to lower IOP in patients with mild to moderate glaucoma while avoiding the morbidity of traditional glaucoma surgery.

CONCLUSION

Although the mechanism is unclear, cataract surgery appears to lower IOP in glaucoma patients. Traditionally, cataract surgery has been thought to lower IOP about 2 mm Hg; however, emerging data indicate that while the average IOP reduction after cataract surgery is 2 mm Hg, the IOP reduction is greater in those with an elevated IOP. Additionally, the IOP-lowering effect appears to be sustained at 5 years. Given the favorable risk–benefit profile of cataract surgery and its low morbidity, cataract surgery provides a good IOP-lowering option for patients with mild to moderate glaucoma.

KEY POINTS

1. Cataract surgery alone lowers IOP.
2. The IOP reduction of cataract surgery appears sustained at 5 years.
3. IOP is reduced more in patients with a higher baseline IOP.
4. Because cataract surgery has a favorable risk–benefit profile, it may be a good option to lower IOP in mild to moderate glaucoma.

REFERENCES

1. West S. Epidemiology of cataract: accomplishments over 25 years and future directions. *Ophthalmic Epidemiol.* 2007;14(4):173-178.
2. Quigley HA. Number of people with glaucoma worldwide. *Br J Ophthalmol.* 1996; 80(5):389-393.
3. Foroozan R, Levkovitch-Verbin H, Habot-Wilner Z, Burla N. Cataract surgery and intraocular pressure. *Ophthalmology.* 2008;115(1):104-108.
4. Poley BJ, Lindstrom RL, Samuelson TW. Long-term effects of phacoemulsification with intraocular lens implantation in normotensive and ocular hypertensive eyes. *J Cataract Refract Surg.* 2008;34(5):735-742.
5. Hansen MH, Gyldenkerne GJ, Otland NW, et al. Intraocular pressure seven years after extracapsular cataract extraction and sulcus implantation of a posterior chamber intraocular lens. *J Cataract Refract Surg.* 1995;21(6):676-678.
6. Friedman DS, Jampel HD, Lubomski LH, et al. Surgical strategies for coexisting glaucoma and cataract: an evidence-based update. *Ophthalmology.* 2002;109(10):1902-1913.
7. Bowling B, Calladine D. Routine reduction of glaucoma medication following phacoemulsification. *J Cataract Refract Surg.* 2009;35(3):406-407.
8. Leelachaikul Y, Euswas A. Long-term intraocular pressure change after clear corneal phacoemulsification in Thai glaucoma patients. *J Med Assoc Thai.* 2005;88(Suppl 9): S21-S25.
9. Hayashi K, Hayashi H, Nakao F, Hayashi F. Effect of cataract surgery on intraocular pressure control in glaucoma patients. *J Cataract Refract Surg.* 2001;27(11):1779-1786.
10. Meyer MA, Savitt ML, Kopitas E. The effect of phacoemulsification on aqueous outflow facility. *Ophthalmology.* 1997;104(8):1221-1227.
11. Vass C, Menapace R. Surgical strategies in patients with combined cataract and glaucoma. *Curr Opin Ophthalmol.* 2004;15(1):61-66.

Endoscopic Cyclophotocoagulation

Steven R. Sarkisian Jr, MD

The surgical management of glaucoma has evolved in recent years to go beyond procedures that make a hole in the eye to bypass the trabecular meshwork to small-incision microsurgical techniques. These trends are similar to trends we have seen in cataract surgery, as well as in general surgery that are distinguished by smaller incisions, shorter procedure times, fewer complications, and faster recovery. In the cataract surgery realm, this can be seen with the ever-decreasing incision sizes for microincisional phacoemulsification and the development that follows with more sophisticated injectors and more flexible foldable lenses. In the general surgical realm, this evolution has been best demonstrated by the ubiquitous utilization of endoscopy, laparoscopy, or arthroscopy, technologies that afford the surgeon direct intraoperative visualization of focal pathology with incisions that are a mere fraction of the size compared with the large open incisions of the past. Endoscopic cyclophotocoagulation (ECP) builds on this idea by having one of the smallest endoscopes manufactured to visualize the ciliary processes within the eye and treat the end organ with minimal, if any, collateral damage.

This chapter will review the physical aspects of the endoscopic cyclophotocoagulator, the rationale for surgery using the device, the surgical technique, and my method for performing ECP. Also reviewed will be indications for surgery, preoperative and postoperative issues, and postoperative management, as well as special situations in which the endoscope can be utilized.

The Endoscopic Cyclophotocoagulation Device and Historical Perspective

The machine used to perform ECP is manufactured by Endo Optiks Inc (Little Silver, New Jersey). It is a microprobe diode laser endoscopy system

Kahook M.
Essentials of Glaucoma Surgery (pp 139-148).
© 2012 SLACK Incorporated.

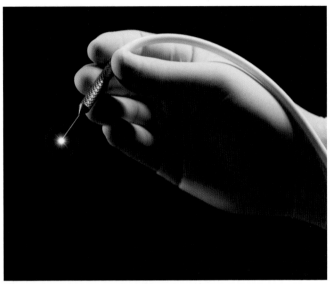

Figure 15-1. 20-gauge straight endoprobe.

that combines illumination, a video imager, and laser in a single handpiece. The endolaser probe has a 20-gauge diameter and can be used at the limbus or through pars plana to treat most types of glaucoma. Most frequently, it is used in combination with phacoemulsification. Transscleral cycloablation has been performed for many years using a variety of techniques, currently the most common being the Nd:YAG or diode lasers. Conventionally, these treatments have been used as a last resort for eyes that have failed multiple glaucoma surgeries, including trabeculectomy, and perhaps multiple glaucoma drainage devices. They also have been used to treat blind, painful eyes or eyes that have poor visual potential. Transscleral cycloablative procedures are nearly impossible to titrate, and it is unclear what the intraocular pressure (IOP)-lowering results will be. They are also blind procedures, because the end organ that you wish to treat is not visualized and the procedures can be associated with high instances of hypotony, visual loss, pain, and inflammation.

Alternatively, ECP does not cause collateral tissue damage because it targets the end organ tissue and treats the ciliary body alone. The endoscope itself has a tripartite construction and includes an image fiber, a light fiber, and a laser fiber that joins in a 20-gauge endoprobe, which is attached with a fiber optic cord to a console (Figures 15-1 and 15-2). The laser provides a 110-degree field of view and depth of focus from 1 mm to 30 mm. The console contains a plug-in for each element of the laser probe, including the video camera, light source, video monitor, and a video recorder. The laser

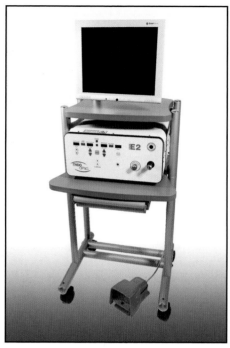

Figure 15-2. Endocyclophotoco-agulation console.

itself is a semiconductor diode tuned to 810 nm in wave length. The console allows you to adjust the strength of the laser power, the brightness of the light, and the brightness of the aiming beam, as well as the focus and orientation of the image. It also allows the laser to have a continuous burn versus an intermittent burn depending on the preference of the surgeon.

INDICATIONS FOR ENDOSCOPIC CYCLOPHOTOCOAGULATION

Endoscopic Cyclophotocoagulation Combined With Cataract Surgery

The vast majority of patients undergoing ECP are patients who have a cataract with concomitant glaucoma, and the ECP is performed at the time of cataract surgery. There is no fixed algorithm for choosing to do ECP in a patient with a cataract. One must consider that cataract surgery alone will likely lower the eye pressure several points; however, the longevity of this effect is uncertain. If the patient is on 1 to 3 glaucoma medications and is well controlled on medications, but wishes to have a lower medication burden or is intolerant to medications these patients may get ECP in combination with cataract surgery to be on fewer medications. Another subgroup is those patients who have marginally controlled IOP on medications, and the surgeon and patient wish to get the IOP closer to the target pressure without changing any medications.

As a glaucoma specialist, I especially find ECP useful in patients who have had previous glaucoma surgery—either trabeculectomy, an Ex-Press shunt, or a conventional tube shunt—but need additional pressure lowering and happen to also have a visually significant cataract.

Plateau Iris Syndrome

Plateau iris syndrome poses an interesting situation in which the peripheral angle is narrow due to anterior rotation of the ciliary body. In plateau iris syndrome, even after peripheral iridotomy, the pressure may remain elevated because the mechanism of angle closure is not pupillary block but narrow peripheral angle due to anterior rotation of the ciliary processes.

In plateau iris, ECP combined with cataract surgery can be a very useful technique to definitively improve the angle of rotation of the ciliary body. During ECP, the shrinking of the ciliary processes rotates the ciliary body posteriorly. This technique has been referred to as endocylcoplasty.[1]

Pseudophakic and Aphakic Glaucoma

Patients who have had previous cataract surgery and have an in-the-bag intraocular lens (IOL) can undergo ECP. Although, the long-term results are less satisfactory than when ECP is combined with cataract surgery, this can be a useful technique in patients with scarred conjunctiva due to chemical injuries or in patients who have had multiple glaucoma surgeries in nearly every quadrant.

In aphakic glaucoma, ECP can be successfully performed; however, extra steps must be taken to prevent the eye from deflating during surgery, and typically an infusion port is required. ECP in an aphakic eye is typically not going to be a first option and typically would be performed after some form of glaucoma drainage implant has been unsuccessful and the eye has good vision. Therefore, it is desirable in those cases to avoid transscleral cyclophotocoagulation and the risk of decreased vision after the procedure.

The Phakic Eye

Endoscopic cyclophotocoagulation in a phakic eye has been described; however, it is my opinion that ECP in a phakic eye is rarely if ever appropriate, especially in an eye with good visual potential because of the degree of inflammation that will likely occur in a phakic eye and the risk of causing trauma to the lens with the instrumentation. In almost every case in which an eye is phakic with elevated IOP, it is better to consider other options besides ECP. ECP in a phakic eye is most likely going to create a cataract and cause adhesions between the lens capsule and the iris.

TECHNIQUE

The usual technique for cataract surgery combined with ECP starts out essentially the same way as any typical cataract surgery using phacoemulsification. The only exception is I typically make a second incision 180 degrees from my original temporal keratome incision to facilitate a full 360 degrees of treatment. If you are using a curved endoprobe, 270 degrees of ECP can be performed through 1 wound; however, the pressure-lowering effects will not be as significant as 360 degrees of treatment.[2] The ECP probe will fit through the small incision keratome wounds that are currently being used for phacoemulsification. I typically make a 1.8-mm keratome incision; however, the probe will fit through a port as small as 1.5 mm and still allow the flexibility and maneuverability required.

After successful phacoemulsification and implantation of the IOL, it is important to fully remove the viscoelastic from the capsular bag. Viscoelastic is then injected into the sulcus. I typically use Healon GV because it provides superior visualization of the entire ciliary body and also the best view of the posterior ciliary processes. This superior view is created because the Healon not only lifts the iris but it also pushes down the anterior capsule and gives space to aim the laser through the zonules toward the posterior processes to get a maximum IOP-lowering effect.

It should be noted that ECP can be performed before implanting the IOL, but great care must be taken not to rupture the capsular bag. The advantage of doing ECP prior to implanting the lens is that it allows the surgeon to laser through the bag and get the very posterior aspects of the ciliary body; however, I rarely perform this technique because I have found that the Healon GV allows for excellent visualization of this area with the IOL in place.

Combined Endoscopic Cyclophotocoagulation and Cataract Surgery

I prefer to first treat the area of the ciliary processes that are 180 degrees from the temporal wound, treating from left to right with a curved probe. Once the aiming beam is over the center of the ciliary process, the foot pedal is depressed and the laser is used to "paint" the ciliary processes in one smooth motion from left to right, treating not only the center but also the valleys in between. Great care is given to avoid treating the iris itself and also from overtreating the processes causing a "pop." Avoiding this overtreatment minimizes postoperative inflammation, making the procedure similar or slightly more inflammatory than what is seen with standard cataract surgery.

After the first 180 to 270 degrees are treated, I then take the viscoelastic and viscodilate the subincisional temporal sulcus and repeat the steps above to get a full 360-degree treatment. Once this has been completed, the probe is slowly removed from the eye, taking care to visualize its path as it exits the eye. The viscoelastic must then be carefully removed. If it is not fully removed there will be a high likelihood of a postoperative IOP spike. Because of the risk of postoperative IOP spikes, it may be appropriate to use either a direct- or indirect-acting injection of a miotic agent in the anterior chamber to improve postoperative aqueous outflow.

Endoscopic Cyclophotocoagulation in Pseudophakes and Aphakes

If the patient is pseudophakic undergoing ECP, the technique is essentially identical to when it is combined with cataract surgery. If the patient has an anterior chamber IOL, ECP is not going to be possible, and likely if there is an iris-fixated or scleral-fixated IOL, ECP will also be contraindicated because of the risk of disrupting the iris sutures. However, in most cases of pseudophakia, one can viscodilate the sulcus and the viscoelastic can often break any adhesions that might be found.

Aphakic glaucoma poses an entirely different problem because often aphakic eyes are unicameral, and when you enter the eye, it will deflate. Typically, an anterior chamber maintainer is required. I use a Lewicky (Beaver-Visitec, Waltham, Massachusetts), which is attached to the phacoemulsification machine and is inserted through a paracentesis placed in a different quadrant from the wound. Usually viscoelastic is unnecessary in an aphakic eye unless a remnant of the capsular bag is opacified. The anterior chamber maintainer serves to constantly irrigate balanced salt solution into the eye to provide chamber stability and an adequate view. If any anterior vitreous is visible, this must be removed by vitrectomy prior to the ECP.

It is possible that due to visibility issues in an aphakic patient, an anterior incision may be impossible and the pars plana approach may be needed. Moreover, the pars plana approach may also be preferred in eyes with anterior chamber IOLs. In the presence of a crystalline lens, ECP is contraindicated for both the anterior and pars plana approach. During the pars plana approach, you also must be certain that vitreous is not present and the laser endoscope is inserted through the pars plana at 3.5 to 4 mm posterior to the limbus.

Pediatric Glaucoma

Endoscopic cyclophotocoagulation can be performed in the pediatric patient population.[3] However, unlike the adult population, ECP in the pediatric patient is typically reserved for refractory glaucoma in which the patient is already aphakic or pseudophakic and has had the maximum amount of the usual anterior segment glaucoma surgery (ie, goniotomy, trabeculotomy, 360-degree trabeculotomy, and/or 1 or 2 tube shunts).

ECP may be used in a child's eye with good visual potential after multiple glaucoma surgeries, especially in eyes with pediatric glaucoma secondary to congenital cataracts. I have not attempted ECP in eyes with primary congenital glaucoma; however, one could argue that after these children reach adulthood and develop cataracts, cataract surgery combined with ECP may be an option for them.

Other Refractory Glaucoma

ECP has also been described for the treatment of refractory glaucomas;[4] however, ECP should be avoided in patients with uveitic glaucoma because ECP will likely worsen the inflammation.

POSTOPERATIVE CONSIDERATIONS

Postoperative medications after ECP mirror those which are used for cataract surgery alone. These include a nonsteroidal anti-inflammatory drop, as well as a fourth-generation fluoroquinolone. With the advent of Durezol (difluprednate) I have found that treatment with this medication 4 to 6 times daily has greatly reduced postoperative inflammation with ECP. I typically taper the Durezol over a 4- to 6-week period; however, care must be taken to avoid a steroid response. Moreover, due to the more dispersive action of the viscoelastic used during ECP and the high risk for IOP spikes, I typically will give patients acetazolamide after the procedure.

Typically, at the first postoperative visit, if the patient is on 1 to 3 glaucoma medicines, I will stop 1 medication, and continuing the other medications, depending on the IOP that day. Then I have the patients follow up in 5 to 7 days and titrate the medications depending on the IOP.

CONCLUSION

Endoscopic cyclophotocoagulation is an effective treatment for lowering IOP, but it has been surrounded by some controversy. I do not perform ECP on every patient in my practice with a cataract and concomitant glaucoma who is on medications. Cataract surgery combined with ECP in patients who are poor candidates for glaucoma filtration surgery or who had a poor experience with glaucoma filtration surgery in 1 eye and need a procedure in their other eye, can be extremely satisfying for both the patient and the surgeon. ECP is also a helpful option in monocular patients or patients who have a bleeding diathesis due to anticoagulants, whereas in the later situation, hyphema can often occur with glaucoma filtration surgery.

A major benefit of ECP is that it avoids the complications that are associated with transscleral cyclophotocoagulation, namely hypotony, severe inflammation, and phthisis. Due to the fact that only the anterior third of the ciliary processes are treated with ECP, hypotony is an extreme rarity.

It should be noted that patients with advanced glaucoma and concomitant cataract who are on multiple glaucoma medications most often require combined phacoemulsification with the Ex-Press mini glaucoma device or phacotrabeculectomy. I typically perform cataract surgery combined with the Ex-Press mini glaucoma shunt in these cases.[5] Phaco combined with ECP is typically reserved for patients with mild glaucoma, as indicated above. However, as previously mentioned, monocular eyes can be considered for ECP in advanced glaucoma; however, the patient must be counseled that they may need some sort of filtration surgery or a nonpenetrating surgery, such as canaloplasty, because the effects of the combined cataract surgery and ECP may not be adequate to keep the patient at target IOP.

The endoscopic laser can also be used for a variety of other things such as anterior chamber visualization to perform synechialysis. Therefore, rather than doing goniosynechialysis, one can perform endosynechialysis. The endolaser is also very helpful in cases of traumatic glaucoma in which there might be issues with visibility. Recently, using the endolaser to close a cyclodialysis cleft has been described.[6]

In this modern age of glaucoma surgery in which there are multiple innovations to improve patient results and lower complication rates, it is helpful to have a broad palette of options to cater the treatment of glaucoma to the individual patient. Endoscopic cyclophotocoagulation is one more vivid color on the surgical palette for the treatment of glaucoma.

KEY POINTS

1. ECP is primarily used in conjunction with cataract surgery to lower IOP in patients with glaucoma.
2. ECP is safe and effective if performed in the proper manner and only causes minimal inflammation if the surgeon does not "over-treat."

3. ECP can be especially useful in patients with plateau iris syndrome, aphakic glaucoma if an infusion port is used, and in other refractory glaucomas after more conventional glaucoma surgery has been performed.

4. The endoscope can be used for visualization of the angle during synechialysis, during cyclodialysis repair, or perhaps to assist with visualization during minimally invasive glaucoma surgery (MIGS) such as trabecular bypass into Schlemm's canal or the suprachoroidal space, in lieu of a goniolens.

REFERENCES

1. Podbielski DW, Devesh K. Varma DK, Tam DY, Ahmed IK. Endocycloplasty. A new technique for managing angle-closure glaucoma secondary to plateau iris syndrome. *Glaucoma Today.* October 2010.

2. Kahook MY, Lathrop KL, Noecker RJ. One-site versus two-site endoscopic cyclophotocoagulation. *J Glaucoma.* 2007;16(6):527-530.

3. Carter BC, Plager DA, Neely DE, Sprunger DT, et al. Endoscopic diode laser cyclophotocoagulation in the management of aphakic and pseudophakic glaucoma in children. *JAAPOS.* 2007;11(1):34-40.

4. Lin SC. Endoscopic and transcleral cyclophotocoagulation for the treatment of refractory glaucoma. *J Glaucoma.* 2008;17(3):238-247.

5. Kanner E, Netland PA, Sarkisian SR, Du H. Ex-Press miniature glaucoma device implanted under a scleral flap alone or combined with phacoemulsification cataract surgery. *J Glaucoma.* 2009;18(6)488-491.

6. Caronia RM, Sturm RT, Marmor MA, Berke SJ. Treatment of a cyclodialysis cleft by means of ophthalmic laser microendoscope endophtocoagulation. *Am J Ophthalmol.* 1999;128(6):760-761.

COMBINED PHACOEMULSIFICATION AND TRABECTOME

Michael B. Horsley, MD and Douglas J. Rhee, MD

The current standard for surgical treatment of glaucoma remains trabeculectomy ab externo. Although an excellent procedure, the potential for intraoperative, perioperative, and long-term complications and side effects has led to the search for safer and less invasive filtration procedures. One of these, trabeculectomy ab interno, also known as Trabectome (NeoMedix Corp, Tustin, California), was approved for clinical use in the United States in 2004.

Using thermal energy similar to bipolar cautery, the Trabectome removes a strip of the trabecular meshwork and the inner wall of Schlemm's canal for 60 to 140 degrees in the nasal angle, thus providing a direct communication between the anterior chamber and collecting channel. Recent studies regarding the intraocular pressure (IOP)-lowering effect of cataract surgery alone have led glaucoma surgeons to include this surgery in their treatment algorithms as well.[1,2] This chapter focuses on the technique of combined phacoemusification and ab interno trabeculectomy (Trabectome) and briefly presents initial clinical data for this technique.

DEVICE DESCRIPTION

The Trabectome utilizes gravity-driven infusion and automated aspiration. The handpiece consists of a 19.5-gauge infusion sleeve handle, a 25-gauge aspiration port, and coupling for the ablation unit at the tip. The 25-gauge shaft is 5 mm longer than the infusion sleeve and this distal end is bent approximately 90 degrees, creating a triangular footplate (Figure 16-1).[3,4] This footplate has a sharp point to facilitate penetration into Schlemm's canal and insulating material over its surface to help protect the canal's outer wall. The meridional diameter of the footplate varies between 350 and 500 μm.

Kahook M.
Essentials of Glaucoma Surgery (pp 149–152).
© 2012 SLACK Incorporated.

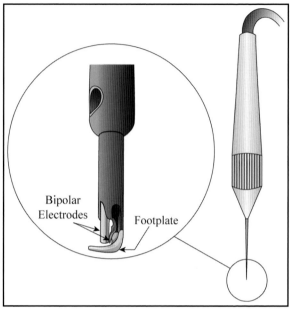

BASIC SURGICAL TECHNIQUE

The typical preoperative dilating, nonsteroidal anti-inflammatory, and antibiotic regimen for cataract surgery is used. Sitting temporally, the surgeon rotates the patient's head away from himself or herself, and the microscope is rotated away from the surgeon approximately 30 to 45 degrees, giving a direct gonioscopic view of the nasal angle. The microscope is at an approximate 45-degree angle and combined with the tilt is approximately 70 to 80 degrees from the eye in primary gaze. The Trabectome is generally performed prior to cataract surgery to allow the use of a smaller clear corneal incision, allowing for better chamber maintenance, and maximize corneal clarity.

A 1.7-mm keratome blade is used to create a beveled temporal corneal incision. Hydroxypropyl methylcellulose 2% (OcuCoat) is then injected into the anterior chamber. The Trabectome handpiece is inserted and advanced to the nasal angle through the anterior chamber with the infusion on. Through direct visualization, using a Trabectome goniosurgical lens (a modified Swan-Jacobs lens), the pointed tip of the footplate is then inserted through the trabecular meshwork and into Schlemm's canal. After seated appropriately, the footswitch is activated to the cautery position and the surgeon advances the handpiece for approximately 90 to 110 degrees of treatment. Some advocate initially starting in a clockwise fashion for the first portion of ablation then re-engaging the canal and completing the treatment counterclockwise.

We prefer a single treatment pass. The initial power setting that we advocate is 0.9 W, although others have suggested 0.7 to 0.8 W.[5] The power should be titrated depending on the desire to ablate a wider strip of trabecular meshwork or to minimize the treatment's effects. The Trabectome handpiece is then removed from the eye and the temporal incision is enlarged using a 2.65 mm or 2.85 mm cataract keratome blade. A standard cataract phacoemulsification is then completed. If the temporal incision does not have a leak at the conclusion of the case, a 10-0 nylon suture is not required.

The postoperative drop regimen consists of an antibiotic 4 times daily for 1 week and a topical steroid 4 times daily tapered over 3 to 4 weeks. Topical glaucoma drops are resumed as needed.

INITIAL RESULTS

Results from a retrospective review of 1127 Trabectome procedures (738 Trabectome-only and 366 Trabectome-phacoemusification surgeries) show a reduction of IOP in Trabectome-phacoemusification of 18% (20.0 ± 6.2 mm Hg to 15.9 ± 3.3 mm Hg) at 12 months, with a 40% reduction (25.7 ± 7.7 mm Hg to 16.6 ± 4.0 mm Hg) for Trabectome alone at 24 months.[6] The most common complication was intraoperative reflux bleeding (77.6%). No cases of wound leak, sustained hypotony, choroidal hemorrhage, or decrease of visual acuity (more than 2 lines) were noted in this series. Another recent prospective case series (304 consecutive eyes) analyzing combined cataract extraction and Trabectome reported similar results in both IOP lowering (20.0 ± 6.3 mm Hg to 15.5 ± 2.9 mm Hg) at 1 year, as well as safety profile.[5]

CONCLUSION

Combined phacoemulsification and ab interno trabeculectomy (Trabectome) has good initial results. This technique offers the ability to lower IOP without precluding the ability of future traditional incisional glaucoma surgeries by sparing the conjunctiva.[7] In addition, due to its minimally invasive nature, Trabectome has a good safety profile with low risk of endophthalmitis, hypotony, vision loss, and choroidal hemorrhage as compared with trabeculectomy ab externo.[5,6] Further prospective studies with long-term follow-up are underway to further determine the role of Trabectome coupled with phacoemulsification in the management of glaucoma.

KEY POINTS

1. Trabectome lowers IOP while maintaining the ability to perform future incisional glaucoma procedures by sparing the conjunctiva.
2. Trabectome has a good safety profile compared with trabeculectomy ab externo.

REFERENCES

1. Tong JT, Miller KM. Intraocular pressure changes after suture-less phacoemulsifica-tion and foldable posterior chamber lens implantation. *J Cataract Refract Surg.* 1998; 24(2):256-262.
2. Mathalone N, Hyams M, Neiman S, Buckman G, Hod Y, Geyer O. Long-term intraocular pressure control after clear corneal phacoemulsification in glaucoma patients. *J Cataract Refract Surg.* 2005;31(3):479-483.
3. Minckler DS, Baerveldt G, Alfaro MR, Francis BA. Clinical results with the Trabec-tome for treatment of open-angle glaucoma. *Ophthalmology.* 2005;112(6):962-967.
4. Francis BA, See RF, Rao NA, Minckler DS, Baerveldt G. Ab interno trabeculectomy: development of a novel device (Trabectome) and surgery for open-angle glaucoma. *J Glaucoma.* 2006;15(1):68-73.
5. Francis BA, Minckler D, Dustin L, et al. Combined cataract extraction and trabeculotomy by the internal approach for coexisting cataract and open-angle glau-coma: initial results. *J Cataract Refract Surg.* 2008;34(7):1096-1103.
6. Minckler D, Mosaed S, Dustin L, Ms BF; Trabectome Study Group. Trabectome (trabec-ulectomy-internal approach): additional experience and extended follow-up. *Trans Am Ophthalmol Soc.* 2008;106:149-159.
7. Jea SY, Mosaed S, Vold SD, Rhee DJ. Effect of a failed trabectome on subsequent trabeculectomy. *J Glaucoma.* 2012;21(2):71-75.

17

GLAUCOMA FILTRATION SURGERY COMBINED WITH CATARACT EXTRACTION

Matthew Rouse, MD and Mahmoud A. Khaimi, MD

Cataracts and glaucoma are common ophthalmic maladies whose incidence increases with age. Therefore, visually significant cataracts often present as a concomitant issue with glaucoma in older patients. This combined presentation can also occur secondary to the effects of glaucoma medications or other ocular diseases.[1-3]

Combined surgery may be indicated in the following scenarios:

- Visually significant cataract with advanced glaucomatous optic neuropathy.
- Visually significant cataract in a patient who cannot tolerate topical medical therapy for glaucoma or in patients burdened by multiple topical medications.
- Visually significant cataract in a patient who has failed prior glaucoma laser or surgical treatment.
- Patients with a phacomorphic component to their glaucoma.

PHACOEMULSIFICATION COMBINED WITH TRABECULECTOMY

Cataract surgery at the time of trabeculectomy has been the most commonly performed glaucoma–cataract combination procedure. The most recent studies have shown that although intraocular pressure (IOP) reduction in a combined surgery may be either equal to or less than with trabeculectomy alone,[4,5] this advantage may be lost with a sequential surgery to remove the cataract at a later date. In addition, there has been a great deal

Kahook M.
Essentials of Glaucoma Surgery (pp 153-162).
© 2012 SLACK Incorporated.

Figure 17-1. Conjunctival dissection.

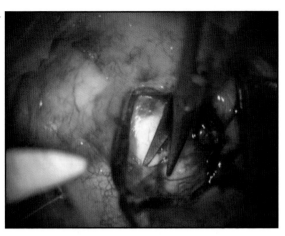

of discussion over whether 1-incision site combination surgery or 2-incision site combination surgery is preferred. The most recent meta-analysis of this discussion indicates that there is no significant difference in IOP reduction, number of glaucoma medications used, or visual acuity between these 2 choices.[6] Ultimately, the best choice may come down to the surgeon's preference based on comfort and experience.

Our preference is for a 2-site combination phacoemulsification with trabeculectomy. A 6-0 Vicryl suture is passed through the superior cornea to be used as a traction suture throughout the entire case. Attention is then turned to the creation of the conjunctival flap superiorly. This can be completed with either a fornix- or limbal-based flap. In our technique, Westcott scissors are carefully used to create a fornix-based peritomy through the conjunctiva and Tenon's capsule, which is carefully dissected forward to the scleral bed at the corneal limbus (Figure 17-1) . After light cauterization of the scleral bed, a 15-degree blade is then used to create a triangular scleral flap dissected forward to the clear cornea. The shape of the scleral flap may vary depending on surgeon preference, but it is important that it is dissected completely to clear cornea. Mitomycin C (MMC)-soaked Weck-Cel sponges are then applied underneath Tenon's capsule and around the scleral flap for approximately 3 minutes (Figure 17-2). The concentration of MMC applied is titrated depending on the appearance of the conjunctiva and Tenon's capsule in each individual case. Our most common dosage of MMC is 0.3 mg/mL with a 3-minute duration of exposure. After removal of the MMC sponges, balanced salt solution is used to vigorously irrigate the ocular surface as well as underneath all edges of the conjunctival-Tenon's flap.

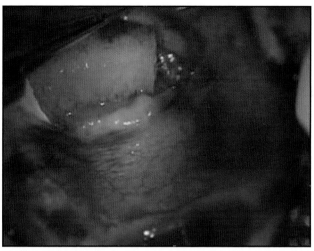

Figure 17-2. Mitomycin C-soaked Weck-Cel sponges applied under Tenon's capsule.

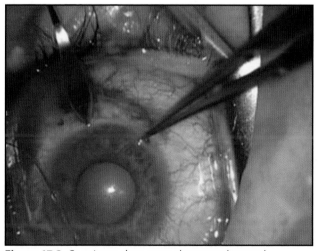

Figure 17-3. Creating a clear corneal temporal wound.

At this point, the surgeon repositions temporally for the beginning of the phacoemulsification. A clear corneal wound is used for the phacoemulsification and placement of the intraocular lens (IOL) as with standard phacoemulsification surgery (Figures 17-3 and 17-4). At the end of the cataract portion of the surgery, a 10-0 Vicryl suture is placed through the small corneal wound for chamber stability. The advantage to

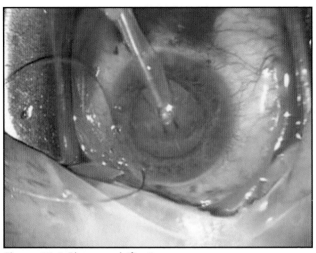

Figure 17-4. Phacoemulsification.

postponing the cataract portion of the surgery until the completion of the early steps of the trabeculectomy is less of a concern for ocular chamber stability during these steps. If the cataract had been completed prior to all steps of the trabeculectomy, this would have allowed for more opportunity for shallowing of the chamber and other intraocular complications. This approach also decreases the chance of MMC exposure inside the eye, as an opening into the anterior chamber is not present until after MMC has been removed from the ocular surface. In addition, the smaller corneal wound is typically less visually significant for the patient astigmatically than would a full scleral cataract wound.

The surgeon next returns to a superior position for the completion of the trabeculectomy portion of the surgery. The scleral flap is carefully lifted and a blade or needle is used to make a small sclerostomy, which is typically enlarged with a Kelly punch (Figure 17-5). The size of the ostomy controls the amount of flow out of the eye. If there is a larger ostomy with less overlap from the scleral flap, more flow is typical. The reverse is true with more overlap from the scleral flap. Next, Vannas scissors are used to create a small iridectomy to reduce the risk of iris closure of the ostomy created. Although there have been some advocates of not using an iridectomy due to the risks of hyphema, any bleeding is typically manageable with light cautery. Three to 5 interrupted 10-0 nylon sutures are then used to close the scleral flap over the sclerostomy to prevent early hypotony in the eye. These sutures can be released with argon laser over the following weeks after surgery to titrate the IOP to the desired level.

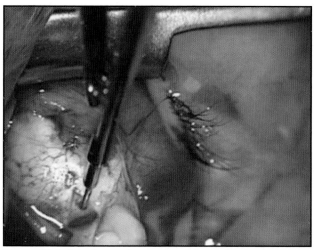

Figure 17-5. Creating a sclerostomy with a Kelly punch.

In this technique, an 8-0 Vicryl suture is then used to complete a double-layered running closure of the Tenon's capsule and conjunctiva. It is important to assure that this wound is watertight at the end of the surgery with an appropriately formed anterior chamber and IOP.

PHACOEMULSIFICATION COMBINED WITH EX-PRESS MINI GLAUCOMA SHUNT

The Ex-Press (Alcon Laboratories Inc) mini glaucoma shunt is a biocompatible, nonvalved stainless steel device with a small internal lumen that has recently gained favor as an alternative to traditional trabeculectomy with or without cataract surgery. Whether the shunt is used in combination with cataract surgery or alone, it has been found to significantly reduce IOP with high surgical success rates.[7]

The Ex-Press mini shunt is indicated in similar settings as described for traditional trabeculectomy. The initiation of the surgery is identical with creation of conjunctival and scleral flaps as well as use of antifibrotics as described above (Figure 17-6). After completion of the phacoemulsification portion of the combined procedure, the scleral flap is lifted and the trabecular meshwork is identified. Next, a 25-gauge needle, aligned parallel to the iris plane, is inserted just posterior to the trabecular meshwork into the anterior chamber (Figure 17-7). Being aware of location and control with the needle are important factors at this point. Too much movement may make a larger opening than required for the implant and lead to excessive aqueous leak around the implant. A poor angle of insertion

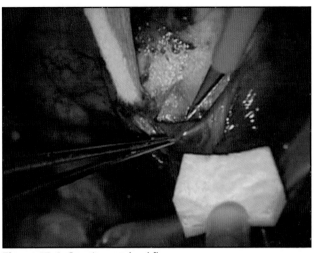

Figure 17-6. Creating a scleral flap.

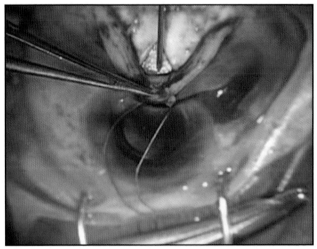

Figure 17-7. Entering the anterior chamber with a 25-gauge needle.

may also place the implant too posterior with the tip buried in the iris or too anterior with the tip causing damage to the endothelial surface of the cornea.

Next, the implant is inserted through the opening created just posterior to the trabecular meshwork. It is important to insert the implant at the same angle of approach that was used with the 25-gauge needle in the previous step. The shunt is injected using a preloaded inserter, which releases the shunt with depression of the inserter button. Prior to inserting the shunt, the surgeon should familiarize himself or herself with the release mechanism on the preloaded inserter to allow for smooth and uncomplicated insertion. Care is taken to make sure that the plate of the implant is flush with the scleral bed and the opening of the lumen is directed posteriorly towards the apex of the scleral flap. Closure of the scleral and conjunctival flaps progresses as indicated for a standard trabeculectomy. An advantage of the Ex-Press implant as compared with traditional trabeculectomy is that there is less intraocular manipulation of tissue required after creating the scleral flap. No creation of an iridectomy is required. In addition, there tends to be less hypotony postoperatively with the glaucoma Ex-Press shunt compared with standard trabeculectomy[8] and it appears to be a successful alternative for combined surgery.

Phacoemulsification Combined With Glaucoma Drainage Device

In eyes that may not be indicated for or have failed trabeculectomy, glaucoma drainage devices have been successfully used to lower IOP. In some of these patients, visually significant cataracts are also present and in need of removal. Although it has not been our practice to do so, some have advocated a combined phacoemulsification and glaucoma drainage device procedure.

This combined procedure typically begins with creation of a fornix-based flap in the superotemporal or inferonasal quadrants[9] for placement of the glaucoma drainage device of choice (Baerveldt, Ahmed, Molteno, etc.). The plate of the glaucoma drainage device is then secured to the scleral bed 9 to 10 mm behind the limbus using 2 interrupted sutures. If a Baerveldt implant is used, the shunt is then ligated with an additional suture around the tube, and fenestrations are made in the tube using the suture needle.

At this stage of the procedure, attention is turned to a clear corneal phacoemulsification. After completing the cataract portion of the procedure, an interrupted 10-0 Vicryl suture is placed through the cataract wound. The tube is then trimmed to an appropriate length and inserted into the anterior chamber through an opening created with a 23-gauge needle (Figure 17-8). An interrupted suture is then used to secure the tube and prevent any inappropriate bending underneath the conjunctiva. A patch graft of donor sclera, cornea, or pericardium is then sutured into place over the exposed tube. The conjunctival flap is then sutured closed with the suture of the surgeon's choice.

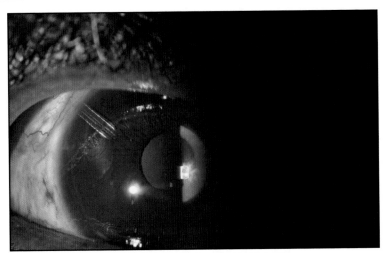

Figure 17-8. Glaucoma drainage tube in anterior chamber.

It is important with the placement of any glaucoma drainage device that careful attention is paid to the anterior chamber depth before surgical incision. This will allow for understanding of whether the tube will be well-positioned in the anterior chamber without being covered by the iris or causing damage to the corneal endothelium. This may be one of the more difficult determinations to be made when combining this surgery with a cataract extraction, as the standard anterior chamber depth typically changes after cataract surgery. Although the few studies addressing combined glaucoma drainage device and cataract surgery have indicated promising IOP reduction and safety profiles, some incidence of corneal decompensation has been indicated as well.[10] Other complications may include choroidal effusion, retraction of the tube, recurrent iritis, cystoid macular edema, corneal edema, fibrin plugging of the tube, and macular striae.

CONCLUSION

Glaucoma and cataracts coexist in the elderly patient population and will continue to present challenges to the ophthalmic surgeon when combination surgery is undertaken. A combined approach to both pathologies may be worthwhile, and perfecting these techniques both individually and combined will lead to improved patient outcomes. Newer approaches with minimally invasive glaucoma surgery, such as the iStent or suprachoroidal devices, are covered elsewhere in this book and may lessen the complications associated with combined surgical procedures. Ultimately, the decision for combined surgery must be undertaken with the individual patient in mind as well as a full understanding of the surgeon's experience and comfort level in combination approaches to both cataract and glaucoma.

KEY POINTS

1. Glaucoma and cataracts are common comorbidities in an aging population and often must be managed together.

2. Intraocular pressure reduction is more profound with trabeculectomy alone, but the advantage of this IOP reduction may be dissipated by a secondary cataract surgery.[4,5]

3. Trabeculectomy with Ex-Press mini glaucoma shunt may provide some advantage over traditional trabeculectomy by reducing intraocular tissue manipulation and postoperative hypotony.[8]

4. One- versus 2-site combined glaucoma procedures have not shown a clear advantage in either direction.[6] The operating physician should proceed with the type of procedure with which they are most comfortable and experienced completing.

5. Care should be taken to evaluate anterior chamber depth before surgical incision when inserting a glaucoma drainage device. This aids in the understanding of the best position of the tube within the eye.

REFERENCES

1. Sabri K, Saurenmann RK, Silverman ED, Levin AV. Course, complications, and outcome of juvenile arthritis-related uveitis. *J AAPOS.* 2008;12(6):539-545.

2. Benjamin KW. Toxicity of ocular medications. *Int Ophthalmol Clin.* 1979;19(1):199-255.

3. Velilla S, Dios E, Herreras JM, Calonge M. Fuchs heterochromic iridocyclitis: a review of 26 cases. *Ocul Immunol Inflamm.* 2001;9(3):169-175.

4. Murthy SK, Damji KF, Pan Y, Hodge WG. Trabeculectomy and phacotrabeculectomy with Mitomycin-C, show similar two-year target IOP outcomes. *Can J Ophthalmol.* 2006;41(1):51-59.

5. Chang L, Thiagarajan M, Moseley M, et al. Intraocular pressure outcome in primary 5-FU phacotrabeculectomies compared with 5-FU trabeculectomies. *J Glaucoma.* 2006;15(6):475-481.

6. Gdih GA, Yuen D, Yan P, Sheng L, Yin YP, Buys, YM. Meta-analysis of 1- versus 2-site phacotrabeculectomy. *Ophthalmology.* 2011;118(1):71-76.

7. Kanner E, Netland PA, Sarkisian SR, Du H. Ex-Press miniature glaucoma device implanted under a scleral flap alone or in combination with phacoemulsification cataract surgery. *J Glaucoma.* 2009;18(6):488-491.

8. Maris PJ, Jr, Ishida K, Netland PA. Comparison of trabeculectomy with Ex-Press miniature glaucoma device implanted under scleral flap. *J Glaucoma.* 2007;16(1):14-19.

9. Sidoti PA. Inferonasal placement of aqueous shunts. *J Glaucoma.* 2004;13(6):520-523.

10. Hoffman KB, Feldman RM, Budenz DL, Gedde SJ, Chacra GA, Schiffman JC. Combined cataract extraction and Baerveldt glaucoma drainage implant: indications and outcomes. *Ophthalmology.* 2002;109(10):1916-1920.

18

CANALOPLASTY COMBINED WITH CATARACT EXTRACTION

Ben J. Harvey, MD and Mahmoud A. Khaimi, MD

Traditionally, glaucoma has been managed medically until disease progression necessitates incisional glaucoma procedures. The trabeculectomy, considered by many to be the gold standard incisional glaucoma procedure, although repeatedly shown to be effective at lowering intraocular pressure (IOP), carries lifelong risks often associated with the necessary conjunctival bleb created during the procedure. These bleb-related risks include bleb leak, bleb encapsulation, bleb dysesthesia, blebitis, and bleb-associated endophthalmitis.[1-4] Other potential complications intra- and postoperatively include hypotony, hyphema, and choroidal detachment.

Such complications have encouraged many glaucoma specialists to seek out a less invasive IOP-lowering surgery. Recently, circumferential viscodilation and tensioning of Schlemm's canal using a flexible microcatheter (canaloplasty) has gained popularity in the treatment of open-angle glaucoma in adults. Lewis et al[5] have shown a significant lowering of IOP and medication usage via canaloplasty at 2 years with results similar to trabeculectomy.[6] At 24 months, canaloplasty lowers IOP from 23.3 ± 4.0 mm Hg to 16.3 ± 3.7 mm Hg and decreases the average number of medications from 2.0 ± 0.8 to 0.6 ± 0.8. Combining clear corneal cataract extraction via phacoemulsification with canaloplasty results in an even greater decrease in IOP. Phacocanaloplasty decreases IOP from 23.1 ± 5.5 mm Hg to 13.4 ± 4.0 mm Hg at 24 months and average number of medications drops from 1.7 ± 1.0 to 0.2 ± 0.4.

Combining cataract and glaucoma surgery is often necessary, as glaucoma surgery can cause cataract progression.[7] In addition, cataract surgery alone has been shown to lower IOP anywhere from 1 to 5 mm Hg.[8-10] Furthermore, phacocanaloplasty shows a lower IOP trend than canaloplasty alone[4]; therefore, combining the 2 has gained popularity.

Kahook M.
Essentials of Glaucoma Surgery (pp 163-170).
© 2012 SLACK Incorporated.

SURGICAL PROCEDURE

Clear corneal cataract extraction via phacoemulsification is performed using traditional methods. A side-port paracentesis is performed followed by introduction of ophthalmic viscosurgical device (OVD) into the anterior chamber. Planning paracentesis placement is important when glaucoma surgery is expected to follow. The surgeon must place the side-port incision in a position such that it will not intersect the anticipated corneal traction suture needed during canaloplasty. If working on a right eye, a right-handed surgeon may place his or her side-port incision at approximately 10 o'clock and skew the clear corneal incision inferotemporally. Clear corneal incisions may vary in size and architecture. A continuous curvilinear capsulorrhexis follows with subsequent hydrodissection and hydrodelineation. Removing the nucleus may be achieved via divide-and-conquer, phaco-chop techniques, or whatever the anterior chamber surgeon favors keeping in mind certain risk factors present in glaucoma patients such as zonular weakness in psuedoexfoliates (Figure 18-1). Epinuclear material may be removed with the phacoemulsification handpiece, and the irrigation and aspiration hand piece is then used to remove remaining cortical material. After insertion of the IOL within the capsule and removal of the remaining OVD, it is important to suture the clear corneal incision wound closed with 10-0 Vicryl (Figure 18-2). Placing a suture through the clear corneal incision promotes anterior chamber stability, which is crucial during canaloplasty and other glaucoma procedures. Be sure all remaining OVDs are removed prior to suturing the wound, as remaining OVD, may cause unsafe IOP elevation postoperatively.

Canaloplasty involves conjunctival exposure to enable a superficial, then deep, scleral flap creation followed by meticulous unroofing of Schlemm's canal, which is then catheterized. A microcatheter tipped with an illuminating optical fiber and an ophthalmic viscosurgical device delivery system is then used to cannulate and viscodilate Schlemm's canal 360 degrees. Finally this same catheter is used to introduce polypropylene suture into Schlemm's canal for tension application and canal distension.

Typically, anesthesia and akinesia is achieved with a retrobulbar block. A corneal traction suture is placed superiorly next to the limbus. Next, a fornix-based conjunctival incision is created followed by careful dissection of conjunctiva and Tenon's capsule down to bare sclera. The authors favor a superonasal approach during this step, as it leaves the superior and superotemporal conjunctiva undisturbed should future incisional surgeries be necessary. Hemostasis is achieved with wet-field cautery. No antifibrotics, such as mitomycin C (MMC), are necessary.

After bare sclera is exposed, a superficial one-third to one-half-thickness scleral flap is created at the limbus. A 5 mm × 5 mm parabolic shape

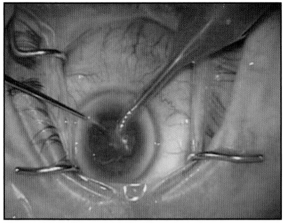

Figure 18-1. Phacoemulsification.

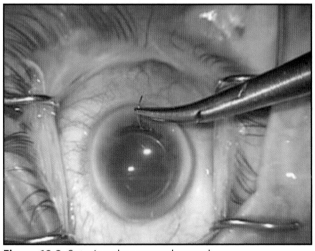

Figure 18-2. Suturing clear corneal wound.

may be used; however, the authors favor a triangular scleral flap. Within the base of the superficial scleral flap, a deep scleral flap is created with a dissection plane just superficial to the choroid. A 4 mm × 4 mm parabolic deep scleral flap may suffice, or a triangular deep scleral flap smaller than the superficial flap may be preferred. The choroid may be slightly visible beneath the deep scleral flap. The deep scleral flap is dissected anteriorly to unroof Schlemm's canal. While dissecting forward, pay close attention to identifying the cross striations of the scleral spur. This assures the surgeon has reached the correct depth and plane while fashioning the deep flap.

Figure 18-3. Securing Prolene suture to catheter.

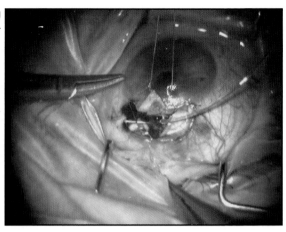

Identifying the cross striations of the scleral spur also anatomically orients the surgeon to the location of Schlemm's canal, which is immediately anterior.

At this point, the IOP should be lowered to the mid- to high-single digits by burping the pre-fashioned paracentesis wound. This serves to decompress the eye and decrease the risk of perforating into the anterior chamber while isolating Schlemm's canal and creating Descemet's window. After the canal is identified, the deep flap is carefully further dissected anteriorly to detach Schwalbe's line and to create an appropriately sized Descemet's window, which should be a minimum of 500 µm. Aqueous usually, but not always, percolates through the Descemet's window. The iTrack microcatheter (iTrack-250, iScience Interventional, Menlo Park, California) is then inserted through 1 of the canal ostiae. The lights are dimmed to allow visualization of the lighted tip of the microcatheter as it is advanced through Schlemm's canal. If an obstruction is encountered during cannulation, the microcatheter may be retracted, inserted into the opposite ostium, and cannulated the other direction to achieve successful passage. After circumferential cannulation is completed, a 10-0 polypropylene (Prolene) suture is tied to the distal end of the catheter, which is retracted, introducing the suture into Schlemm's canal (Figure 18-3). As the suture is pulled through, OVD is injected at a rate of 0.5 mL/2 hours (1/8th turn of the OVD injector every 2 clock hours). The suture is tied, allowing appropriate tension to be placed on the canal without inadvertently performing a trabeculotomy (Figure 18-4). Suture tensioning is critically important, as this allows for transmission of tension 360 degrees on Schlemm's canal and the trabecular meshwork, thereby restoring natural aqueous outflow.

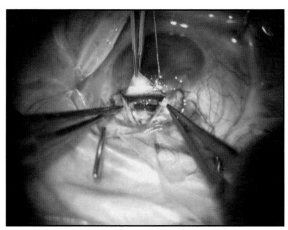

Figure 18-4. Applying tension on Prolene suture.

Excision of the deep scleral flap is followed by watertight closure of the superficial scleral flap with interrupted 10-0 nylon sutures. The conjunctiva and Tenon's capsule is reapproximated with 8-0 Vicryl at the limbus, and subconjunctival antibiotics are given along with topical antibiotic-steroid ointment.

SUMMARY

Canaloplasty has become an appealing alternative to traditional incisional glaucoma therapies. It is less invasive, blebless, no mitomycin C is necessary, and it rejuvenates the natural drainage system. Although canaloplasty is effective in lowering IOP and medication dependence, it still has limitations. Canaloplasty may be contraindicated in patients with chronic angle closure, narrow angles, angle recession, neovascular glaucoma, and in eyes that have undergone previous glaucoma procedures that preclude adequate cannulation of Schlemm's canal.[11] If pressure lowering below mid- to low-teens is desired, then a trabeculectomy with antifibrotics or glaucoma drainage implant may be more optimal than canaloplasty, which may not be the best option in patients with advanced glaucoma in need of very low IOP. A learning curve is necessary for successful catheterization of Schlemm's canal, and certain anatomical variations may prohibit successful catheterization such as the microcatheter tip entering a large collector channel or meeting unknown resistance.[12] Canaloplasty is designed to be a blebless procedure; however, laser goniopuncture was necessary in 4.7% and blebs occurred in only 3.8% of patients at 24 months in the study by Lewis et al.[5] More common complications listed in this study were microhyphema (less than 1.0 mm layered blood; 7.9%), early-elevated IOP (0 to 3 months postoperative; 7.9%), and hyphema (≥1.0 mm layered blood; 6.3%). All hyphemas and microhyphemas resolved by 1 month, which was consistent with other studies.[5,13] Early IOP elevation was also transient and resolved spontaneously by the next office visit. Other less common complications include late IOP elevation (more than 3 months postoperative; 2.4%), wound hemorrhage (2.4%), Descemet's membrane detachment (1.6%), gross hyphema (1.6%), suture extrusion through trabecular meshwork (1.6%), and hypotony (0.8%).[5,12,13] Probably the most significant advances canaloplasty offers are the lack of choroidal detachments, blebitis, or bleb-related endophthalmitis observed in any eyes treated with canaloplasty or phacocanaloplasty.[5,12,13]

Ideal patient selection is key when contemplating phacocanaloplasty. A patient with a visually significant cataract and mild-to-moderate open-angle glaucoma with desired IOP in the low- to mid-teens would be an ideal candidate for phacocanaloplasty. Additionally, one may consider combining phacoemulsification with canaloplasty if cataract surgery is anticipated in the near future or if a phacomorphic glaucoma component exists. Cataract surgery and canaloplasty have also been shown to lower IOP more than canaloplasty alone. The difference was significant at 1 year; however, although there was a trend for lower IOP with phacocanaloplasty versus canaloplasty alone, there was no significant difference at 2 years.[5] In conclusion, phacocanaloplasty is a viable option for treating open-angle glaucoma in patients with cataracts.

KEY POINTS

1. Ideal patient selection includes the following:
   - Mild to moderate open-angle glaucoma with IOP desired in the mid- to low-teens.
   - Ocular hypertension uncontrolled with maximal medical management.
   - Visually significant cataract.

2. Contraindications for canaloplasty include patients with chronic angle closure, narrow angles, angle recession, neovascular glaucoma, and in eyes that have undergone previous glaucoma procedures that preclude adequate cannulation of Schlemm's canal.

3. Do not overlap side-port or clear corneal incisions with the corneal traction suture.

4. Thoroughly remove all OVD after cataract surgery in order to avoid postoperative IOP spikes.

5. Suture the clear corneal incision after completion of cataract surgery to maintain control of the anterior chamber.

6. To identify Schlemm's canal, dissect the deep scleral flap anteriorly, identify cross striations of scleral spur—Schlemm's canal is immediately anterior.

7. Lower the IOP prior to unroofing Schlemm's canal via burping the paracentesis wound, which decreases the risk of perforating the anterior chamber.

REFERENCES

1. Greenfield DS, Suner IJ, Miller MP, Kangas TA, Palmberg PF, Flynn HW. Endopthalmitis after filtering surgery with mitomycin. *Arch Opthalmol.* 1996;114(8):943-949.
2. Prasad N, Latina MA. Blebitis and endopthalmitis after glaucoma filtering surgery. *Int Ophthalmol Clin.* 2007;47:850-897.
3. Radhakrishnan S, Quigley HA, Jampel HD, et al. Outcomes of surgical bleb revision for complications of trabeculectomy. *Ophthalmology.* 2009;116:1713-1718.
4. Azuara-Blanco A, Katz LJ. Dysfunctional filtering blebs. *Surv Ophthalmol.* 1998;43: 93-126.
5. Lewis RA, von Wolff K, Tetz M, et al. Canaloplasty: circumferential viscodilation and tensioning of Schlemm's canal using a flexible microcatheter for the treatment of open-angle glaucoma in adults: Two-year interim clinical study results. *J Cataract Refract Surg.* 2009;35:814-824.
6. Feiner L, Piltz-Seymour JR. Collaborative Initial Glaucoma Treatment Study: a summary of results to date. *Curr Opin Ophthalmol.* 2003;14:106-111.
7. Advanced Glaucoma Intervention Study Investigators. The Advanced Glaucoma Intervention Study; 8. Risk of cataract formation after trabeculectomy. *Arch Ophthalmol.* 2001;119:1771-1779.
8. Shingleton BJ, Paternack JJ, Hung JW, O'Donoghue MW. Three and five year changes in intraocular pressure after clear corneal phacoemulsification in open angle glaucoma patients. *J Glaucoma.* 2006;15:494-498.
9. Hayashi K, Hayashi H, Nakao F, Hayashi F. Effect of cataract surgery on intraocular pressure control in glaucoma patients. *J Cataract Refract Surg.* 2001;27:1779-1786.
10. Mathalone N, Hyam M, Neiman S, Buckman G, Hod Y, Geyer O. Long-term intraocular pressure control after clear corneal phacoemulsification in glaucoma patients. *J Cataract Refract Surg.* 2005;31:479-483.
11. Khaimi MA. Canaloplasty using iTrack 250 microcatheter with suture tensioning on Schlemm's canal. *Middle East Afr J Opthalmol.* 2009;19:127-129.
12. Shingleton B, Tetz M, Korber N. Circumferential viscodilation and tensioning of Schlemm's canal (canaloplasty) with temporal clear corneal phacoemulsification cataract surgery for open-angle glaucoma and visually significant cataract: one-year results. *J Cataract Refract Surg.* 2008;34:433-440.
13. Grieshaber MC, Fraenkl S, Schoetzau A, Flammer J, Orgul S. Circumferential visco-canalostomy and suture canal distension (canaloplasty) for whites with open-angle glaucoma. *J Glaucoma.* 2011;20(5):298-302.

19

CATARACT EXTRACTION PLUS ISTENT

John P. Berdahl, MD

Traditionally, patients with cataract and progressive glaucoma would be candidates for combined cataract surgery plus trabeculectomy or insertion of a glaucoma drainage device (GDD). Although often successful, these combined surgeries carry significant comorbidities and delayed visual recovery.

Cataract surgery alone can decrease intraocular pressure (IOP); however, many times cataract surgery alone is not sufficient to lower the IOP adequately in patients with progressive glaucoma. The mechanism by which cataract surgery lowers IOP remains unclear, but numerous studies demonstrate a sustained reduction of IOP after cataract surgery.[1]

New devices, such as the iStent (Trabecular Micro-Bypass; Glaukos Corp, Laguna Hills, California), aim to lower IOP more than cataract surgery alone while decreasing the comorbitidies associated with traditional glaucoma surgeries.[2,3]

TECHNOLOGY OVERVIEW

The iStent device is an ab interno bypass of the trabecular meshwork (Figure 19-1). The device is smaller than 1 mm in length and 0.5 mm in width, making it the smallest device ever implanted into humans. The titanium stent is placed through the trabecular meshwork and into Schlemm's canal, bypassing the high resistance trabecular meshwork. Implanting the device is typically performed in conjunction with cataract surgery. Direct visualization of the trabecular meshwork is accomplished with a gonioprism and an operating microscope. Under direct visualization, the device is implanted using an injector through the trabecular meshwork.

Kahook M.
Essentials of Glaucoma Surgery (pp 171-176).
© 2012 SLACK Incorporated.

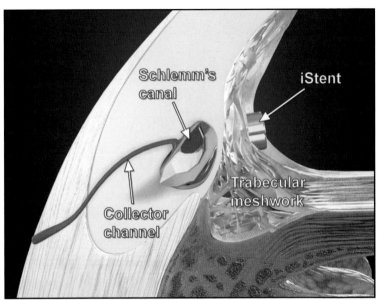

Figure 19-1. Schematic representation of the Glaukos iStent in the trabecular meshwork. The stent allows aqueous to bypass the high resistance trabecular meshwork and pass directly into Schlemm's canal. (Reprinted with permission of Glaukos.)

CATARACT CONSIDERATIONS

Typically, surgeons do not need to alter their standard cataract approach when coupled with the iStent. However, a couple of important points should be considered. First, it is important that the capsular bag remain intact during the surgery and that there is no vitreous present in the anterior chamber. Because the lumen of the device is only 120 μm, it may be prone to obstruction by vitreous. If vitreous is encountered during planned cataract extraction plus an iStent, the surgeon should consider delaying the stent portion of the surgery. The surgeon can then return a couple of months later to place the iStent under more stable considerations and avoid vitreous obstructing the stent. Additionally, it is important to maintain a stable anterior chamber in the early postoperative period. For this reason, there should be no wound leak at the time of surgery. If stromal hydration is insufficient to create a watertight seal, the surgeon should consider placing a 10-0 nylon suture through the incision to ensure a stable anterior chamber. This would prevent anterior chamber collapse in which the iris could obstruct the lumen of the device. Furthermore, all remaining viscoelastics should be completely evacuated at the end of the surgery to ensure stent patency.

Many types of intraocular lenses (IOLs) can be placed in conjunction with an iStent. Standard monofocal, toric, multifocal, or accommodating IOLs are all acceptable in combination with the iStent. Single-piece or 3-piece lenses are also acceptable. It is important that the patient have adequate capsulorrhexis coverage of the anterior optic to prevent prolapse or dislocation of the lens anteriorly. When considering a multifocal IOL in a glaucoma patient, the surgeon should ensure that the visual field deficit is not bad enough to limit the patient's ability to function with a multifocal lens. Additionally, the surgeon could consider contrast sensitivity testing in patients considering a multifocal IOL because both the lens and the glaucoma can cause decreased contrast sensitivity and lead to a patient who is unsatisfied with the postoperative visual results.

SURGICAL CONSIDERATIONS

A surgeon can perform his or her routine cataract surgery through either a clear corneal incision or a scleral tunnel. After the standard cataract surgery is performed and the IOL is placed, the viscoelastic is left in the eye. The patient's head is tilted away from the temporally positioned surgeon by approximately 30 degrees, and the operating microscope is tilted approximately 30 degrees toward the surgeon to allow for the best visualization of the trabecular mesh work through the gonioprism. Viscoelastic is placed on the cornea to act as a coupling agent between the gonioprism and the eye. A gonioprism is placed on the eye and used to directly visualize the trabecular meshwork. It is helpful if the IOP is not too high (less than 15 mm Hg) when visualizing the trabecular meshwork because back flow of blood can be seen in Schlemm's canal as an important landmark to identify the posterior trabecular meshwork. If blood is not seen in Schlemm's canal, then identification of the typical gonioscopic landmarks, such as the scleral spur, Schwalbe's line, or pigment in the posterior trabecular meshwork can assist the surgeon in determining the proper stent placement (Figure 19-2). The surgeon holds the gonioprism in the nondominant hand and uses the insertion device in the dominant hand through the cataract incision to place the iStent device into the trabecular meshwork. Injector systems help facilitate this for the surgeon. As the trabecular meshwork is engaged, the surgeon should be conscientious of not burying the device all the way into the trabecular meshwork, thereby limiting its effectiveness. Oftentimes, after the device is implanted, a bit of blood is noticed coming out from the stent, which indicates that it is properly positioned through the trabecular meshwork. Multiple devices can be placed to help decrease the IOP even further.

The viscoelastic is then removed from behind the lens and the anterior chamber, ensuring that no remaining viscoelastic could obstruct the lumen of the stent. The wounds are hydrated to ensure that they are watertight. If a watertight seal is not obtained, a suture should be placed.

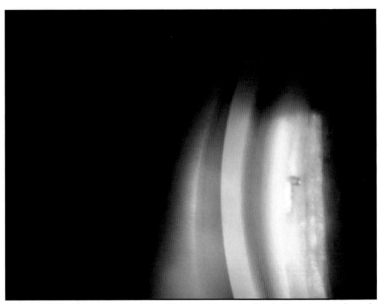

Figure 19-2. Photograph of the Glaukos iStent in the trabecular meshwork. (Reprinted with permission of Thomas W. Samuelson, MD.)

POSTOPERATIVE CONSIDERATIONS

The postoperative recovery is typically very similar to standard cataract surgery. Occasionally, some red blood cells are present in the anterior chamber as blood has back-washed from Schlemm's canal into the anterior chamber through the iStent at the time of surgery. This blood typically reabsorbs quickly. The standard regimen of cataract drops includes antibiotics, steroids, and possibly nonsteroidal anti-inflammatory drugs. Depending on the patient's preoperative IOP, glaucoma medications may be stopped immediately to determine the new baseline IOP.

It is important to note that unlike a trabeculectomy or glaucoma drainage device, the remaining trabecular meshwork continues to provide significant outflow for the patient, and placing him or her on steroids may decrease this outflow, leading to a steroid-induced elevation of IOP.

It is also important to remember that Schlemm's canal is not a continuous chamber that encircles the eye 360 degrees. There are 20 to 35 collector channels present in Schlemm's canal, and by placing an iStent typically only 1 or 2 of these collector channels is accessed. This is the most likely reason that multiple stents would lower the IOP further. It is also important to remember that Schlemm's canal drains into the episcleral veins and therefore subject to the episcleral venous pressure. Episcleral venous pressure represents the lowest obtainable IOP by devices that access Schlemm's canal. The glaucomas that result from elevated episcleral venous pressure, such as Sturge-Weber, are not good candidates for the iStent.

CONCLUSION

The iStent is a promising alternative to lowering IOP further than cataract surgery alone and provides a minimally invasive elegant option for lowering IOP at the time of cataract surgery. The device could also be used in patients who are pseudophakic, but it would be more challenging to perform in patients who retain their natural crystalline lens.

Although the iStent likely will not lower IOP as much as trabeculectomy or other glaucoma drainage devices, the less invasive approach and the lower morbidity make it an appealing option for early intervention in mild to moderate glaucoma. Hopefully, early intervention will decrease the need for more invasive glaucoma surgery such as trabeculectomy or glaucoma drainage devices.

KEY POINTS

1. The iStent provides a direct communication from the anterior chamber to Schlemm's canal, bypassing the trabecular meshwork.
2. More than one stent can be placed.
3. There is minimal morbidity.
4. IOP reduction is limited by episcleral venous pressure.
5. Because the procedure is completely intraocular, the conjunctiva remains undisturbed and available for future procedures.
6. The iStent provides a good option for mild to moderate glaucoma, given its risk–benefit profile.

REFERENCES

1. Poley BJ, Lindstrom RL, Samuelson TW. Long-term effects of phacoemulsification with intraocular lens implantation in normotensive and ocular hypertensive eyes. *J Cataract Refract Surg.* 2008;34(5):735-742.
2. Spiegel D, Wetzel W, Neuhann T, et al. Coexistent primary open-angle glaucoma and cataract: interim analysis of a trabecular micro-bypass stent and concurrent cataract surgery. *Eur J Ophthalmol.* 2009;19(3):393-399.
3. Samuelson TW, Katz LJ, Wells JM, et al. Randomized evaluation of the trabecular micro-bypass stent with phacoemulsification in patients with glaucoma and cataract. *Ophthalmology.* 2011;118(3):459-467.

V

LASERS

20

Argon Laser Trabeculoplasty

Elizabeth T. Viriya, MD and Joseph R. Zelefsky, MD

Argon laser trabeculoplasty (ALT) is a treatment option for open-angle glaucoma, involving the application of laser energy to the trabecular meshwork (TM) to lower intraocular pressure (IOP). It can be performed as first-line therapy or in conjunction with medical therapy. ALT can be used to lower pressure either before or after filtering surgery as demonstrated by the Advanced Glaucoma Interventional Study (AGIS).[1]

Efficacy

On average, ALT reduces IOP by 25% from baseline.[2] This reduction, however, wanes over time. Failure—defined as IOP reduction from baseline of less than 3 mm Hg, IOP greater than 20 mm Hg, or anatomical or visual field progression—occurs nearly 25% of the time in the first year after treatment and at a rate of 7% to 10% per year afterwards.[3]

Mechanism of Action

The exact mechanism of action for ALT is unknown, although ALT increases aqueous outflow up to 50%.[4] Two popular theories as to how ALT lowers IOP are the mechanical theory and the biological theory. The mechanical theory states that the thermal energy delivered by the laser leads to coagulative necrosis and mechanical stretching of trabecular meshwork, thereby improving aqueous outflow.[5] The biological theory states that upregulation of macrophage activity, as well as the release of inflammatory cytokines (IL-1a, IL-1b, TNF-alpha),[6] leads to remodeling of the extracellular matrix of the trabecular meshwork, thereby improving aqueous outflow facility.

Preoperative Evaluation

Because argon laser treatment is applied directly to the trabecular meshwork, it is important to perform gonioscopy to visualize and evaluate

Kahook M.
Essentials of Glaucoma Surgery (pp 179–184).
© 2012 SLACK Incorporated.

the TM preoperatively. Chronic angle-closure glaucoma and other conditions involving angle obscurations, such as media opacities and iridocorneal endothelial (ICE) syndrome, are contraindications for ALT. Laser iridoplasty may be indicated in cases of narrow angles if it allows better access to an open angle.

Active uveitis is another contraindication because ALT can exacerbate intraocular inflammation. Because IOP spikes can occur after the procedure, ALT must be used with caution in cases of end-stage glaucoma where such sudden changes in IOP can worsen vision or lead to progression of visual field damage.

Patient Consent

As with all surgical procedures, a detailed discussion involving the risks and benefits of the procedure must be done prior to performing ALT. Patients should be advised that reduction of IOP may not occur until 4 to 6 weeks after the ALT. During this time period, patients must continue using all of their ocular antihypertensive medications. Patients must also be aware that even with effective ALT, the IOP reduction wanes over time, and continued follow-up will be necessary.

Procedure

IOP should be measured prior to performing ALT. Some advocate that this measurement of IOP should be performed without the instillation of fluorescein on the ocular surface because the fluorescein may absorb laser energy.[7]

Topical antihypertensive medications should be administered 30 to 60 minutes before ALT to blunt post-ALT IOP spikes. Commonly used prophylactic medications include apraclonidine, pilocarpine, and brimonidine.[8,9]

A topical anesthetic should be instilled into the operative eye and the patient is positioned comfortably at the slit lamp. A gonioscopy lens, such as a 3-mirror Goldmann lens, the Ritch trabeculoplasty lens, or Karickhoff lens, should be applied to the operative eye using a coupling gel. Care should be taken to prevent formation or retention of an air bubble between the lens and the eye.

Although the laser settings vary from surgeon to surgeon, commonly used parameters are 50 μm spot size, 800 mW, 0.1 seconds of exposure, and 50 to 100 total burns.[10,11] Care should be taken to ensure that the laser burns are equally spaced. The wavelength most commonly used in multiple trials ranged from 488 to 514 nm, within the green light component of the visible spectrum.[12,13]

Laser spots are targeted at the junction of nonpigmented TM and the pigmented TM posterior to it. Coagulation of posterior TM results in formation of peripheral anterior synechiae and more severe postoperative inflammation. A well-focused laser beam is achieved when the front plane of the goniolens is perpendicular to the laser delivery path. The aiming beam should appear small and round. If the aiming beam is not focused properly, the laser strikes a larger area and coagulates less effectively.

The power of the laser burns should be titrated to the level required to induce slight blanching of the TM or formation of small bubbles. Typically, one starts with a low power, such as 700 mW, and the power can be adjusted by 50- to 100-mW intervals to achieve the desired effect.[14] If large bubbles form, the power should be reduced. The amount of energy required tends to be inversely proportional to the degree of TM pigmentation; heavier pigmented TM requires less power than lighter pigmented ones.

How much trabecular meshwork needs to be treated? Multiple trials have demonstrated that applying 50 burns to 180 degrees of TM is as effective in achieving IOP control and preventing progression of glaucoma as compared to applying 100 burns to 360 degrees of TM.[15-17] Based on this, most clinicians treat a maximum of 180 degrees of TM when performing ALT.

It is common practice to instill one drop of a topical steroid, such as prednisolone acetate 1%, immediately after completing the ALT treatment. IOP should be checked at approximately 1 to 2 hours after the procedure.

POSTOPERATIVE CARE

Topical steroids should be administered during the first postoperative week to limit postoperative inflammation. Various trials involving the use of fluorometholone 0.25%, prednisolone acetate 1%, or loteprednol 0.5% postoperatively for 1 week or less revealed no differences between the type of steroids used with respect to long-term outcomes.[18,19]

The frequency of follow-up is at the clinician's discretion. Given the fact that the maximal effect of the ALT may not manifest until 4 to 6 weeks postoperatively, clinicians should wait at least 6 weeks before declaring the procedure a success or failure.

COMPLICATIONS

The most common adverse effect associated with ALT is inflammation. Postlaser inflammation is generally mild, localized to the anterior chamber, and occasionally associated with mild hyperemia and photophobia. Treatment with a short course of topical steroids or NSAIDs effectively resolves the inflammation in most cases.[20] This treatment can be supplemented with oral analgesics if patients remain symptomatic.

Acute IOP spikes can occur after ALT. The incidence of an IOP spike of at least 10 mm Hg is 12%.[21] When IOP spikes occur, they tend to transpire within the first hour postoperatively. IOP spikes occur more frequently in cases of higher power burns, higher total administered power, greater pigmentation in the trabecular meshwork, placement of laser burns more posteriorly, and treatment of 360 degrees in one session.[22]

Peripheral anterior synechiae can develop as a result of ALT. This can be minimized by careful placement of the laser burns and avoiding treatment posterior to the pigmented TM.

Corneal epithelial or endothelial thermal burns can develop from improper focusing of the laser beam. Additionally, corneal decompensation with subsequent corneal edema may develop. Typically, this is associated with higher power settings and/or pre-existing corneal disease such as Fuchs' endothelial dystrophy or Chandler's syndrome.

Hyphema, resulting from laser-induced damage to the TM, is a rare complication of ALT.[23] Hyphema can be managed intraoperatively by applying pressure to the globe with the goniolens to minimize the bleeding.

TREATMENT SUCCESS AND FAILURE

Occasionally, ALT is not successful at achieving the expected IOP reduction by 6 weeks postoperatively. Factors that contribute to decreased ALT efficacy include age less than 50 years, higher preoperative IOP, and previous failed laser trabeculoplasty.[24] Patients with traumatic glaucoma and juvenile or congenital glaucoma tend to respond poorly to ALT. Factors associated with better response to ALT include heavier pigmentation of the trabecular meshwork and African descent. Patients with pigmentary glaucoma and exfoliative glaucoma respond very well to ALT.

RETREATMENT

In the event that further IOP reduction is needed after ALT is performed, reapplication of ALT can be considered. In patients who were previously treated with 180 degrees of ALT, the other 180 degrees should be treated. ALT can even be considered after 360 degrees of TM has been treated, but the success rate of retreatment is low. The majority of patients do not respond well to ALT retreatment.[25,26]

CONCLUSION

ALT is an effective treatment for open-angle glaucoma. It can be used either as first-line therapy or in conjunction with medical therapy. When successful, the effects can last years and potentially reduce the amount of medication needed by the patient, thereby improving compliance and limiting side effects. As with any procedure, careful follow-up is critical in identifying short- or long-term adverse effects, the nonresponders, and those whose initial reduction in IOP from ALT become inadequate over time.

KEY POINTS

1. ALT can be performed at any stage of glaucoma, ranging from primary therapy to treatment after filtering surgery.

2. Preoperative gonioscopy is imperative to visualize the angle and determine the likelihood of response to ALT.

3. Use caution when applying the argon beam so that treatment does not extend posterior to the junction of the nonpigmented and pigmented trabecular meshwork.

4. Use prophylactic medications to blunt IOP spikes and inflammation that commonly occur postoperatively.

5. Continued follow-up after ALT is necessary because the effect of ALT wanes over time.

REFERENCES

1. Ederer F, Gaasterland DA, Dally LG, et al. The Advanced Glaucoma Intervention Study (AGIS): 13. Comparison of treatment outcomes within race: 10-year results. *Ophthalmology.* 2004;111:651-664.
2. Spaeth GL. *Ophthalmic Surgery: Principles and Practice.* Philadelphia, PA: WB Saunders; 1990:309-312.
3. Shingleton BJ, Richter CU, Bellows AR, et al. Long-term efficacy of argon laser trabeculoplasty. *Ophthalmology.* 1987;94:1513-1518.
4. Wilensky JT, Jampol LM. Laser therapy for open angle glaucoma. *Ophthalmology.* 1981;88:213-217.
5. Wise JB, Witter SL. Argon laser therapy for open-angle glaucoma. A pilot study. *Arch Ophthalmol.* 1979;97:319-322.
6. Stein JD, Challa P. Mechanisms of action and efficacy of argon laser trabeculoplasty and selective laser trabeculoplasty. *Curr Opin Ophthalmol.* 2007;18:140-145.
7. Stamper RL, Lieberman MF, Drake MV. *Becker-Shaffer's Diagnosis and Therapy of the Glaucomas.* 8th ed. St. Louis, MO: Mosby; 2009:447-452.
8. Barnes SD, Campagna JA, Dirks MS, et al. Control of intraocular pressure elevations after argon laser trabeculoplasty: comparison of brimonidine 0.2% to apraclonidine 1.0%. *Ophthalmology.* 1999;106:2033-2037.
9. The Brimonidine-ALT Study Group. Effect of brimonidine 0.5% on intraocular pressure spikes following 360% argon laser trabeculoplasty. *Ophthalmic Surg Lasers.* 1995;26:404-409.
10. Rouhiainen HJ, Teräsvirta ME, Tuovinen EJ. The effect of some treatment variables on the results of trabeculoplasty. *Arch Ophthalmol.* 1988;106:611-613.
11. Rolim de Moura CR, Paranhos Jr A, Wormald R. Laser trabeculoplasty for open angle glaucoma. *Cochrane Database Syst Rev.* 2007;(4):CD003919.
12. Gupta D. *Glaucoma Diagnosis and Management.* Philadelphia,PA: Lippincott Williams & Wilkins; 2005:255-266.

13. Smith J. Argon laser trabeculoplasty: comparison of bichromatic and monochromatic wavelengths. *Ophthalmology.* 1984;91:355-360.

14. Rouhiainen HJ, Teräsvirta ME, Tuovinen EJ. The effect of some treatment variables on the results of trabeculoplasty. *Arch Ophthalmol.* 1988;106:611-613.

15. Schwartz LW, Spaeth GL, Traverso C, et al. Variation of techniques on the results of argon laser trabeculoplasty. *Ophthalmology.* 1983;90:781-784.

16. Eguchi S, Yamashita H, Yamamoto T, et al. Methods of argon laser trabeculoplasty, complications and long-term followup of the results. *Jpn J Ophthalmol.* 1985;29:198-211.

17. Klein HZ, Shields MB, Ernest JT. Two-stage argon laser trabeculoplasty in open angle glaucoma. *Am J Ophthalmol.* 1985;99:392-395.

18. Kim YY, Glover BK, Shin DH, et al. Effect of topical anti-inflammatory treatment on the long-term outcome of laser trabeculoplasty. Fluorometholone-Laser Trabeculoplasty Study Group. *Am J Ophthalmol.* 1998;126:721-723.

19. Shin DH, Frenkel RE, David R, et al. Effect of topical anti-inflammatory treatment on the outcome of laser trabeculoplasty. The Fluorometholone-Laser Trabeculoplasty Study Group. *Am J Ophthalmol.* 1996;122:349-354.

20. Herbort CP, Mermoud A, Schnyder C, et al. Anti-inflammatory effect of diclofenac drops after argon laser trabeculoplasty. *Arch Ophthalmol.* 1993;111:481-483.

21. Glaucoma Laser Trial Research Group. The Glaucoma Laser Trial. I. Acute effects of argon laser trabeculoplasty on intraocular pressure. *Arch Ophthalmol.* 1989;107: 1135-1142.

22. Rosenblatt MA, Luntz MH. Intraocular pressure rise after argon laser trabeculoplasty. *Br J Ophthalmol.* 1987;71:772-775.

23. Shields MB, Krupin T, Ritch R. *Glaucomas.* St. Louis, MO: Mosby; 1996:1582.

24. AGIS Investigators. The Advanced Glaucoma Intervention Study (AGIS): 11. Risk factors for failure of trabeculectomy and argon laser trabeculoplasty. *Am J Ophthalmol.* 2002;134:481-498.

25. Richter CU, Shingleton BJ, Bellows AR, et al. Retreatment with argon laser trabeculoplasty. *Ophthalmology.* 1987;94:1085-1089.

26. Feldman RM, Katz LJ, Spaeth GL, et al. Long-term efficacy of repeat argon laser trabeculoplasty. *Ophthalmology.* 1991;98:1061-1065.

21

Selective Laser Trabeculoplasty

Denise A. John, MD, FRCSC and Jennifer Somers Weizer, MD

Laser photocoagulation to the trabecular meshwork has been in use since the early 1970s.[1] First described by Worthen and Wickham in 1974, laser trabeculoplasty was initially performed using an argon laser.[2] It was not until 1979, when Wise and Witter[3] modified the argon laser trabeculoplasty (ALT) technique, that the procedure became widely accepted as a modality for the treatment of primary OAG and some forms of secondary OAG. The Glaucoma Laser Trial demonstrated that ALT is at least as effective as timolol in the treatment of OAG, and thus may be used as either a primary or adjunctive method to lower the intraocular pressure (IOP).[4] Numerous histologic studies have shown that coagulative damage occurs to the trabecular meshwork with ALT. It is believed that this structural damage to the trabecular meshwork limits the success of retreatment with ALT.

Selective laser trabeculoplasty (SLT), based on the concept of selective photothermolysis, selectively targets pigmented trabecular meshwork cells while avoiding thermal and mechanical damage to neighboring cells.[5] Approved for use by the United States Food and Drug Administration in March 2001, SLT has gained acceptance among ophthalmologists as a safe and effective alternative to ALT for lowering IOP.

Background and Mechanism of Action

In 1983 Anderson and Parrish selectively targeted pigmented structures in vivo by manipulating optical radiation parameters.[5] In 1995 Latina and Park[6] conducted a study using various lasers to selectively target the pigmented trabecular meshwork cells while sparing the adjacent nonpigmented cells. These studies led to the development of the current 532-nm, frequency-doubled, Q-switched Nd:YAG SLT laser.

Kahook M.
Essentials of Glaucoma Surgery (pp 185–196).
© 2012 SLACK Incorporated.

The precise mechanisms of action of the ALT and SLT lasers remain poorly understood. However, 3 theories have been proposed to explain how these lasers lower IOP.

Mechanical Theory

Electromagnetic energy produced by the argon laser is transformed into thermal energy when it comes into contact with the trabecular meshwork. This thermal energy results in collagen shrinkage and tissue contraction, which leads to mechanical stretching of the surrounding uveoscleral tissue and widening of Schlemm's canal. This structural change increases the passage of aqueous humor through the meshwork and into Schlemm's canal, thus lowering the IOP.[7,8] Histological evidence exists to support this theory only for ALT.

Biologic Theory

Thermal energy generated by the laser stimulates increased cellular activity.[9] Studies involving both the ALT and SLT lasers have shown an upregulation of various cytokines, including interleukin (IL)-1 and tumor necrosis factor (TNF)-α, which leads to the recruitment of macrophages into the trabecular meshwork and upregulation of matrix metalloproteinase expression with subsequent remodeling of the extracellular matrix and increased aqueous outflow.[10,11] Studies involving SLT have not shown scarring or contraction of the trabecular meshwork tissue (which is inconsistent with the mechanical theory) but rather favors the biologic theory.[12]

Repopulation Theory

One study specifically examining the ALT laser suggested the laser energy stimulates increased cell division and trabecular meshwork repopulation. These new cells were found to repopulate the burn sites where aqueous filtration occurs.[13]

METHOD OF TREATMENT FOR SELECTIVE LASER TRABECULOPLASTY

As described above, the SLT is a 532-nm, frequency-doubled, Q-switched Nd:YAG laser. It has a 3-ns pulse duration and a spot size of 400 μm. Postlaser IOP spikes may possibly be reduced with pretreatment with a topical alpha-agonist (apraclonidine 0.5% or brimonidine tartrate 0.2%). After topical anesthesia is accomplished, either a Goldmann 3-mirror lens or Latina SLT lens (Ocular Instruments Inc, Bellevue, Washington) is used to focus the aiming beam onto the trabecular meshwork. The large spot size covers the entire width of the trabecular meshwork, making application of the laser beam easier. Studies have not conclusively demonstrated how much of the angle should be treated to achieve the maximum IOP lowering effect. However, ophthalmologists tend to apply either 50 nonoverlapping spots to 180 degrees (the superior, inferior, nasal, or temporal 180 degrees can be treated) of the angle or treat the full 360 degrees with 100 spots. The initial energy setting is 0.8 mJ per pulse, which is titrated to achieve the end point of visible "champagne bubbles" with 50% or more of the applications. In eyes with heavily pigmented meshwork, it is recommended to lower the initial setting (to 0.6 to 0.7 mJ) to prevent a postlaser IOP spike; the amount of angle treated or the number of laser spots may also be reduced in these eyes. After the procedure is completed, the same pretreatment glaucoma medications may be instilled into the eye. The IOP is typically checked 30 to 60 minutes after laser. A corticosteroid or nonsteroidal anti-inflammatory agent may be given to the patient to be used approximately 4 times a day for several days following SLT, depending on the treating physician's preference. The prescribed glaucoma medications the patient was taking prior to the laser are typically continued until the efficacy of the laser is determined. The effect of the laser can be seen as early as the first week, but generally at least 4 to 6 weeks are allowed before determining the success of the laser.[14-16]

INDICATIONS AND CONTRAINDICATIONS FOR SELECTIVE LASER TRABECULOPLASTY

Indications[17]

1. Primary open-angle glaucoma, exfoliation glaucoma, or pigmentary glaucoma.
2. Glaucoma with medically uncontrolled IOP.
3. Previously failed ALT.
4. Patients with poor glaucoma medication compliance.
5. Patients who cannot afford glaucoma medications.
6. Patients who would like to reduce the number of glaucoma medications they are taking.
7. Patients who do not tolerate glaucoma medications.

Contraindications[17]

1. Inadequate visualization of the trabecular meshwork.
2. Neovascular glaucoma.

3. Active uveitis or history of uveitis (relative contraindication; see Further Study Needed section on page 192).

4. Traumatic glaucoma (relative contraindication; see Further Study Needed section on page 192).

5. Congenital or early childhood glaucoma (relative contraindication; see Further Study Needed section on page 192).

6. Primary or secondary angle-closure glaucoma (relative contraindication; see Further Study Needed section on page 192).

EFFICACY RATES

Selective Laser Trabeculoplasty Versus Argon Laser Trabeculoplasty

Several studies, both retrospective and prospective, have compared the IOP-lowering efficacy of ALT to SLT in open-angle glaucoma. In these studies, some eyes had been previously treated with ALT. Most of these initial studies involved a follow-up period of 6 to 12 months and demonstrated that both lasers produce a statistically equivalent IOP reduction at both 6 and 12 months postlaser.[14,17-19] Longer-term follow-up ranging to 60 months also describes similar rates of IOP reduction between the two laser types.[20]

Selective Laser Trabeculoplasty After Failed Argon Laser Trabeculoplasty

In one study, patients with prior failed ALT received treatment with 180 degrees of SLT and their IOP reduction was compared with patients who received SLT as an initial treatment.[17] No difference in IOP reduction was observed between the 2 groups. Another study found a greater IOP reduction (6.8 mm Hg) in a failed prior ALT group treated with SLT versus repeat ALT (3.6 mm Hg).[21] These studies suggest that SLT can effectively reduce the IOP even after failed ALT.

Selective Laser Trabeculoplasty Versus Glaucoma Medications

The SLT MED Study,[22] which is a prospective, randomized trial comparing SLT to topical medications as initial glaucoma therapy, showed after at least 8 months of follow-up that patients randomized to receive SLT achieved a mean IOP reduction of 6.7 mm Hg, whereas those in the medication group achieved a mean IOP reduction of 7.6 mm Hg. One study observed that after 12 months, SLT provided a mean IOP reduction of 31%, whereas topical latanoprost had a mean IOP reduction of 30.6%.[23] It has also been shown that 360 degrees of SLT provides an equivalent IOP reduction as latanoprost 0.005% once daily at night, whereas medication provides superior IOP lowering compared with 90- or 180-degree SLT treatments.[24]

Repeatability of Selective Laser Trabeculoplasty

It has been suggested that SLT can be repeated due to the apparent lack of structural damage to the trabecular meshwork from this laser. The repeatability of the SLT laser, in addition to its easier technical use, would give SLT some advantage compared with ALT. However, long-term prospective studies evaluating the repeatability of SLT have yet to be performed. One published study showed that SLT can lower IOP successfully in the short-term after prior SLT treatment.[25] Other results suggesting similar findings are as of yet unpublished.[26] Although these reports involve small patient populations, their results are encouraging and further exemplify the need for further studies in this area.

SELECTIVE LASER TRABECULOPLASTY'S EFFECT IN SPECIFIC PATIENT SUBGROUPS

Type of Glaucoma

1. Exfoliation glaucoma: Just as ALT has been shown to be at least as effective in exfoliation glaucoma as in primary open-angle glaucoma eyes, studies comparing SLT in these 2 groups of patients show similar findings with comparable success rates. There is some minor evidence that the effects of SLT in exfoliation glaucoma patients may last somewhat longer than in primary open-angle glaucoma patients.[16,27]

2. Pigmentary glaucoma: For SLT in pigmentary glaucoma, please see the following section.

Degree of Trabecular Meshwork Pigmentation

Most studies have not found a relationship between the degree of trabecular meshwork pigmentation and the success rates of SLT. These studies have included a small number of pigmentary glaucoma patients who have had similar SLT success rates when compared with patients with less trabecular meshwork pigment.[16,27]

The literature does contain case series of pigmentary glaucoma patients who have experienced sustained post-SLT IOP spikes, however. Some of these patients required trabeculectomy shortly after SLT to control the IOP.

The authors of these series suggest that the SLT parameters be altered for pigmentary glaucoma patients. For instance, lower energy levels, fewer laser spots, or treating a smaller circumference of the angle at each session should be considered. The treating ophthalmologist should monitor the post-SLT IOP especially carefully in these patients.[28]

Level of Preoperative Laser Intraocular Pressure

Several studies suggest that SLT tends to be more successful in eyes with higher preoperative laser IOPs, at least when SLT success is measured as a percentage of IOP lowering from baseline.[29,30] This finding is similar to the published evidence that glaucoma medications also tend to reduce IOP more significantly in eyes with higher pretreatment pressures. One published study involving normal tension glaucoma patients who underwent SLT suggests that SLT does lower IOP in these patients to some degree and may also help reduce the amount of IOP fluctuation in this disease.[31]

Race

A paucity of studies exists regarding race in relation to SLT success, but one article did find that SLT and ALT had similar success rates in black and white patients.[20] Some studies performed in Asian populations showed that SLT had good success rates in these groups.[32,33]

Lens Status

Phakic and pseudophakic eyes seem to have similar responses to SLT, in terms of amount of IOP lowering and success rates.[34]

Prior Trabeculoplasty Treatment

1. ALT: As described above, studies have shown that the efficacy of ALT and SLT are similar when comparing results up to 60 months after laser treatment.[16,20] There is no clear evidence that eyes with previous ALT have more adverse effects from SLT when compared with laser-naïve eyes undergoing SLT.

2. SLT: The issue of SLT's efficacy when repeated needs further study. One published article reports that repeat 360-degree SLT lowers pressure equally well to the first SLT treatment when performed at least 6 months after the original treatment has failed.[35]

Other Patient Subgroups

1. Several studies in the literature have shown that SLT can be a useful adjunctive treatment in eyes that experience an IOP elevation after intravitreal triamcinolone injection. These eyes tend to also require topical glaucoma medications to control the IOP.[16,36,37]

2. One study of SLT in diabetic versus nondiabetic eyes showed similar levels of efficacy.[38]

3. One study described IOP lowering after SLT in eyes with chronic primary angle closure that had already been treated with laser iridotomy. In these eyes, SLT was applied to the portions of the trabecular meshwork that were visible on gonioscopy.[39]

ADVERSE EFFECTS OF SELECTIVE LASER TRABECULOPLASTY

Fortunately, the vast majority of reported adverse reactions to SLT have been transient and without lasting sequelae. The most common reactions are described below.

Early Postoperative Intraocular Pressure Elevation

The most commonly reported adverse reaction after SLT is an early postlaser IOP elevation. Most studies report a significant pressure elevation as >5 mm Hg compared with pre-SLT levels. The occurrence rate of this pressure elevation ranged from 0% to 30%, depending on the study. Some study patients received a prophylactic pressure-lowering eye drop perioperatively (usually apraclonidine 0.5% or brimonidine tartrate 0.2%), whereas others did not. In several studies,[18,21,30] use of a prophylactic pressure-lowering eyedrop did not seem to affect the rate of postlaser pressure elevation. The majority of patients with a significant pressure elevation post-SLT respond well to additional topical medications and/or watchful waiting, with resolution of the pressure elevation. The exception to this was 3 reported patients with heavily pigmented trabecular meshwork who had severe, prolonged IOP elevation after SLT and underwent trabeculectomy.[16,27,28]

Anterior Chamber Reaction

Although numerous studies report no anterior chamber reaction after SLT, some studies have described mild to moderate level of cells and flare. In all published studies, the anterior chamber inflammation was self-limited and resolved without long-term sequelae. No peripheral anterior synechiae were reported after these episodes of anterior chamber reaction.[16]

Pain

A few studies have noted small numbers of patients who experienced pain with SLT treatment.[18,24,40] There is a suggestion that of patients who felt pain with SLT, the pain level was significantly lower when compared with patients undergoing ALT.[40] One study described more patients experiencing pain during SLT when a larger circumference of the angle was treated compared to a smaller treatment area.[24]

Other Adverse Reactions

Other adverse reactions from SLT are rare. One case report is in the literature of self-limited hyphema occurring during SLT; this resolved spontaneously.[41] Four case reports were published indicating corneal edema, haze, and thinning. The corneal thinning persisted long-term in these cases.[42]

FURTHER STUDY NEEDED

More work needs to done regarding the long-term effect of SLT, as well as its repeatability. Given the fact that SLT has few adverse effects, and if it is shown over time to be successful with repeated treatments, it may help influence the glaucoma treatment paradigm in our aging patient population. Regarding aging, investigating the efficacy of SLT in patients of different ages would be helpful. Studies addressing the interaction and possible synergy of SLT with medical glaucoma therapy also need to be performed. With more recognition and emphasis placed on the diurnal nature of IOP fluctuation, SLT's effect on possibly blunting the pressure curve should be investigated.

Establishing optimal treatment parameters for SLT would help the thousands of ophthalmologists who currently perform this treatment. Currently, we do not know whether treating 90 versus 180 or 360 degrees of the angle is best. Also, the effect of the number of applications and pulse duration has not been well studied. Postlaser anti-inflammatory treatment varies widely across practitioners, and although it is suggested in the literature that using topical steroids short-term after SLT does not affect its success, the efficacy or necessity of this is not clearly known.[43]

SLT has not been well studied in eyes in which ALT has not been considered useful. For instance, it is not known whether SLT is safe and effective in eyes with uveitic, angle recession, or congenital glaucoma. More studies addressing the efficacy of SLT in normal tension glaucoma, particularly with regard to diurnal fluctuation, are also needed.

CONCLUSION

SLT is a procedure that is gaining increasingly wider popularity due to its efficacy, favorable side-effect profile, technical ease, and potential repeatability. Ophthalmologists can consider SLT as primary or adjunctive treatment for elevated IOP. The evidence is clear that lowering IOP can effectively slow glaucoma disease progression and vision loss, and thus SLT is a useful tool in the armamentarium against this widespread disease. Further studies will clarify its role in terms of longer-term follow-up, repeatability, and usefulness in secondary glaucomas.

KEY POINTS

1. SLT can be useful as primary or adjunctive therapy for elevated IOP.
2. SLT is relatively straightforward to perform and may yield benefits even when performed more than once.
3. Side effects from performing SLT tend to be mild and self-limited; however, transient pressure spikes shortly after SLT have been reported, especially in eyes with heavy trabecular meshwork pigment.
4. More research is needed to determine SLT's usefulness in long-term follow-up, in certain secondary glaucoma populations, and in terms of repeatability.

REFERENCES

1. Van der Zypen E, Frankhauser F. Lasers in the treatment of chronic simple glaucoma. *Trans Ophthalmol Soc UK.* 1982 Apr;102(1):147-153.
2. Worthen DM, Wickham MG. Argon laser trabeculotomy. *Trans Am Acad Ophthalmol Otolaryngol.* 1974;78(2):OP371-OP375.
3. Wise JB, Witter SL. Argon laser therapy for open-angle glaucoma: a pilot study. *Arch Ophthalmol.* 1979;97(2):319-322.
4. The Glaucoma Laser Trial Research Group. The Glaucoma Laser Trial (GLT). 2. Results of argon laser trabeculoplasty versus topical medications. *Ophthalmology.* 1990;97(11):1403-1413.
5. Anderson RR, Parrish JA. Selective photothermolysis: precise microsurgery by selective absorption of pulsed radiation. *Science.* 1983;220(4596):524-527.
6. Latina MA, Park C. Selective targeting of trabecular meshwork cells: in vitro studies of pulsed and CW laser interactions. *Exp Eye Res.* 1995;60(4):359-372.
7. Melamed S. Argon laser trabeculoplasty: how does it work? In: Epstein DL, Allingham RR, Schuman JS, eds. *Chandler and Grant's Glaucoma.* 4th ed. Baltimore, MD: Lippincott Williams & Wilkins; 1997:466-469.
8. Melamed S, Pei J, Epstein DL. Delayed response to argon laser trabeculoplasty in monkeys: morphological and morphometric analysis. *Arch Ophthalmol.* 1986;104(7): 1078-1083.
9. Stein JD, Challa P. Mechanisms of action and efficacy of argon laser trabeculoplasty and selective laser trabeculoplasty. *Curr Opin Ophthalmol.* 2007;18(2):140-145.
10. Melamed S, Pei J, Epstein DL. Short-term effect of argon laser trabeculoplasty: studies of mechanism of action. *Arch Ophthalmol.* 1985;103(10):1546-1552.

11. Ruddat MS, Alexander JR, Samples JR, et al. Early changes in trabecular metallopro-teinase mRNA levels in response to laser trabeculoplasty are induced by media bome factors. *Invest Ophthalmol Vis Sci.* 1989;30(Suppl):280.

12. Kramer TR, Noecker RJ. Comparison of the morphologic changes after selective laser trabeculoplasty and argon laser trabeculoplasty in human eye bank eyes. *Ophthalmol-ogy.* 2001;108(4):773-779.

13. Bylsma SS, Samples JR, Acott TS, Van Buskirk EM. Trabecular cell division after argon laser trabeculoplasty. *Arch Ophthalmol.* 1988;106(4):544-547.

14. Latina MA, de Leon JMS. Selective laser trabeculoplasty. *Ophthalmol Clin N Am.* 2005;18(3):409-419.

15. Zao JC, Grosskreutz CL, Pasquale LR. Argon versus selective laser trabeculoplasty in the treatment of open angle glaucoma. *Int Ophthalmol Clin.* 2005;45(4):97-106.

16. Barkana Y, Belkin M. Selective laser trabeculoplasty. *Surv Ophthalmol.* 2007;52(6):634-654.

17. Damiji K. Selective laser trabeculoplasty: a better alternative. *Surv Ophthalmol.* 2008;53(6):646-651.

18. Latina MA, Sibayan SA, Shin DH, et al. Q-switched 532 nm Nd:YAG laser trabeculoplasty (selective laser trabeculoplasty): a multicenter pilot, clinical study. *Ophthalmology.* 1998;105(11):2082-2088.

19. Pirnazar JR, Kolker A, Way M, et al. The efficacy of 532 nm laser trabeculoplasty. *Invest Ophthalmol Vis Sci.* 1998;39(4):S5.

20. Juzych MS, Chopra V, Banitt MR, et al. Comparision of long-term outcomes of selec-tive laser trabeculoplasty versus argon laser trabeculoplasty in open-angle glaucoma. *Ophthalmology.* 2004;111(10):1853-1859.

21. Damji KF, Shah KC, Rock WJ, et al. Selective laser trabeculoplasty versus argon laser trabeculoplasty: a prospective randomized clinical trial. *Br J Ophthalmol.* 1999;83(6):718-722.

22. Katz LJ, Steinmann WC, Marcellino GR; The SLT MED Study Group. Comparison of selective laser trabeculoplasty vs. medical therapy from intial therpay for glaucoma or ocular hypertension. Presented at: American Academy of Ophthalmology Annual Meet-ing; November 2006; Las Vegas, NV. Presentation #PO108.

23. McIlraith I, Strasfeld M, Colev G, Hutnik CM. Selective laser trabeculoplasty as initial and adjunctive treatment for open-angle glaucoma. *J Glaucoma.* 2006;15(2):124-130.

24. Nagar M, Ogunyomade A, O'Brart DP, et al. A randomized, prospective study comparing selective laser trabeculoplasty with latanoprost for the control of intraocular pressure in ocular hypertension and open angle glaucoma. *Br J Ophthalmol.* 2005;89(11):1413-1417.

25. Lai J, Bournias TE. Repeatability of selective laser trabeculoplasty (SLT). *Invest Ophthalmol Vis Sci.* 2005;46:E-Abstract 119.

26. Nagar M. SLT—effect of enhancement and repeatability on IOP. Unpublished American Academy of Ophthalmology 2006 poster presentation.

27. Realini T. Selective laser trabeculoplasty: a review. *J Glaucoma.* 2008 Sep;17(6):497-502.

28. Harasymowycz PJ, Papamatheakis DG, Latina M, et al. Selective laser trabeculoplasty (SLT) complicated by intraocular pressure elevation in eyes with heavily pigmented trabecular meshworks. *Am J Ophthalmol.* 2005;139(6):1110-1113.

29. Hodge WG, Damji KF, Rock W, et al. Baseline IOP predicts selective laser trabeculoplasty success at 1 year post-treatment: results from a randomized clinical trial. *Br J Ophthalmol.* 2005;89(9):1157-1160.

30. Song J, Lee PP, Epstein DL, et al. High failure rate associated with 180 degrees selective laser trabeculoplasty. *J Glaucoma.* 2005;14(5):400-408.

31. El Mallah MK, Walsh MM, Stinnett SS, Asrani SG. Selective laser trabeculoplasty reduces mean IOP and IOP variation in normal tension glaucoma patients. *Clin Ophthalmol.* 2010;4:889-893.

32. Lai JS, Chua JK, Tham CC, Lam DS. Five-year follow up of selective laser trabeculoplasty in Chinese eyes. *Clin Experiment Ophthalmol.* 2004;32(4):368-372.

33. Shibata M, Sugiyama T, Ishida O, et al. Clinical results of selective laser trabeculoplasty in open-angle glaucoma in Japanese eyes: comparison of 180 degree with 360 degree SLT. *J Glaucoma.* 2010;21(1):17-21.

34. Werner M, Smith WM, Doyle JW. Selective laser trabeculoplasty in phakic and pseudophakic eyes. *Ophthalmic Surg Lasers Imaging.* 2007;38(3):182-188.

35. Hong BK, Winer JC, Martone JF, Wand M, Altman B, Shields B. Repeat selective laser trabeculoplasty. *J Glaucoma.* 2009;18(3):180-183.

36. Pizzimenti JJ, Nickerson MM, Pizzimenti CE, et al. Selective laser trabeculoplasty for intraocular pressure elevation after intravitreal triamcinolone acetonide injection. *Optom Vis Sci.* 2006;83(7):421-425.

37. Rubin B, Taglienti A, Rothman RF, Marcus CH, Serle JB. The effect of selective laser trabeculoplasty on intraocular pressure in patients with intravitreal steroid-induced elevated intraocular pressure. *J Glaucoma.* 2008;17(4):287-292.

38. Leung EH. Modulation of SLT response in patients with diabetes—six month follow-up of the University of Chicago SLT study. Paper presented at: Annual Meeting of the Association for Research in Vision and Ophthalmology; May 2005; Fort Lauderdale, FL.

39. Ho CL, Lai JS, Aquino MV, et al. Selective laser trabeculoplasty for primary angle closure with persistently elevated IOP after iridotomy. *J Glaucoma.* 2009;18(7):563-566.

40. Martinez-de-la-Casa JM, Garcia-Feijoo J, Castillo A, et al. Selective vs argon laser trabeculoplasty: hypotensive efficacy, anterior chamber inflammation, and postoperative pain. *Eye.* 2004;18(5):498-502.

41. Rhee DJ, Krad O, Pasquale LR. Hyphema following selective laser trabeculoplasty. *Ophthalmic Surg Lasers Imaging.* 2009;40(5):493-494.

42. Regina M, Bunya RM, Orlin SE, Ansari H. Corneal edema and haze after selective laser trabeculoplasty. *J Glaucoma.* 2011;20(5):327-329.

43. Realini T, Hettlinger CJ. The impact of anti-inflammatory therapy on IOP reduction following selective laser trabeculoplasty. *Ophthalmic Surg Lasers Imaging.* 2010;41(1): 100-103.

22

COMPARISON OF ARGON LASER TRABECULOPLASTY AND SELECTIVE LASER TRABECULOPLASTY

Fiorella Saponara, MD and Joshua D. Stein, MD, MS

Although previous chapters in this book describe in detail the indications, safety profile, effectiveness, risks, and complications of argon laser trabeculoplasty (ALT; Chapter 20) and selective laser trabeculoplasty (SLT; Chapter 21), in this chapter we compare and contrast these surgical procedures with one another.

EFFICACY OF ARGON LASER TRABECULOPLASTY AND SELECTIVE LASER TRABECULOPLASTY

A few studies have compared the efficacy of ALT and SLT at lowering intraocular pressure (IOP).[1-4,10,15] With sample sizes ranging from 36 to 60 patients, and follow-up times ranging from 3 months to 5 years, these studies have demonstrated that ALT and SLT achieve a relatively similar level of IOP reduction. The series with the longest length of follow-up, by Juzych et al,[1] found a 24% reduction of IOP among patients with primary open-angle glaucoma who underwent ALT, and a 27% reduction in IOP among those who received SLT—a difference in pressure lowering that was not statistically significant. Table 22-1 shows the findings from the studies in the literature comparing the efficacy of these 2 lasers.

REPEATABILITY OF ARGON LASER TRABECULOPLASTY AND SELECTIVE LASER TRABECULOPLASTY

Several studies have assessed the repeatability of ALT and SLT. Most studies of patients undergoing repeat ALT have found that only approximately one-third of those who underwent retreatment experienced

Kahook M.
Essentials of Glaucoma Surgery (pp 197-202).
© 2012 SLACK Incorporated.

TABLE 22-1. SUMMARY OF SELECTED STUDIES THAT COMPARE ARGON LASER TRABECULOPLASTY WITH SELECTIVE LASER TRABECULOPLASTY

Author	Glaucoma	# of Eyes	Follow-Up	ALT Preop IOP (mm Hg)	ALT Postop IOP (mm Hg)	ALT Reduction (%)	SLT Preop IOP (mm Hg)	SLT Postop IOP (mm Hg)	SLT Reduction (%)	P Value
Damji et al[2]	POAG	18 ALT 18 SLT	6 months	22.5 ± 3.6	17.7 ± 3.3	21.3	22.8 ± 3.0	17.8 ± 4.8	21.9	.97
Popiela et al[3]	Mixed	27 ALT 27 SLT	3 months	20.3 ± 4.0	17.6 ± 3.6	13.0	21.3 ± 4.8	18.4 ± 4.6	13.4	.84
Martinez-de-la-casa et al[4]	POAG	20 ALT 20 SLT	6 months	23.6 ± 3.8	19 ± 3.2	19.5	24.0 ± 4.7	18.6 ± 4.2	22.2	.74
Juzych et al[1]	POAG	40 ALT 20 SLT	5 years	24.3 ± 4.1		23.5 ± 25.2	23.9 ± 2.6		27.1 ± 21.4	.58

ALT indicates argon laser trabeculoplasty; SLT, selective laser trabeculoplasty; IOP, intraocular pressure; POAG, primary open angle glaucoma; SD, standard deviation; preop, preoperative; postop, postoperative.

additional pressure lowering at 6 to 12 months following the repeat procedure.[5-8] Not only was retreatment with ALT ineffective in the majority of patients in these studies, one study also found that nearly one-fifth of those who received a second ALT experienced an acute rise in IOP of 10 mm Hg or higher following the repeat procedure.[9] Because one of the proposed mechanisms of action of ALT is that the laser creates scar tissue at the site of application, with contraction and opening of the adjacent trabecular meshwork tissue to improve outflow, repeat treatment may result in further scarring of the trabecular meshwork, resulting in a reduced ability for aqueous to exit through the trabecular meshwork and a subsequent increase in IOP.[10] Thus, it is generally not recommended to perform repeat ALT.

Little is known about the success of repeating SLT. Unlike with ALT, because SLT does not induce significant scarring of the trabecular meshwork, retreatment offers a greater potential for achieving an additional IOP-lowering effect relative to ALT without as great a risk for complications. A study by Shah et al[11] of patients who underwent repeat SLT demonstrated a 70% and 53% success rate at 1 and 2 years, respectively. Although more studies are underway that will further elucidate the efficacy and risks of repeat SLT, we feel that it is reasonable to consider retreating patients who had achieved a good response to their first treatment with SLT. However, if the patient had a limited response the first time SLT was performed, it is unlikely he or she will achieve a better response with additional treatment, and, often, one should look for other options for lowering the IOP, such as filtering surgery.

Various studies have reported success with SLT in patients who had previously undergone ALT.[2,12,13] Given that the mechanism of action of ALT and SLT differ from one another, it is not surprising that a subset of patients who do not respond to ALT achieve a pressure-lowering effect from SLT. In patients who have undergone previous ALT, if the IOP is close to target, it is reasonable to try SLT to further reduce the IOP before proceeding with more invasive incisional surgical procedures.

Complications of Argon Laser Trabeculoplasty and Selective Laser Trabeculoplasty

Few reports are in the literature comparing the rates of complications associated with ALT and SLT. The 2 most common adverse events associated with both of these lasers are an acute postoperative rise in IOP following the procedure and postoperative inflammation. Marked elevations in IOP have been reported in patients with heavily pigmented trabecular meshwork following both lasers, some eventually requiring trabeculectomy.[14] Martinez-de-la-casa et al[4] reported greater rates of transient anterior chamber reaction at 1 hour post-treatment and pain with ALT as compared with SLT. By contrast, Damji et al[15] found that overall there was no significant difference between these 2 lasers in terms of frequency of postoperative IOP spikes, pain, and peripheral anterior synechiae formation. Overall, the complications associated with both of these lasers are usually mild, transient, and self-limiting.

COSTS OF THE LASERS USED TO PERFORM ARGON LASER TRABECULOPLASTY AND SELECTIVE LASER TRABECULOPLASTY

Purchasing a laser to perform trabeculoplasty can be expensive. ALT is performed using an argon laser, which costs approximately $30,000 to $50,000. By comparison, the cost of a laser to perform SLT is approximately $80,000. When comparing the costs of these lasers, one should also consider the capability of using these lasers to perform other procedures besides trabeculoplasty. In addition to performing ALT with the argon laser, this laser can be used to perform panretinal photocoagulation, focal laser to treat macular edema, retinopexy for retinal tears, as well as peripheral iridotomy and iridoplasty procedures. Some lasers that can be used for SLT are also capable of being used for YAG iridotomy and capsulotomy procedures. Thus, if a practice can afford to purchase only one laser, the argon laser may be a better option given its cheaper price and its ability to be used for multiple purposes in addition to simply trabeculoplasty.

TEACHING TRAINEES HOW TO PERFORM ARGON LASER TRABECULOPLASTY AND SELECTIVE LASER TRABECULOPLASTY

When comparing and contrasting these 2 lasers, it is worth noting that it is easier to teach trainees and clinicians who have a limited knowledge of angle anatomy how to perform SLT because the 400-μm spot size of this laser fills up the entire angle. By comparison, with ALT, the spot size is considerably smaller and it is necessary to apply the laser in a precise location to achieve the desired effect.

KEY POINTS

1. Current evidence suggests that ALT remains a safe and effective treatment for ocular hypertension and open-angle glaucoma.
2. Most studies show similar efficacy at lowering IOP with ALT and SLT.
3. Risk of complications is relatively low with both procedures.

4. Although most agree that the potential risks outweigh the potential benefits when it comes to retreatment with ALT, it is possible to perform retreatment with SLT.

REFERENCES

1. Juzych MS, Chopra V, Banitt MR, et al. Comparison of longterm outcomes of selective laser trabeculoplasty versus argon laser trabeculoplasty in open-angle glaucoma. *Ophthalmology.* 2004;111(10):1853-1859.
2. Damji KF, Shah KC, Rock WJ. Selective laser trabeculoplasty v argon laser trabeculoplasty: a prospective randomised clinical trial. *Br J Ophthalmol.* 1999;83(6):718-722.
3. Popiela G, Muzyka M, Szelepin L, et al. Use of YAG-Selecta laser and argon laser in the treatment of open angle glaucoma [Polish]. *Klinika Oczna.* 2000;102(2):129-133.
4. Martinez-de-la-Casa JM, Garcia-Feijoo J, Castillo A, et al. Selective vs argon laser trabeculoplasty: hypotensive efficacy, anterior chamber inflammation, and postoperative pain. *Eye.* 2004;18(5):498-502.
5. Feldman RM, Katz LJ, Spaeth GL, et al. Long-term efficacy of repeat argon laser trabeculoplasty. *Ophthalmology.* 1991;98(7):1061-1065.
6. Richter CU, Shingleton BJ, Bellows AR, et al. Retreatment with argon laser trabeculoplasty. *Ophthalmology.* 1987;94(9):1085-1089.
7. Weber PA, Burton GD, Epitropoulos AT. Laser trabeculoplasty retreatment. *Ophthalmic Surg.* 1989;20(10):702-706.
8. Grayson DK, Camras CB, Podos SM, Lustgarten JS. Long-term reduction of intraocular pressure after repeat argon laser trabeculoplasty. *Am J Ophthalmol.* 1988;106(3):312-321.
9. Starita RJ, Fellman RL, Spaeth GL, et al. The effect of repeating full-circumference argon laser trabeculoplasty. *Ophthalmic Surg.* 1984;15(1):41-43.
10. Stein JD, Challa P. Mechanisms of action and efficacy of argon laser trabeculoplasty and selective laser trabeculoplasty. *Curr Opin Ophthalmol.* 2007;18(2):140-145.
11. Shah N, Yadav R, Nagar M. Selective laser trabeculoplasty: the effect of enhancement and retreatment on IOP control. Paper presented at: XXIV Congress of the European Cataract and Refractive Surgeons (ESCRS); 2006; London, UK.
12. Latina MA, Sibayan SA, Shin DH, et al. Q-switched 532-nm Nd :YAG laser trabeculoplasty (selective laser trabeculoplasty): a multicenter, pilot, clinical study. *Ophthalmology.* 1998;105(11):2082-2088.
13. Kano K, Kuwayama Y, Mizoue S, Ito N. Clinical results of selective laser trabeculoplasty [Japanese]. *Nippon Ganka Gakkai Zasshi.* 1999;103(8):612-616.
14. Harasymowycz PJ, Papamatheakis DG, Latina M. et al. Selective laser trabeculoplasty (SLT) complicated by intraocular pressure elevation in eyes with heavily pigmented trabecular meshworks. *Am J Ophthalmol.* 2005;139(6):1110-1113.
15. Damji KF, Shah KC, Rock WJ et al. Selective laser trabeculoplasty versus argon laser trabeculoplasty: results from a 1-year randomized clinical trial. *Br J Ophthalmol.* 2006;90(12):1490-1494.

LASER PERIPHERAL IRIDOTOMY

Christopher K. S. Leung, MD

Laser peripheral iridotomy (LPI) is a laser procedure that creates an aperture in the peripheral iris. It is an effective treatment for relieving pupil block in eyes with acute primary angle-closure (APAC) and a prophylactic measure indicated for protecting the fellow eyes from APAC. Prophylactic LPI is also commonly considered in eyes with occludable angles (usually defined as an angle in which at least 270 degrees of the posterior trabecular meshwork cannot be visualized).

PRINCIPLE

In relative pupil block, there is an increase in resistance to the flow of aqueous humor at the pupillary margin, resulting in a pressure gradient between the posterior and anterior chambers. With a greater pressure posterior to the iris, the iris assumes a characteristic forward-bowing appearance (Figure 23-1A). LPI provides a communication between the posterior and anterior chambers, thereby eliminating the pressure gradient, flattening the iris, and opening up the anterior chamber angle (Figure 23-1B).

INSTRUMENTATION

LPI can be performed with slit lamp-mounted Nd:YAG laser alone or with sequential argon Nd:YAG laser. A contact lens (eg, Abraham iridotomy lens) is useful to keep the eyelids separated and the globe stable.

TECHNIQUE

1. Perform a complete ophthalmic examination. Review the risks and benefits of the procedure with the patient and obtain a signed informed consent.

2. Instill 1 drop of brimonidine 0.15% (to reduce the risk of a post-LPI intraocular pressure [IOP] rise) and pilocarpine 2% (to thin the peripheral iris and widen the angle; Figure 23-2) 30 minutes prior to LPI.

Kahook M.
Essentials of Glaucoma Surgery (pp 203-206).
© 2012 SLACK Incorporated.

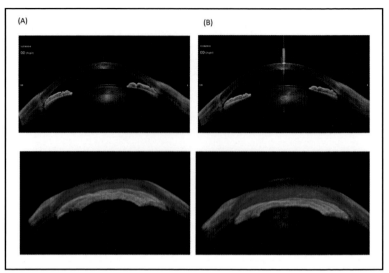

Figure 23-1. Effect of LPI on the configuration of the iris and the anterior chamber angle. Optical coherence tomography imaging (CASIA OCT, Tomey Corp, Nagoya, Japan) of an eye with primary angle closure before (A) and after (B) LPI. In primary angle closure, the iris assumes an anterior convex configuration. LPI eliminates the pressure gradient, widens the anterior chamber angle (above) and flattens the iris (below).

3. Instill one drop of topical anesthesia (eg, proparacaine 0.5%).

4. Apply a contact lens to the globe and identify a suitable location for laser application. The treatment site is preferably located at the peripheral third of the superior iris from 10 to 2 o'clock position (12 o'clock is usually avoided as gas bubble formation may hamper completion of the procedure) and completely covered by the eyelid (some patients with iridotomy partially covered by the eyelid have reported glare and double vision). In an aphakic eye with silicone oil, LPI is performed at the inferior iris. An area of thin iris or a crypt is preferable as less laser energy is required to penetrate the iris.

5. Laser treatment:
   a. Nd:YAG laser alone: 4 to 6 mJ, 1 to 3 pulses per shot for 1 to 3 applications.
   b. Sequential argon Nd:YAG laser: (1) Argon laser—size: 50 μm, duration: 0.05 to 0.1 second, energy: 700 to 1000 mW. (2) Nd:YAG laser: 1 to 3 mJ, 1 to 2 pulses per shot.

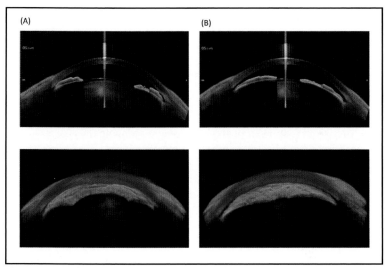

Figure 23-2. Effect of pilocarpine on the configuration of the iris and the anterior chamber angle. Optical coherence tomography imaging (CASIA OCT) of an eye with primary angle closure before (A) and 20 minutes after (B) application of 1 drop of pilocarpine 2%. Pilocarpine facilitates laser peripheral iridotomy by thinning the iris (below) and creating a space between the cornea and the peripheral iris (above).

The actual laser energy required and the treatment chosen depend on the color and the thickness of the iris. For example, sequential argon Nd:YAG laser may be more effective than Nd:YAG laser alone in dark brown iris with thick stroma; argon laser can minimize bleeding and create a stromal crater for subsequent penetration by Nd:YAG laser application. The size of iridotomy is usually 150 to 200 μm.

6. Measure the IOP 1 hour after the procedure to check for IOP rise.

7. Topical steroid (eg, dexamethasone 0.1% or prednisolone acetate 1%) is commonly prescribed for 5 to 7 days to reduce intraocular inflammation after the procedure.

COMPLICATIONS

The most common complications following LPI are anterior uveitis and transient IOP elevation. Anterior uveitis is usually self-limiting and resolves in 1 to 2 weeks with topical steroid treatment. A rise in IOP >6 mm Hg 1 to 2 hours after LPI has been reported in 40% of patients with narrow angles or chronic angle-closure glaucoma. One drop of brimonidine 0.15% before or after LPI is often effective in preventing IOP spike. Although lens opacity formation beneath an iridotomy may occur following LPI, published data on cataract progression are conflicting. Visual symptoms including ghost images and shadows can occur in up to 4% of patients. Hyphema, damage to the corneal endothelium, retinal injury, and malignant glaucoma are other potential but rare complications.

FOLLOW-UP

Although LPI has been proven effective in reducing the risk of APAC, a significant number of patients may still develop chronic elevation of IOP in the presence of a patent iridotomy. Therefore, patients should be monitored for development of peripheral anterior synechia and angle-closure glaucoma in the follow-up visits.

SUGGESTED READINGS

de Silva DJ, Gazzard G, Foster P. Laser iridotomy in dark irides. *Br J Ophthalmol.* 2007;91(2):222-225.

Drake MV. Neodymium:YAG laser iridotomy. *Surv Ophthalmol.* 1987;32(3):171-177.

Saw SM, Gazzard G, Friedman DS. Interventions for angle-closure glaucoma: an evidence-based update. *Ophthalmology.* 2003;110(10):1869-1878.

Argon Laser Peripheral Iridoplasty

Clement C. Y. Tham, FRCS(Glasgow), FCOphth(HK);
Dennis S. C. Lam, MD(HK), FRCS(Edin), FRCOphth(UK), FCOphth(HK);
and Robert Ritch, MD

Argon laser peripheral iridoplasty (ALPI) is a procedure in which long-duration, low-power contraction burns placed circumferentially on the peripheral iris open an appositionally closed anterior chamber drainage angle (Figure 24-1). Iris stromal contraction and compaction mechanically pull open the appositionally closed drainage angle, creating a space where none existed before (Figure 24-2). ALPI is not effective at breaking peripheral anterior synechiae, nor does it replace laser iridotomy in eliminating pupil block.

INDICATIONS

ALPI is effective in acute primary angle closure (APAC),[1] acute phacomorphic angle closure (phacomorphic glaucoma),[2] plateau iris syndrome,[3] secondary and malignant glaucomas with a component of appositional angle closure, as an adjunct to facilitate laser trabeculoplasty, and to reduce the chance of angle reclosure after goniosynechialysis (GSL).[4]

ALPI is remarkably effective at breaking attacks of acute angle closure, safely and effectively reducing intraocular pressure (IOP), at a time when more definitive treatment (eg, laser iridotomy or cataract extraction) cannot be performed due to corneal edema, very shallow anterior chamber, and significant ocular inflammation. It can be done prior to any medical treatment of the angle closure, and the days in which acute angle closure was treated with hospitalization and infusions of mannitol, along with prolonged medical therapy, in an attempt to break an attack belong to the past.

TECHNIQUES[5]

ALPI is performed using an Abraham iridotomy lens (Ocular Instruments, Inc., Bellevue, Washington) under topical anesthesia. Diode laser

Kahook M.
Essentials of Glaucoma Surgery (pp 207-212).
© 2012 SLACK Incorporated.

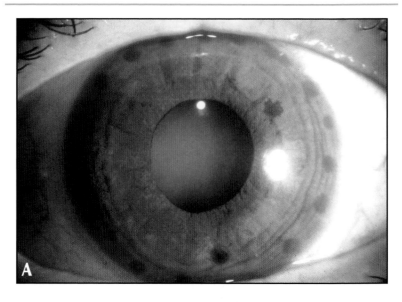

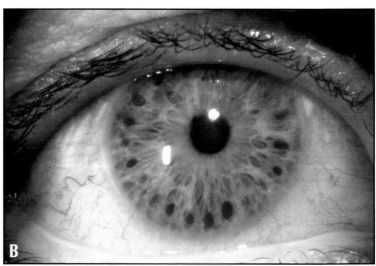

Figure 24-1. (A) Laser peripheral iridoplasty marks on the peripheral iris. (B) Burns placed too centrally.

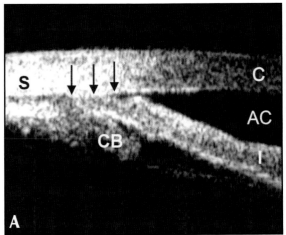

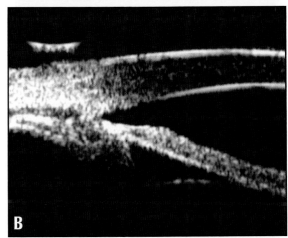

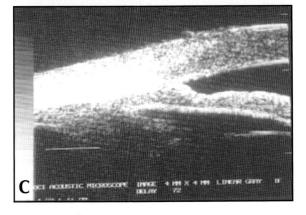

Figure 24-2. (A) Ultrasound biomicroscopy (UBM) image showing an appositionally closed angle in an eye with plateau iris syndrome (S indicates sclera; AC, anterior chamber; I, iris; CB, ciliary body; C, cornea; arrows indicate position of laser application.) (B) After ALPI, the angle is open. (C) When ALPI is not applied peripherally enough (laser applied at position of dimple in iris), the angle remains appositionally closed.

is also effective. For brown irides, we start with a laser power of 200 mW (240 mW for lighter irides), 500-μm spot size (can be reduced to 200 μm for lighter irides, if there is no contraction even with a power of 360 mW or more), and 0.5 to 0.7 second duration. ALPI is successful even when corneal edema and a very shallow anterior chamber are present. The laser is aimed at the far periphery of the iris. The aiming beam may have to slightly overlap the sclera at the limbus to reach the far iris periphery. A total of 20 to 24 laser spots over the 360 degrees is sufficient. The laser power should be titrated against the observed iris response. If there is no or insufficient iris contraction, the laser power can be increased in steps of 20 mW. On the contrary, the laser power should be reduced if there is bubble formation, iris charring, pigment release from the iris, or if there is a "pop" sound. The endpoint is visible iris contraction and slight deepening of the anterior chamber at the point of laser application.

IOP should be rechecked 1 hour afterward to exclude an IOP spike. Topical steroid 4 times a day should be prescribed to control post-laser iritis. At a subsequent visit, darkroom gonioscopy should be repeated, and further iridoplasty should be added if there are still areas of appositional angle closure.

PRECAUTIONS

Irreversible iris changes indicate too much power and should be avoided. Radial iris vessels, if visible, should be avoided. Iris necrosis or atrophy may occur if too many laser spots are placed too closely together.

CONCLUSION

Laser peripheral iridoplasty is a safe and effective technique for mechanically opening appositionally closed drainage angles and in situations in which the closed angle results in significant ocular hypertension, and definitive treatments, such as laser iridotomy, cannot be safely performed.

KEY POINTS

1. Laser peripheral iridoplasty mechanically pulls open appositionally closed drainage angles and is effective in breaking acute attacks of angle closure.

2. Laser peripheral iridoplasty is not effective in synechial angle closure and does not replace laser iridotomy in eliminating pupil block.

3. Laser peripheral iridoplasty is useful in APAC, phacomorphic glaucoma, plateau iris syndrome, secondary and malignant glaucomas with a component of appositional angle closure, as an adjunct to facilitate laser trabeculoplasty, and as an adjunct to reduce the chance of angle reclosure after GSL.

4. Laser peripheral iridoplasty can be safely performed even in situations in which laser iridotomy is not safe due to corneal edema and/or very shallow anterior chamber.

5. When performing laser peripheral iridoplasty, we are aiming for just iris stromal contraction. Bubble formation, iris charring, pigment release from the iris, or a "pop" sound signify too much power and should be avoided.

REFERENCES

1. Lam DS, Lai JS, Tham CC, et al. Argon laser peripheral iridoplasty versus conventional systemic medical therapy in treatment of acute primary angle-closure glaucoma: a prospective, randomized, controlled trial. *Ophthalmology.* 2002;109(9):1591-1596.

2. Tham CC, Lai JS, Poon AS, et al. Immediate argon laser peripheral iridoplasty (ALPI) as initial treatment for acute phacomorphic angle-closure (phacomorphic glaucoma) before cataract extraction: a preliminary study. *Eye.* 2005;19(7):778-783.

3. Ritch R, Tham CC, Lam DS. Long-term success of argon laser peripheral iridoplasty in the management of plateau iris syndrome. *Ophthalmology.* 2004;111(1):104-108.

4. Lai JS, Tham CC, Chua JK, Lam DS. Efficacy and safety of inferior 180 degrees goniosynechialysis followed by diode laser peripheral iridoplasty in the treatment of chronic angle-closure glaucoma. *J Glaucoma.* 2000;9(5):388-391.

5. Ritch R, Tham CC, Lam DS. Argon laser peripheral iridoplasty (ALPI): an update. *Surv Ophthalmol.* 2007;52(3):279-288.

25

Transscleral Cyclophotocoagulation

Douglas E. Gaasterland, MD

Transscleral cyclophotocoagulation (TSCPC) is a laser procedure to reduce intraocular pressure (IOP) by slowing aqueous humor formation. The surgeon applies laser energy through the conjunctiva, Tenon's fascia, and sclera with the goal to coagulate proteins in cells of the ciliary body and processes. After treatment, reduced aqueous humor inflow lowers fluid load to poorly functioning outflow pathways, similar to the effect of various medications (eg, beta-blockers). Response depends on the treatment method and amount of pretreatment aqueous humor outflow impediment.

INDICATIONS AND CONTRAINDICATIONS

Refractory glaucoma is the usual indication for TSCPC.[1] This includes failures of previous filtering surgery, eyes with limited vision potential and excessively high IOP despite maximum acceptable medical treatment, painful glaucomatous eyes with both highly elevated IOP and little or no vision potential, eyes with severe surface scarring precluding additional filtration procedures, or eyes with recent onset (open-angle stage) of neovascular glaucoma. TSCPC may be helpful in eyes with refractory glaucoma after penetrating keratoplasty, uveitic glaucoma, intravitreal silicone oil, refractory pediatric glaucoma, and failure of previous tube-shunt surgery. Patients with medical contraindications or who refuse invasive surgery may be able to have TSCPC.

Eyes with recalcitrant glaucoma are often at risk of imminent loss of vision from glaucoma. Eyes with good vision are not excluded, but approximately 25% of eyes with serious glaucoma problems have postoperative vision worse than the pretreatment level, whereas some eyes have slightly improved vision.[2]

Kahook M.
Essentials of Glaucoma Surgery (pp 213–220).
© 2012 SLACK Incorporated.

TSCPC is not for eyes with total occlusion of outflow, as complete cessation of inflow would be required for IOP to be reduced to acceptable levels, and labile IOP reduction would likely result.

TSCPC is often performed in an office setting or a minor surgery facility. The procedure usually requires retrobulbar anesthesia, but it can be done with general anesthesia.

BENEFITS

The surgeon can perform TSCPC expeditiously in urgent situations. TSCPC does not preclude alternative procedures if it fails. Reported success of the first step of TSCPC after 1 to 2 years varies from 50% to more than 90%.[1,3]

RISKS

Postoperative pain is common during the first 48 hours. Rarely, there is hyphema or fibrinous reaction. TSCPC is not incisional, so risk of postoperative intraocular infection is absent. The procedure may fail to control the IOP elevation sufficiently, requiring a second or third step of TSCPC.

SURGERY

Preparation

Patients should be aware of the plan, requirements, benefits, risks, and alternatives; all questions should be addressed. Warn patients about potential for postoperative pain, possible reduced vision, and possibility of need for more than one step of treatment to achieve control. Surgery is done with infrared, 810-nm diode laser irradiation delivered with a fiber optic handpiece (G-Probe, Iridex Corp, Mountain View, California). The surgeon assures the Iridex OcuLight SLx system or the Iridex IQ 810 system is ready to use and working prior to anesthesia.

Anesthesia

Local peribulbar and retrobulbar anesthesia is the usual method. Subconjunctival anesthesia may be adequate, yet TSCPC requires a thorough block; lesser amounts of anesthesia are seldom sufficient. Gentle touching of the perilimbal conjunctiva with forceps allows testing for sufficient numbness.

TABLE 25-1. Power and Duration Settings for Slow Coagulation Transscleral Cyclophotocoagulation Technique			
Iris Color	Power (W)	Duration (s)	Energy Per Application (J)
Brown	1.25	4.0 to 4.5	5.0 to 5.6
All others	1.5	3.5 to 4.0	5.25 to 6.0

Methods

Two approaches for laser delivery with the G-Probe are as follows:

Slow Coagulation Technique

For eyes with dark and medium brown iris color, use 1.25-W power and 4.0- to 4.5-s duration (5.0 to 5.6 J per application). For eyes with lesser degrees of iris pigmentation (light brown, hazel, or blue) use 1.5-W power and 3.5- to 4.0-s duration (5.25 to 6.0 J per application) (Table 25-1). "Pops," as described below, rarely occur when using this technique.

Original Technique

Start with 1.75-W power and 2.0-s duration (3.5 J per application); adjust power downward or upward in 0.25-W increments according to whether there are excessive tissue "pops" (evidence of boiling of intracellular water and aqueous) during applications. Eyes with darker pigmentation require slightly lower power and energy per application to obtain equivalent results. With this technique, occasional "pops" will occur. If they occur with every application, the power is too high and should be reduced. Consider lengthening the duration of the laser applications at lower power.

DETAILS OF TREATMENT

Eye Protection

The G-Probe is ready for use on opening its sterile package. Cleaning is not necessary; however, if it becomes contaminated with tissue debris during the procedure, clean the G-Probe tip. Discard the probe if debris or discoloration on the tip is not removed by cleaning. Conjunctival or scleral burns are not typical and indicate contamination at the tip.[4] Retinal irradiation due to laser transmission during TSCPC with the G-Probe is well within safety guidelines.

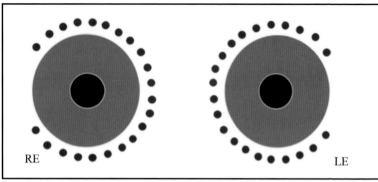

Figure 25-1. First step of TSCPC treatment showing locations for applications in right eye (RE) or left eye (LE). Surgeon makes approximately 21 to 23 applications (7 applications per quadrant), omitting the temporal quadrant.

Keep the eye surface moist during treatment to enhance probe-tip-to-eye mating. This is especially true if the surgeon uses a lid retractor that inhibits blinking.

Delivery

Extent

With the slit-lamp biomicroscope or other magnified observation, treat 3 quadrants, making approximately 7 applications per quadrant. Omit the temporal quadrant for the first step of treatment (Figure 25-1). For a second step on a later date, if needed, again treat 3 quadrants but turned 45 degrees, thus omitting either the upper or lower temporal quadrant.

Treatment is facilitated by having the slit lamp biomicroscope oriented 45 degrees from the visual axis on the temporal side with the illuminating light coaxial while the fiber optic is parallel to the visual axis (Figure 25-2).

The location and spacing of applications are guided by the footplate of the G-Probe (Figures 25-2 and 25-3). The protruding fiber optic tip is hemispherical in shape. It indents conjunctiva, Tenon's fascia, and sclera during treatment, increasing clarity to infrared photons.

During applications, the footplate is positioned with the curved anterior edge on the anterior border of the limbus. Each application blanches 3 to 4 ciliary processes. Each subsequent application is spaced one-half width of the footplate. The rounded fiber optic tip, protruding 0.7 mm from the footplate, causes a slight indentation at each treatment site. This

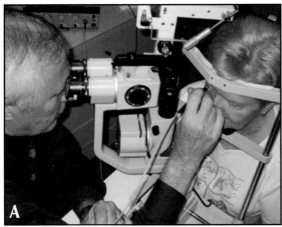

Figure 25-2. (A) Patient sitting at the slit-lamp biomicroscope with surgeon applying G-Probe to eye parallel to visual axis while observing approximately 45 degrees off the visual axis, from the temporal side. Illuminating light coaxial with microscope. (B) Left eye treatment showing alignment of the inner surface of the G-Probe at the anterior edge of limbus.

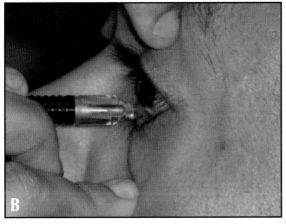

is a marker for the next application (ie, during the next application, the trailing edge of the footplate bisects the indention at the site of the previous application).

POSTOPERATIVE MANAGEMENT

Apply a strong, long-lasting cycloplegic and a topical steroid after the procedure and patch the eye. Continue cycloplegic twice daily and steroid drops 3 or 4 times daily for at least 2 weeks and longer if required.

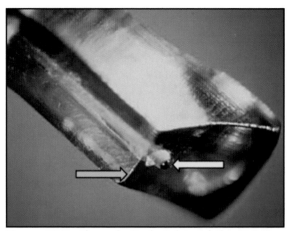

Figure 25-3. Clear plastic footplate of the G-Probe. Hemispherical tip of fiberoptic (yellow arrow) protrudes 0.7 mm from curved mating surface that matches sclera curvature. Anterior edge (green arrow) matches curvature of limbus. When lid speculum is not used, the back surface of the G-Probe can retract the lid.

POTENTIAL POSTOPERATIVE PROBLEMS

Change of Visual Acuity

Decrease of 2 or more Snellen lines has been reported in various studies in anywhere from 12% to 40% of eyes treated with TSCPC (mean: approximately 25%).[2,3] Eyes with pre-existing poor vision appear more likely to experience a decrease in visual function. The decrease of vision, which sometimes improves with healing, has to be considered compared with the expected deterioration that would occur in the absence of intervention. Although it is seldom discussed, improved vision has also been observed after TSCPC.[1,2]

Sympathetic Ophthalmia

This serious problem has occurred in a small number of fellow eyes after ciliary destructive procedures.[5] According to anecdotal reports, one case followed diode laser TSCPC in a child and another occurred in an adult.

Phthisis

In one series of 206 eyes, phthisis occurred in 4 (1.9%) eyes after TSCPC.[2] There are anecdotal reports of additional cases, usually in eyes with severe problems.

Outcomes

The IOP will often dip during the first weeks. Often, as inflammation clears, IOP slowly rises to a new plateau lower than the pretreatment level. Starting after approximately 6 weeks, provided a substantial decrease of IOP has occurred and has been maintained, medications for glaucoma may be reduced while monitoring to assure IOP stays within target. Patients are often able to reduce slightly topical or systemic medical glaucoma treatment after TSCPC, yet most eyes continue to need some medical treatment.

REFERENCES

1. Kosoko O, Gaasterland DE, Pollack IP, Enger CL; The Diode Laser Ciliary Ablation Study Group. Long-term outcome of initial ciliary ablation with contact diode laser transscleral cyclophotocoagulation for severe glaucoma. *Ophthalmology.* 1996;103(8):1294-1202.

2. Wilensky JT, Kammer J. Long-term visual outcome of transscleral laser cyclotherapy I: eyes with ambulatory vision. *Ophthalmology.* 2008;111(7):1389-1392.

3. Pastor SA, Singh K, Lee DA, et al. Cyclophotocoagulation. A report by the American Academy of Ophthalmology. *Ophthalmology.* 2001;108(11):2130-2138.

4. Gaasterland D, Pollack I. Initial experience with a new method of laser transscleral cyclophotocoagulation for ciliary ablation in severe glaucoma. *Trans Am Ophthalmol Soc.* 1992;90:225-246.

5. Bechrakis NE, Müller-Stolzenburg NE, Helbig H, et al. Sympathetic ophthalmia following laser cyclocoagulation. *Arch Ophthalmol.* 1994;112(1):80-84.

26

ENDOCYCLOPHOTOCOAGULATION

Nathan M. Radcliffe, MD and Malik Y. Kahook, MD

As described in Chapter 25 on transscleral cyclophotocoagulation (TSCPC), destruction of ciliary body tissue reduces aqueous humor formation and lowers intraocular pressure (IOP). Because the ciliary tissue cannot be directly visualized with this approach, the titration of the dose can be difficult, resulting in overtreatment (hypotony) or undertreatment, often necessitating multiple laser procedures. While this chapter is focused on the use of endocyclophotocoagulation (ECP) with cataract extraction (CE), this chapter also delves into the specifics of ECP and offers pearls for practice from our experience.

ECP is an ab interno (rather than transscleral) approach for cycloablation that utilizes the E2 microprobe laser and endoscopy system (Endo Optiks Inc, Little Silver, New Jersey) with an 810-nm diode laser, a 175-W xenon light source, and a helium neon laser-aiming beam. The single probe contains an endoscope attached to the laser, and this endoscope can also be used as a diagnostic tool because it allows for direct visualization of intraocular structures. Two probe sizes are available: the 20-gauge probe can provide a 70-degree field of view and a depth of focus ranging from 0.5 to 15.0 mm, whereas the 18-gauge system provides a field of view of 110 degrees, with a depth of focus ranging from 1 to 30 mm. Also, there are options between straight and curved probes, with the curved option providing greater ability to access more ciliary processes through a single incision.

MECHANISM OF ACTION

ECP causes coagulative necrotic damage to the ciliary body epithelium along with tissue contraction, sparing of the ciliary muscle, and minimal vascular destruction.[1] In contrast, TSCPC causes more profound destruction of ciliary body architecture, including the ciliary body muscle.

Kahook M.
Essentials of Glaucoma Surgery (pp 221–226).
© 2012 SLACK Incorporated.

Rationale

EPC (through a transcorneal approach) is one of a few incisional glaucoma surgeries that does not sacrifice conjunctiva that could be used for future filtration surgeries. Additionally, ECP does not invade Schlemm's canal and does not eliminate future canal-based surgery (eg, canaloplasty). Furthermore, because hypotony and other severe complications seen with TSCPC are rarely seen with ECP, and because ECP can be combined with cataract surgery with minimal additional time and manipulation, ECP may have a role for glaucoma management earlier in the glaucoma spectrum than many other incisional surgeries.

Common Indications

1. Patients undergoing phacoemulsification who use 2 or more topical glaucoma medications with or without controlled IOP.
2. Patients with poorly controlled glaucoma despite maximal medical therapy and IOP under 35 mm, particularly in the presence of extensive conjunctival scarring from previous glaucoma surgery.
3. Eyes with opaque and failed corneas or keratoprostheses in which the ECP probe may be valuable for diagnosis and treatment.
4. Plateau iris syndrome with elevated IOPs and persistent angle closure after cataract extraction in which endocycloplasty has the potential to correct the ciliary malposition.

Relative Contraindications

1. Active uveitic glaucoma
2. IOP greater than 40 mm Hg

Necessary Equipment and Materials

1. Twenty- or 18-gauge endoprobe with 810-nm diode laser, a 175-W xenon light source, and a helium neon laser-aiming beam
2. Healon GV ophthalmic viscoelastic device (or other cohesive viscoelastic)
3. 15-degree paracentesis blade
4. Irrigation and aspiration unit
5. Balanced salt solution on a cannula
6. 10-0 nylon suture

PROCEDURE

Obtain Informed Consent

In addition to a discussion of the patient's glaucoma prognosis and the risks, benefits, and alternatives of continuing present management or alternative procedures, such as incisional surgery, the patient should be informed that he or she may experience mild discomfort during the procedure; that the surgery is not guaranteed to be effective; and that complications, such as anterior segment inflammation and hyphema, are possible; in addition to other rare complications of incisional surgery, such as endophthalmitis or choroidal hemorrhage. Theoretically these risks are already present if the eye is being incised for cataract surgery at the same sitting.

Anesthesia

ECP may be performed with topical/intracameral anesthesia or after retrobulbar block (RBB). While RBB tends to provide exceptional intra- and postoperative pain control, the standard risks associated with RBB are present and must be considered. Topical anesthesia is performed in 2 stages, with topical lidocaine jelly applied to the cornea and into the superior and inferior fornices prior to preparing and draping the patient, followed by an intracameral injection of unpreserved lidocaine 1% into the anterior chamber for ciliary anesthesia just prior to ophthalmic viscoelastic device (OVD) placement and cyclophotocoagulation. Both RBB and topical approaches are performed with monitored anesthesia care with conscious sedation.

Surgical Approach

A clear corneal incision is created with a 15-degree paracentesis blade. The phacoemulsification main wound may also be employed. Prior to the entry of the ECP probe, the anterior chamber is filled and the ciliary sulcus is inflated with Healon GV, depressing the capsule (or intraocular lens [IOL] and capsule if the patient is already pseudophakic) and elevating the iris with the cohesive OVD. Three probes are available: straight, curved (preferred by the authors), or hockey stick-shaped. In the case of combined ECP and cataract extraction, ECP is performed just prior to IOL insertion. ECP treatment with a curved probe is then performed for 270 degrees with 0.25-W of energy set on continuous mode, although 360-degrees of treatment can be achieved through 2 corneal incisions (100 degrees apart) for greater treatment effect.[2] The clinical endpoint is blanching/whitening and shrinking of the ciliary processes (Figure 26-1). A slow and deliberate "painting" of the laser along the ciliary processes is preferred, rather than

Figure 26-1. Ciliary processes are in view through the endoscope and appear white and shrunken after treatment.

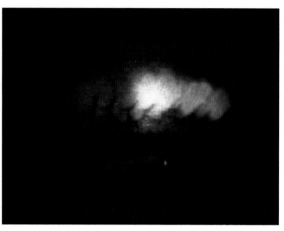

the delivery of discrete applications. The laser is applied to both the anterior and posterior extent of the ciliary processes, and any bubble formation is indicative that too much energy has been applied, either in duration, laser power, or proximity. Optimally, the ECP probe is held within 2 mm of the ciliary processes, and this location will typically allow 6 ciliary processes in the view of the endoscope.[3] In the case of ECP for plateau iris syndrome, the laser is concentrated more on the posterior aspects of the ciliary processes and the clinical endpoint is the above, plus posterior rotation of the ciliary processes with deepening of the peripheral anterior chamber. After the treatment has been performed (and the IOL has been implanted), the OVD is removed and the anterior chamber is appropriately pressurized with balanced salt solution. All wounds are confirmed to be watertight, and standard postcataract medical therapy is initialized, usually with topical steroids, nonsteroidal anti-inflammatory drugs, and topical antibiotic.

EFFICACY

In a head-to-head prospective comparison of ECP and Ahmed valve implantation in 68 eyes of 68 patients with refractory glaucoma, Lima et al[4] found that after 24 months follow-up, the IOP was 14.73 ± 6.44 mm Hg in the Ahmed group and 14.07 ± 7.21 mm Hg in the ECP group (P = .7), with roughly 70% of patients in both groups achieving a successful outcome. Comparing complications between the Ahmed and ECP groups, there was a 17.6% versus 3.0% rate of choroidal detachment, a 17.6% versus 0% rate of flat anterior chamber, and a 14.7 versus 17.6% rate of hyphema, respectively. Gayton et al[5] prospectively randomized 58 eyes of 58 patients to receive phacotrabeculectomy versus phacoemulsification/ECP. They found that 30% of ECP-treated patients achieved IOP below 19 mm Hg without medication and 65% achieved IOP below 19 mm Hg with medication, as opposed to 40% and 52% in the trabeculectomy group, respectively.

CONCLUSION

ECP, particularly when combined with cataract extraction, offers a safe and effective approach for IOP reduction in the glaucoma patient. The surgery is minimally invasive, does not eliminate future surgical options, and likely has a role earlier in the management of glaucoma patients than some other surgical options.

KEY POINTS

1. ECP allows for focused treatment of the ciliary processes with minimal collateral damage.

2. ECP is often combined with cataract surgery but can also be effective as a stand-alone procedure.

3. As with other ab interno procedures, ECP does not cause scarring of the conjunctiva and thus does not negatively influence future filtration surgery if needed.

REFERENCES

1. Pantcheva MB, Kahook MY, Schuman JS, Rubin MW, Noecker RJ. Comparison of acute structural and histopathological changes of the porcine ciliary processes after endoscopic cyclophotocoagulation and transscleral cyclophotocoagulation. *Clin Experiment Ophthalmol.* 2007;35(3):270-274.

2. Kahook MY, Lathrop KL, Noecker RJ. One-site versus two-site endoscopic cyclophotocoagulation. *J Glaucoma.* 2007;16(6):527-530.

3. Yu JY, Kahook MY, Lathrop KL, Noecker RJ. The effect of probe placement and type of viscoelastic material on endoscopic cyclophotocoagulation laser energy transmission. *Ophthalmic Surg Lasers Imaging.* 2008;39(2):133-136.

4. Lima FE, Magacho L, Carvalho DM, Susanna R Jr, Avila MP. A prospective, comparative study between endoscopic cyclophotocoagulation and the Ahmed drainage implant in refractory glaucoma. *J Glaucoma.* 2004;13(3):233-237.

5. Gayton JL, Van Der Karr M, Sanders V. Combined cataract and glaucoma surgery: trabeculectomy versus endoscopic laser cycloablation. *J Cataract Refract Surg.* 1999;25(9):1214-1219.

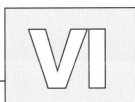

LESS COMMON SURGERIES

27

SURGICAL IRIDECTOMY

Stephen P. Verb, MD, MHSA and Nauman Imami, MD, MHSA

Incisional iridectomy was first introduced by Albrecht von Graefe as a procedure for the treatment of glaucoma in Germany during the period of 1855 to 1860.[1] The iridectomy performed by von Graefe involved excision of the iris through a scleral incision without a conjunctival flap. von Graefe thought that it was the iris tissue itself that, when removed, lowered the intraocular pressure (IOP).[2] At that time, this was the only surgery widely used to treat all forms of glaucoma, and it was plagued with complications.

Today, surgical iridectomy is used to treat angle-closure glaucoma secondary to a pupil block mechanism. In modern practice, laser iridotomy is preferred over incisional iridectomy because it is quick and easy to perform, has a high success rate, has a low complication rate, and has fewer risks when compared with incisional iridectomy.[3] Laser iridotomy is performed by utilizing the Nd:YAG laser and/or argon laser to create a communication between the anterior and posterior chamber, which equalizes the pressure between the 2 compartments, thus reducing the risk of angle-closure glaucoma.

Although largely replaced by laser iridotomy, situations may still arise in which an incisional iridectomy is the preferred technique. Specific situations that may require surgical iridectomy include the following:

- No laser available (such as in developing countries).
- Corneal opacification limiting the view of the anterior chamber.
- Patient unable to cooperate with the laser technique (examples include positioning issues or dementia).
- Repeated closure of the iridotomy secondary to an inflammatory membrane.

Kahook M.
Essentials of Glaucoma Surgery (pp 229-238).
© 2012 SLACK Incorporated.

Figure 27-1. Peripheral iridectomy in conjunction with trabeculectomy.

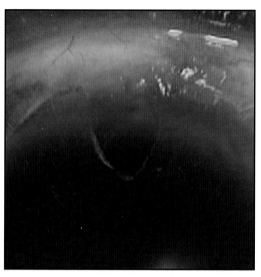

In addition to the previous situations, surgical iridectomy may be combined with other surgical procedures, including the following:

- Trabeculectomy (to avoid occlusion of the sclerostomy by the iris) (Figure 27-1).
- Insertion of phakic[4,5] or anterior chamber intraocular lenses (IOLs) (to avoid pupil block).
- Corneal surgery such as Descemet's stripping endothelial keratoplasty (DSEK; to prevent pupil block from the air bubble).
- Intracapsular cataract extraction (to avoid pupil block by vitreous).
- Vitrectomy with silicone oil placement (inferiorly to prevent pupil block by the oil).

Other less common situations necessitating surgical iridectomy include the following:

- Biopsy or excision of iris or ciliary body lesions.
- Creation of an optical iridectomy in patients with significant corneal opacification.[6,7]

PREOPERATIVE CONSIDERATIONS

A thorough ophthalmic and medical history and a complete ophthalmic examination should be performed prior to surgical iridectomy. Medication history is important to inquire about use of anticoagulants including warfarin and nonsteroidal anti-inflammatory medications, such as aspirin and ibuprofen. Although the urgent or emergent nature of surgical iridectomy often prevents sufficient time off the medication to reverse the anticoagulant effect, anticoagulants should be stopped if medically possible. This is often done in conjunction with the patient's primary care physician. On examination, particular attention should be paid to corneal clarity, presence or absence of conjunctival scarring, the status of the lens, and presence or absence of silicone oil in the eye. Preoperative assessment of these issues is important to determine the location of the planned iridectomy.

Appropriate informed and signed consent should be obtained from the patient or legal guardian. One hour before surgery, one drop of Vigamox (moxifloxacin 0.5%), or an equivalent antibiotic, and one drop of pilocarpine 1% are instilled into the operative eye every 5 minutes for 3 doses. The broad antibiotic spectrum of a fourth-generation fluoroquinolone provides prophylaxis against ocular infections. The direct cholinergic properties of pilocarpine cause miosis, placing the iris on stretch and facilitating formation of a basal iridectomy.

ANESTHESIA

Surgical iridectomy should be performed in the operating room under monitored anesthesia care. A subconjunctival injection of 1% preservative-free lidocaine is usually adequate for anesthesia. This is performed by injecting 0.2 to 0.4 mL of lidocaine through a 30-gauge needle at the planned site of the conjunctival incision.

If anesthesia and akinesia are required, or if there is significant preoperative pain, as can be present with an attack of acute angle-closure crisis, a retrobulbar block with a 50-50 mixture of 4% lidocaine and 0.75% bupivicaine may be considered instead of local anesthesia. The block is performed by injecting 2 to 4 mL of the mixture into the muscle cone with a blunt 23-gauge needle (Atkinson retrobulbar, Eagle Labs, Rancho Cucamonga, California). A retrobulbar block carries with it specific complications, such as retrobulbar hemorrhage and globe perforation. In the rare event that such a complication were to occur, it should be able to be appropriately managed by the surgeon.

Patient situations in which general anesthesia with an endotracheal tube or laryngeal mask airway should be considered include young age, tremor, and dementia.

OPERATIVE TECHNIQUE

Povidone-iodine 5% is used to prepare the eyelids, skin, and conjunctiva. The eyelids are then draped in the standard ophthalmic surgical fashion. An eyelid speculum is used to retract the drape and lashes from the surgical field. Blunt Westcott scissors are used to perform a 3-mm superior conjunctival peritomy. Wet-field cautery is used to provide adequate hemostasis.

A diamond blade set at 375-μm depth is used to create a partial-thickness scleral incision 2 mm behind and tangential to the limbus. Using 0.12-mm toothed forceps to stabilize the globe, a crescent blade is used to create a corneoscleral tunnel just beyond the limbal vessels. Vanass scissors are used to fashion a partial-thickness scleral flap.

If technically possible, a 15-degree paracentesis incision knife is used to create a temporal clear corneal paracentesis (this may be technically challenging due to shallow anterior chamber depth in phakic patients). A syringe containing 1% preservative-free lidocaine on a 30-gauge cannula may be injected into the anterior chamber to provide additional anesthesia. If necessary, a 0.5 to 2 mL acetylcholine chloride (Miochol-E) solution may be injected into the anterior chamber to assist with iris sphincter contraction.

The 15-degree blade is then used to enter the anterior chamber parallel to the iris at the end of the corneoscleral tunnel. The iris is mechanically prolapsed through the incision by gently pushing on the posterior lip of the wound with a blunt instrument. The iris is then grasped with the 0.12-mm forceps and cut with iris scissors. Care must be taken to incise both the stromal and pigment layers of the iris to create a full-thickness iridectomy. The iris is repositioned into the anterior chamber by gently stroking the cornea with a blunt instrument, such as a muscle hook.

The scleral wound is closed with 2 interrupted sutures at the corners of the scleral flap with a 10-0 nylon suture on a spatulated needle (Ethilon TG160-6, Ethicon, Somerville, New Jersey). The conjunctiva is then closed with an 8-0 polyglactin 910 suture on a vascular needle (Vicryl BV130-4, Ethicon).

A subconjunctival injection of 0.1 mL of 1% dexamethasone sodium phosphate may be given. One drop of Vigamox or an equivalent antibiotic is applied to the operative eye. The drapes are removed and a shield is applied. If a block was given, neomycin/polymyxin B/dexamethasone ointment (neomycin-polymyxin-dexamethasone ointment) is applied and the eye is patched and shielded.

Postoperatively, the patient is routinely started on atropine 1% once daily, Vigamox 4 times a day, and prednisolone acetate 1% 4 times a day.

VARIATIONS

We prefer a limbal approach to iridectomy as opposed to a clear corneal approach. The downside of the clear corneal approach is that it may be technically difficult to perform a basal iridectomy. When using a clear corneal approach, the angle of entry into the anterior chamber must be perpendicular to the cornea to allow for a basal iridectomy.[3] Without the benefit of a tunnel, closure of this wound is critical to prevent wound leak, often necessitating 10-0 nylon sutures. Furthermore, corneal sutures may induce astigmatism,

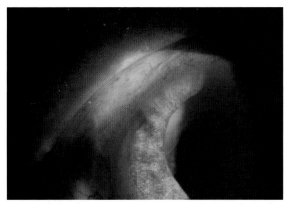

Figure 27-2. Peripheral iridectomy created with the vitrector using a posterior approach in conjunction with pars plana vitrectomy for management of aqueous misdirection.

cause foreign body sensation, and cause corneal infection or abscess. The benefit of a clear corneal incision is that it does not involve manipulation of the conjunctiva, thereby preserving the conjunctiva for future glaucoma surgery.

Some surgeons have used a vitrector to create an iridectomy.[6,8] This has been performed through a clear corneal wound with the benefits of preserving the conjunctiva and avoiding a scleral tunnel. This procedure can be performed with an irrigation port or under a dispersive ophthalmic viscoelastic device (OVD) to maintain the anterior chamber. If the patient is phakic, the OVD should be placed in the ciliary sulcus, allowing for protection against damage to the lens. When positioning the vitrector, the aspiration port should be facing the iris tissue at the site of the planned iridectomy. The vitrector setting should be placed on irrigation-aspiration-cut mode, with the cut rate set at 20 cuts per minute.[9] After the iris is engaged, the vitrector is used to fashion a small peripheral iridectomy. The vitrectomy approach is an ideal method to create a small superior iridectomy after temporal phacoemulsification with placement of an anterior chamber IOL.

The vitrector can also be used from a posterior approach to create an iridectomy if needed in conjunction with pars plana vitrectomy in patients who are pseudophakic or aphakic (Figure 27-2). The pars plana vitrector-assisted iridectomy is used in conjunction with pars plana vitrectomy for the treatment of aqueous misdirection when Nd:YAG lysis of the anterior hyaloid face fails to create a communication between the anterior and posterior chambers.

Sector iridectomy involves excision of the iris near its root up to the pupillary sphincter. Excision of iris tumors may necessitate a sector iridectomy, and this may be performed in conjunction with removal of a portion of the ciliary body (iridocyclectomy). A modified sector iridectomy has been used in the creation of an optical iridectomy in children and adults with corneal opacifications.[6,7]

Figure 27-3. Inferior peripheral iridectomy for management of acute angle closure glaucoma after unsuccessful laser iridotomy.

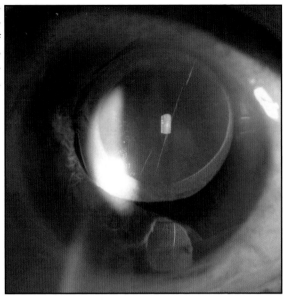

LOCATION OF SURGICAL IRIDECTOMY

The location of the iridectomy is determined by the clinical situation. The 12 o'clock position is the preferred location for iridectomy. The upper lid covers the iridectomy opening, reducing the incidence of visual disturbances. The iridectomy size should be such that it can be completely covered by the upper lid. Theoretically, an iridotomy should be at least 150 to 200 μm to safely prevent angle closure.[10] This should not be an problem when creating a surgical iridectomy because this technique will produce an iridectomy that is larger than 200 μm. Partially exposed iridectomies may have increased risk for visual disturbances such as monocular diplopia, lines, crescents, shadows, and ghost images.[11] After vitrectomy with placement of silicone oil, it is appropriate to place an iridectomy inferiorly to prevent pupil block caused by the oil.[12] Silicone oil (specific gravity: 0.97) floats above the aqueous and can potentially occlude a superior iridectomy. An inferior iridectomy breaks this block, allowing free passage of aqueous between the anterior and posterior chambers. A superior iridectomy may be created if heavy silicone oil is used. An inferior iridectomy may also be considered in situations in which future glaucoma surgery is being contemplated. In this case, anatomical preservation of the superior conjunctiva is important to allow for successful filtering surgery and bleb formation (Figure 27-3).

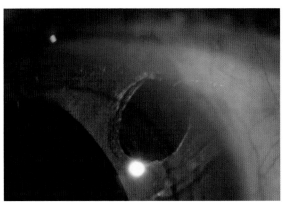

Figure 27-4. Incomplete peripheral iridectomy with remaining posterior pigmented layer of the iris.

COMPLICATIONS

Incomplete iridectomy is caused when only the anterior layers of the iris tissue are removed, leaving the posterior pigmented layer (Figure 27-4). An incomplete iridectomy may lead to occlusion of the sclerostomy and elevation of the IOP. Patency of the iridectomy should be confirmed intraoperatively by observing a red reflex through the iridectomy or by wiping the iris specimen on the surgical drape, demonstrating deposition of pigment. Intraoperatively, the exposed posterior pigmented layer can be aspirated with a 25-gauge cannula as described by Hoffer.[5] If discovered postoperatively, argon or Nd:YAG laser may be used to complete the iridectomy.[13]

Postoperative shallow or flat anterior chamber are also caused by wound leak. Seidel testing should be performed using a moistened fluorescein strip at the end of the procedure to evaluate for the presence of a leaking wound. Meticulous surgical technique and use of a beveled triplanar scleral tunnel helps prevent persistent wound leak and conjunctival bleb formation. Wound leak can be managed pharmacologically with aqueous suppressants, cycloplegics, and topical antibiotics. Additionally, placing a bandage contact lens or patching can help the conjunctiva heal at the limbus, eliminating the leak. Persistent leaks may need to be operatively repaired. In the setting of a shallow or flat anterior chamber, the IOP measurement is important. If the IOP is low, there may be conjunctival bleb formation with overfiltration or wound leak. Choroidal effusion often presents as a shallow flat anterior chamber with low IOP. If the anterior chamber is flat and the IOP is high, one must consider choroidal hemorrhage or aqueous misdirection in the differential diagnosis. After confirmation of patent iridectomy and watertight wound, evaluation of the posterior chamber should be performed by indirect ophthalmoscopy or

B-scan ultrasonography. Choroidal effusion or hemorrhage and aqueous misdirection should be managed appropriately, potentially in conjunction with a retinal surgeon.

Other complications of iridectomy include cataract and hyphema. Cataract may develop from inadvertent injury to the crystalline lens or from disruption of the lens capsule. This can be managed conservatively unless significant inflammation or worsening vision develops, necessitating lens extraction. Hyphema may develop from transection of iris vessels. Although usually not necessary, cautery may be used to help minimize iris bleeding. If hyphema does occur, it is usually minimal and transient, and observation is advised. If necessary, anterior chamber washout with balanced salt solution and injection of OVD can be employed to tamponade the bleeding during the surgery.

CONCLUSION

Although largely replaced by laser iridotomy, incisional iridectomy is necessary in a variety of situations and remains an important component of the glaucoma surgeon's armamentarium. Newer variations of the traditional iridectomy include using a clear corneal approach or employing the use of the vitrector as a cutting instrument. It is imperative for the glaucoma surgeon to understand and be able to manage the potential postoperative complications of iridectomy.

KEY POINTS

1. Although largely replaced by laser iridotomy, situations may arise where an incisional iridectomy is the preferred technique.

2. A partial-thickness scleral flap is the preferred approach compared with a clear corneal technique.

3. A vitrector may also be used to create a surgical iridectomy, especially in the setting of aqueous misdirection.

4. Incomplete iridectomy is the most common complication. The cause of the flat anterior chamber should be determined and managed appropriately, and the IOP is an important component of this evaluation.

REFERENCES

1. Habegger H. Iridectomy—A century of progress. *N Engl J Med.* 1955;252(23):992-993.
2. Albert DM, Edwards DD. *The History of Ophthalmology.* Cambridge, MA: Blackwell Science; 1996.
3. Allingham RR. *Shields' Textbook of Glaucoma.* Philadelphia, PA: Lippincott Willliams & Wilkins; 2005.

4. Huang D, Schallhorn SC, Sugar A, et al. Phakic intraocular lens implantation for the correction of myopia: a report by the American Academy of Ophthalmology. *Ophthalmology.* 2009;116(11):2244-2258.
5. Hoffer KJ. Pigment vacuum iridectomy for phakic refractive lens implantation. *J Cataract Refract Surg.* 2001;27(8):1166-1168.
6. Agarwal T, Jhanji V, Dutta P, et al. Automated vitrector-assisted optical iridectomy: customized iridectomy. *J Cataract Refract Surg.* 2007;33(6):959-961.
7. Sundaresh K, Jethani J, Vijayalakshmi P. Optical iridectomy in children with corneal opacities. *J AAPOS.* 2008;12(2):163-165.
8. Finger PT. Small incision surgical iridotomy and iridectomy. *Graefes Arch Clin Exp Ophthalmol.* 2006;244(3):399-400.
9. Day A, Angunawela RI, Allan BD. Blow-back technique for confirmation of peripheral iridectomy patency. *J Cataract Refract Surg.* 2008;34(11):1832-1833.
10. Fleck BW. How large must an iridotomy be? *Br J Ophthalmol.* 1990;74(10):583.
11. Spaeth GL, Idowu O, Seligsohn A, et al. The effects of iridotomy size and position on symptoms following laser peripheral iridotomy. *J Glaucoma.* 2005;14(5):364-367.
12. Ichhpujani P, Jindal A, Jay Katz L. Silicone oil induced glaucoma: a review. *Graefes Arch Clin Exp Ophthalmol.* 2009;247(12):1585-1593.
13. Tessler HH, Peyman GA, Huamonte F, Menachof I. Argon laser iridotomy in incomplete peripheral iridectomy. *Am J Ophthalmol.* 1975;79(6):1051-1052.

28

REPAIR OF CYCLODIALYSIS CLEFTS

Amy Badger-Asaravala, MD and Robert Stamper, MD

A cyclodialysis cleft is a separation of the circumferential insertion of the meridional ciliary muscle fibers from the scleral spur. It often occurs as a result of blunt or penetrating trauma to the eye.[1] It may also develop as a complication of intraocular surgery, usually through unintentional manipulation of the iris. Inadvertent excision of a block of scleral spur tissue during filtration surgery can also result in a cyclodialysis cleft.[2] Opening of a cleft many years after the original trauma has been described following phacoemulsification, resulting in unexplained hypotony after seemingly uncomplicated surgery.[3] A cleft may also be created when a scleral tunnel is made too deep, or when an anterior chamber intraocular lens (IOL) implant of inappropriate size is used.[2,4] Cyclodialysis has also been used as a surgical procedure for aphakic glaucoma.[5]

EPIDEMIOLOGY

Unintentional cyclodialysis clefts have generally been thought of as being quite rare. The Erlangen Ocular Contusion Registry reported an incidence of 3.4% in patients presenting with ocular contusion or globe rupture.[6] An incidence of 2.6% has been reported in patients undergoing trabeculotomy ab externo for developmental glaucoma.[7] However, a prospective study of 92 patients presenting with closed globe injuries in which every patient underwent ultrasound biomicroscopy (UBM) found a 35% incidence of cyclodialysis clefts in those who did not develop traumatic glaucoma and an 18% incidence in those who did develop traumatic glaucoma.[8] However, not all cyclodialysis clefts result in hypotony. In a large series of cyclodialysis procedures performed for glaucoma, there was a 9% incidence of hypotony in 291 cases.[9] Cyclodialysis procedures are rarely performed today, and so cyclodialysis clefts presently occur more often as a result of trauma than surgery. In a retrospective review of 29 patients who underwent consecutive

Kahook M. *Essentials of Glaucoma Surgery* (pp 239-252). © 2012 SLACK Incorporated.

direct surgical cyclopexy during a 13-year time period, 26 clefts were the result of traumatic injury and 3 were postsurgical.[10]

SIGNS AND SYMPTOMS

The presence of a cyclodialysis cleft should be suspected in any eye with hypotony following recent surgery or trauma after all other causes have been ruled out.[11] Other common causes of postoperative hypotony include wound leaks, overfiltering blebs, choroidal effusions, retinal detachment, and aqueous suppression due to active inflammation or prior use of aqueous suppressants.[2] Free communication between the anterior chamber and the suprachoroidal space is created by the cyclodialysis cleft, often resulting in hypotony. The intraocular pressure (IOP) frequently is quite low (<5 mm Hg), resulting in secondary complications such as shallow anterior chamber, induced hyperopia, cataract progression, choroidal effusion, optic disc edema, and hypotony maculopathy.[1] If untreated, it may result in permanent vision loss or phthisis. The incidence of hypotony is dependent on the flow rate between the anterior chamber and the suprachoroidal space, which is unrelated to the size of the cyclodialysis cleft.[3] Typical presenting symptoms include eye pain, tenderness, and blurred vision.[12]

DIAGNOSIS

Various techniques may be used to identify a cyclodialysis cleft. It is important to identify the full extent of the cyclodialysis cleft and the total number of clefts to achieve complete repair of the cleft or clefts.

Gonioscopy

Using gonioscopy, the cleft appears as a deep-angle recess with a gap between the scleral spur and the ciliary body.[13] Identification of cyclodialysis clefts by gonioscopy can be challenging due to the often concomitant presence of corneal edema, hyphema, peripheral anterior synechiae, and shallow anterior chamber, as well as the softness of the hypotonous eye. Intracameral viscoelastic can improve angle visualization by making the eye firm and deepening the anterior chamber angle. Pilocarpine may also be added to induce miosis and maximally open the anterior chamber angle and cleft. However, visualization may still be poor due to corneal edema. Further, one may wish to avoid such maneuvers in the setting of hyphema by using noncontact diagnostic techniques instead.[1]

Ultrasound Biomicroscopy

UBM can provide a detailed representation of the anterior chamber, iridotrabecular angle, and ciliary body. It has been shown to be highly accurate in detecting cyclodialysis clefts, as well as anterior suprachoroidal effusions.[1] However, it can be difficult to perform in a hypotonous, tender eye.

Anterior Segment Optical Coherence Tomography

This technique has been shown to be accurate and reproducible, correlating well with UBM in the assessment of angle configuration. It has the advantage of being a noncontact technique and having higher resolution than UBM.[14] However, it does not provide visualization of the ciliary body, and thus it may miss some clefts.[1]

Scleral Transillumination

By transilluminating the sclera, a cyclodialysis cleft may be detected as a transillumination defect at the periphery of the iris.[1]

MANAGEMENT

Medical

Patients with cyclodialysis clefts may initially be managed conservatively, with atropine 1% twice daily to encourage apposition of the ciliary body to the sclera. Cycloplegia also deepens the anterior chamber and reduces the patient's discomfort. It has also been suggested that inflammation may be beneficial in promoting adhesion at the cleft site, and so reduction of postoperative steroids may be considered. Filling the anterior chamber with viscoelastic may also help break the vicious cycle of hypotony.[2] However, if medical management fails to close the cleft after 6 to 8 weeks, then more aggressive measures should be considered.

Transscleral Diathermy

In this technique, the pupil is dilated and a partial-thickness scleral flap is made in the area overlying the cleft. Diathermy is then applied in the bed of the flap in the vicinity of the cleft. This induces a localized thermal burn and secondary inflammation, encouraging closure of the cleft. Both scleral ectasia and lens damage have been reported, and no more than 4 clock hours should be treated to prevent these complications.[1,12] Adequate anesthesia with a retrobulbar or sub-Tenon's block should be achieved prior to performing this technique.

Argon Laser Photocoagulation

This technique, unlike the other nonincisional methods, requires an adequate view of the angle structures, without significant corneal edema

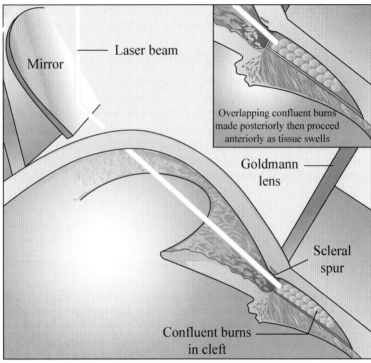

Figure 28-1. Argon laser cleft repair. Heavy confluent laser burns are applied to the scleral aspect of the cleft first, followed by the uveal aspect. (Adapted from Spaeth G, ed. *Ophthalmic Principles and Practice.* 3rd ed. Philadelphia, PA: Saunders; 2003: 384.)

or hyphema. Nevertheless, it is generally considered the first line of therapy when medical management fails. Topical anesthesia is applied, and a Goldmann 3-mirror lens is placed on the ocular surface with a coupling agent. Rows of heavy confluent burns should be placed on the scleral aspect of the cleft first, from the scleral spur toward the depths of the cleft. Then the uveal aspect of the cleft (ie, the undersurface of the ciliary body and choroid) should be treated, starting at the depth of the cleft and working anteriorly to avoid an obscured view due to uveal edema and pigment dispersion (Figure 28-1).[2] Recommended laser settings are as follows:

1. Duration of 0.1 sec.[2,12]
2. 50 to 100 μm spot size.[2,12]
3. 500 to 1500 mW power.[12] Higher powers (1000 to 3000 mW) may be used on the sclera, and lower powers (800 to 1200 mW) should be used on the uvea.[2]
4. Approximately 100 applications should be applied.[12]

Pretreatment with pilocarpine and modest hyperinflation of the anterior chamber with viscoelastic may be used to improve the view into the cleft. However, care must be taken to remove the viscoelastic material after the laser procedure to blunt the IOP elevation that may occur immediately after the procedure.[2] Atropine 1% is continued after treatment. If the initial treatment is unsuccessful, it may be repeated.[12] At higher powers, retrobulbar anesthesia is often needed.[15]

Cryotherapy

Under retrobulbar anesthesia, a curved retinal probe with a diameter of 2.8 mm (CR 3010, Mira Inc, Uxbridge, Massachusetts) is applied transconjunctivally 3 mm posterior to the limbus at the presumed location of the cyclodialysis cleft. Five overlapping applications, each with a duration of 30 seconds and a temperature of –85°C, are applied. Atropine 1% is administered postoperatively.[16] Cryotherapy is useful in the management of smaller clefts when medical management has failed. It is advantageous in that it is noninvasive and applied ab externo. Unlike transscleral diathermy, it does not destroy or thin the sclera; unlike laser photocoagulation, it does not require a clear cornea to visualize the angle.[1]

Incisional Surgery

If more conservative measures fail, then incisional surgery may be attempted. Various techniques have been described. Three methods will be described in detail here.

1. The Direct Cyclopexy Technique[2]

   This method has the advantage of providing direct visualization of the disinserted ciliary body and scleral spur, allowing the most anatomically correct closure. It is more difficult and requires intimate knowledge of limbal anatomy. However, it is often the definitive procedure when other measures have failed.

   a. Anesthesia—Adequate anesthesia should be ensured with a retrobulbar, peribulbar, or sub-Tenon's block.

   b. Anterior chamber formation—A paracentesis should be created and the anterior chamber filled with viscoelastic material to firm the globe and to allow better visualization of the cleft.

   c. Cleft identification—The location of the cleft is confirmed by gonioscopy under the microscope. A disposable cautery unit can be used to mark the extent and location of the cleft by making small burns at the limbus.

   d. Bridle suture—A bridle suture of braided polyglactin or polyester on a spatulated needle may be placed in the limbal cornea adjacent to the cyclodialysis cleft to allow rotation of the globe and adequate visualization.

e. Conjunctival peritomy—This is typically performed with micro Westcott scissors. A small radial cut is made 3 to 4 mm beyond the edge of the cleft, 1 to 2 mm posterior to the limbus. Blunt dissection is used to remove Tenon's membrane and conjunctiva from the globe. The scissor blades are kept parallel to the limbus and one blade is inserted into the sub-Tenon's space. The blades are pulled gently toward the cornea and the conjunctiva is cut. This is repeated until the peritomy extends 3 to 4 mm beyond the opposite edge of the cleft.

f. Cautery—Eraser cautery may be used to achieve hemostasis.

g. Scleral flap—A two-thirds scleral thickness rectangular flap is created extending radially 4 mm from the limbus and 1 to 2 mm beyond the edge of the cleft in length. This may be done by using a crescent blade to create a two-thirds depth scleral groove 4 mm posterior to limbus and extending 1 to 2 mm beyond each edge of the cleft. A pocket blade may be used to create a scleral tunnel extending to the limbus. Vannas scissors may be used to cut at each side of the scleral tunnel, creating the scleral flap.

h. Reattachment of the ciliary body—A full-thickness circumferential incision is made 1.5 mm posterior to the limbus within the scleral bed using a size 67 miniature surgical blade. This should result in entry into the cleft and release of aqueous. Direct visualization of the cleft should be made and light cautery applied to the exposed surface of the ciliary body. The ciliary body is then sutured to the sclera using interrupted 10-0 nylon sutures on a tapered vascular needle, spaced 1 mm apart. Each suture is passed first through the anterior lip of the scleral wound, exiting in the region of scleral spur. The next pass is through ciliary muscle away from the iris root vessels, and then through the posterior lip of the scleral flap. The sutures are then tied after all sutures have been placed (Figure 28-2).

i. Cryotherapy—Light cryotherapy may be applied at the base of the scleral bed to promote adhesion.

j. Flap closure—Simple interrupted 10-0 nylon sutures are placed at each corner of the scleral flap to suture the flap back into the scleral bed. Additional sutures should be placed as needed to securely close the flap.

k. Conjunctival closure—Buried simple interrupted sutures of 8-0 polyglactin are placed at each edge of the peritomy to reapproximate the conjunctiva to the limbus.

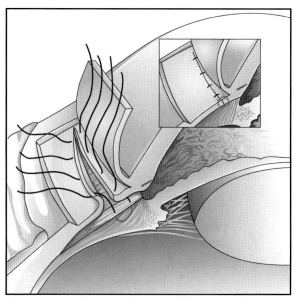

Figure 28-2. Direct cyclopexy. Each suture is passed through the anterior lip of the scleral wound, exiting in the region of the scleral spur, then through the ciliary muscle and out through the posterior lip of the scleral wound. After all sutures have been placed, each one is tied, closing the cleft. (Adapted from Spaeth G, ed. *Ophthalmic Principles and Practice*. 3rd ed. Philadelphia, PA: Saunders; 2003: 385.)

    (l) Viscoelastic removal—Balanced salt solution on a cannula may be used to inject the solution into the anterior chamber and burp the viscoelastic out. Care should be taken to ensure that the paracentesis is watertight and the eye has a physiologic IOP when this is completed.

2. The Cross Chamber Cyclopexy Technique[2]

    This is an indirect method of closure using techniques borrowed from suturing posterior chamber IOLs. It is less difficult than direct cyclopexy but may only be used in aphakic and pseudophakic eyes.

    a. Pupil dilation—Dilating drops should be applied preoperatively.

    b. Administration of anesthesia, anterior chamber formation with viscoelastic, cleft identification by gonioscopy, bridle suture placement, conjunctival peritomy creation, and cautery application are performed as described above.

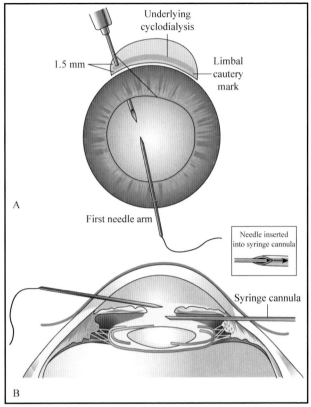

Figure 28-3. Cross chamber cyclopexy. A 27-gauge needle is passed through sclera 1.5 mm posterior to the limbus in the region of the cleft and exits through the ciliary sulcus. (A) One arm of a double-armed 10-0 polypropylene suture is passed through the keratectomy on the side opposite the cleft. (B) The straight needle is inserted into the lumen of the 27-gauge needle. The 27-gauge needle is then pulled out of the eye, together with the suture. (Adapted from Spaeth G, ed. *Ophthalmic Principles and Practice*. 3rd ed. Philadelphia, PA: Saunders; 2003: 385.)

c. Ciliary body reattachment—A 1- to 2-mm corneal keratotomy is created 180 degrees opposite the cleft with a sharp blade. A 27-gauge needle is passed ab externo through the sclera 1.5 mm posterior to the limbus at one end of the cleft, exiting through the ciliary sulcus between the iris and the posterior chamber lens. One arm of a 10-0 double-armed polypropylene suture is introduced through the keratotomy into the anterior chamber and is threaded deep into the barrel of the 27-gauge needle (Figure 28-3). The 27-gauge needle

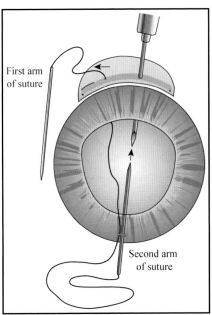

First arm
of suture

Second arm
of suture

Figure 28-4. To continue the cross-chamber cyclopexy, the suturing maneuver (see Figure 28-3) is repeated by reinserting the 27-gauge needle through the sclera 3 mm adjacent to the first pass. The second arm of the polypropylene suture is then passed through the keratectomy into the lumen of the 27-gauge needle and pulled out of the eye. (Adapted from Spaeth G, ed. *Ophthalmic Principles and Practice.* 3rd ed. Philadelphia, PA: Saunders; 2003: 386.)

is pulled along with the straight needle out of the eye, leaving the polypropylene suture passing through the keratotomy, across the anterior chamber, through the ciliary sulcus, across the cleft, and out through the sclera. The 27-gauge needle is reinserted in the same fashion 3 mm adjacent to the previous entry site. The second arm of the suture is passed through the keratotomy and inserted into the barrel of the needle, then the needles are pulled out of the eye (Figure 28-4). The 2 ends of the suture should now both be lying outside the eye on the side with the cyclodialysis cleft. The needles are removed and the suture tightened and tied, pulling the ciliary body up against the scleral wall. This maneuver is repeated as often as needed to close the full length of the cleft (Figure 28-5). The suture knots should be buried.

    d. Cryotherapy—Light cryotherapy can be applied to the sclera posterior to the sutures to promote adhesion.

    e. Viscoelastic removal and conjunctival closure are performed as above.

3. Iris Base Fixation[2,17]

    This is the easiest of the three incisional techniques but is only appropriate for smaller clefts of less than 2 clock hours because it creates broad peripheral anterior synechiae along the length of the cleft.

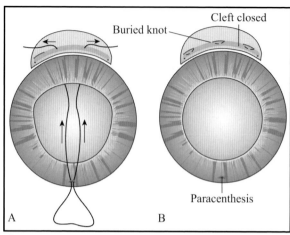

Figure 28-5. Completing the cross-chamber cyclopexy. (A) Both suture ends are pulled out where they exit the sclera, pulling a loop of suture into the anterior chamber toward the cleft. (B) The suture is tightened, pulling the cleft against the scleral wall. This technique is repeated as needed to close the entire length of the cleft. (Adapted from Spaeth G, ed. *Ophthalmic Principles and Practice.* 3rd ed. Philadelphia, PA: Saunders; 2003: 386.)

a. Anesthesia administration, anterior chamber formation with viscoelastic, cleft identification, bridle suture placement, conjunctival peritomy creation, and cautery application are performed as described previously.

b. Keratotomy—A 1- to 2-mm keratotomy is created through peripheral clear cornea 1 mm anterior to the limbus, adjacent to the cleft. For larger clefts, the keratotomy should be 1 mm shorter than the extent of the cleft.

c. Scleral flap—A scleral flap is created as descibed previously.

d. Ciliary body reattachment—One arm of a double-armed 10-0 nylon suture on a curved cutting needle is passed through the keratotomy, through peripheral iris at 1 end of the cleft, and then exits through the scleral bed 0.5 to 1 mm behind the limbus. Care should be taken not to snag the corneal endothelium. This maneuver is repeated with the second arm of the suture, catching iris 1 mm from the first iris pass (Figure 28-6). The suture is pulled taut to pull the peripheral iris against the scleral wall, then the suture is tied down. This often causes the pupil to peak

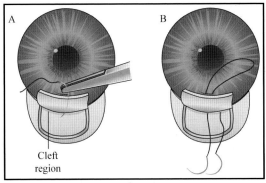

Figure 28-6. Iris base fixation. (A) One arm of the needle is passed through the keratectomy, catches peripheral iris, and exits beneath the scleral flap. (B) This maneuver is repeated with the second arm of the suture. (Adapted from Spaeth G, ed. *Ophthalmic Principles and Practice.* 3rd ed. Philadelphia, PA: Saunders; 2003: 386.)

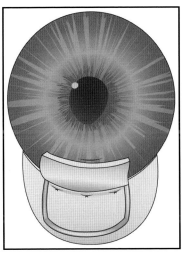

Figure 28-7. Completing the iris base fixation. Additional mattress sutures are placed as needed to close the entire length of the cleft. (Adapted from Spaeth G, ed. *Ophthalmic Principles and Practice.* 3rd ed. Philadelphia, PA: Saunders; 2003: 387.)

somewhat toward the cleft. Additional mattress sutures are placed in the same fashion as needed to span the width of the cleft (Figure 28-7).

e. Light cryotherapy at the base of the scleral flap, viscoelastic removal, scleral flap closure, and conjunctival closure are performed as noted previously.

POSTOPERATIVE CARE

Atropine 1% is used for 2 to 4 weeks, and steroids are avoided, if possible, after any of the previously mentioned surgical techniques. Postoperative topical antibiotics are also recommended after any of the previously described incisional surgical techniques. Sometimes the cleft does not immediately close, and a few weeks may pass before the hypotony is reversed, particularly after the nonincisional techniques.[12] However, after the cleft does close, an extreme spike in IOP and eye pain may occur, requiring treatment with topical and oral aqueous suppressants.[2] Patients should be warned of this possibility, and the surgeon may consider prescribing oral aqueous suppressants ahead of time to be used if the patient develops severe eye pain shortly after surgery. Pilocarpine can facilitate reopening of the cleft and thus should be avoided.[12]

COMPLICATIONS

Potential complications of any of the incisional surgical techniques include endophthalmitis and significant hemorrhage from the ciliary body. IOP elevation frequently accompanies successful cleft closure and can be dramatic. In eyes that have undergone direct cyclopexy, the pressure can rise high enough to dehisce the surgical wound if it has not been closed tightly. In most cases, the IOP can be controlled medically, and long-term treatment is usually not needed unless there has been pre-existing glaucoma.[1] One case series of cyclodialysis clefts repaired by direct cyclopexy found that the extent of the cyclodialysis cleft was positively correlated with the length of time needed for normalization of IOP, as well as with the accelerated development of cataract.[18]

PROGNOSIS

Traumatic and inadvertent surgically induced cyclodialysis clefts seldom close spontaneously, especially more than 6 weeks after the inciting event. Spontaneous closure may occur more often in children.[17] The prognosis of cyclodialysis clefts after surgical intervention is quite good. Although delayed closure may result in permanently reduced visual acuity, some patients have been reported to improve even after prolonged periods of hypotony. In one case report, a patient treated with argon laser photocoagulation improved from 20/200 to 20/30 after 7 years of hypotony.[12,19] In a series of 58 eyes with hypotonous cyclodialysis clefts that had undergone intervention after a period of hypotony ranging from 3 weeks to 3.5 years, all patients without damage to the visual pathways had a postoperative visual acuity of 20/60 or better. However, intervening within 2 months resulted in better postoperative visual acuities of 20/20 to 20/25.[17]

In contrast, a more recent series of 32 eyes showed no correlation between cleft duration and postoperative visual acuity, with durations ranging from 0.1 to 54 months.[18]

Argon laser photocoagulation and direct cyclopexy have each been shown to be highly successful in small case series. In a series of 9 patients with cyclodialysis clefts, 6 of 7 were successfully treated with argon laser photocoagulation, 2 with adjunctive diathermy, and 1 with adjunctive direct cyclopexy. In the same series, an eighth patient closed with conservative management and a ninth closed without treatment.[15] In another case series, the cyclodialysis clefts of 28 of 29 eyes were successfully closed with direct cyclopexy. This and another series demonstrated that 86% to 94% of patients experienced an improvement in visual acuity after direct cyclopexy. Mean postoperative visual acuities were 20/35 to 20/38.[10,18] Many other techniques have also been described as effective in case reports, including anterior scleral buckling, capsular tension rings, polymethyl methacrylate sulcus IOL implants, and gas endotamponade.[1]

CONCLUSION

Although conservative measures may result in closure of cyclodialysis clefts, laser, cryotherapy, or incisional surgical techniques are often required to close these clefts and reverse hypotony. Cryotherapy and laser photocoagulation may work well with smaller clefts, but incisional surgical techniques are generally needed to close larger clefts. These techniques include the direct cyclopexy technique, the cross-chamber cyclopexy technique, and iris base fixation.

KEY POINTS

1. Cyclodialysis clefts should be suspected in any eye with unexplained hypotony and a history of recent ocular surgery or trauma.

2. Identification of cyclodialysis clefts may be assisted by the use of intracameral viscoelastic during gonioscopy, UBM, or anterior segment optical coherence tomography (AS-OCT).

3. The size of the cleft does not correlate with the degree of hypotony.

4. If conservative measures, including atropine 1% and cessation of steroids fail, then cryotherapy or argon laser should be attempted.

5. If these methods also fail, then incisional surgical techniques should be used (eg the direct cyclopexy technique, the cross chamber cyclopexy technique, or iris base fixation technique).

6. Postoperative care includes atropine 1% and avoidance of steroids.

7. Patients should be warned that a dramatic IOP spike may occur immediately following successful closure of a cyclodialysis cleft. These IOP spikes should be treated with topical and oral aqueous suppressants.

REFERENCES

1. Ioannidis AS, Barton K. Cyclodialysis cleft: causes and repair. *Curr Opin Ophthalmol.* 2010;21(2):150-154.
2. Leen MM, Mills RP. Low postoperative intraocular pressure. In: Spaeth G, ed. *Ophthalmic Surgery: Principles and Practice.* Philadelphia, PA: Saunders; 2003:380-387.
3. Mushtaq B, Chiang MY, Kumar V, Ramanathan US, Shah P. Phacoemulsification, persistent hypotony, and cyclodialysis clefts. *J Cataract Refract Surg.* 2005;31(7):1428-1432.
4. Esquenazi S. Management of a displaced angle-supported anterior chamber intraocular lens. *Ophthalmic Surg Lasers Imaging.* 2006;37(1):65-67.
5. Aminlari A, Callahan CE. Medical, laser, and surgical management of inadvertent cyclodialysis cleft with hypotony. *Arch Ophthalmol* 2004;122(3):399-404.
6. Viestenz A, Kuchle M. Retrospective analysis of 417 cases of contusion and rupture of the globe with frequent avoidable causes of trauma: the Erlangen Ocular Contusion-Registry (EOCR) 1985–1995 [German]. *Klin Monbl Augenheilkd.* 2001;218(10):662-629.
7. Akimoto M, Tanihara H, Negi A, Nagata M. Surgical results of trabeculotomy ab externo for developmental glaucoma. *Arch Ophthalmol.* 1994;112(12):1540-1544.
8. Sihota R, Kumar S, Gupta V, et al. Early predictors of traumatic glaucoma after closed globe injury: trabecular pigmentation, widened angle recess, and higher baseline intraocular pressure. *Arch Ophthalmol.* 2008;126(7):921-926.
9. Viikari K, Tuovinen E. On hypotony following cyclodialysis surgery. *Acta Ophthalmol (Copenh).* 1957;35(5):543-549.
10. Kuchle M, Naumann GO. Direct cyclopexy for traumatic cyclodialysis with persisting hypotony. Report in 29 consecutive patients. *Ophthalmology.* 1995;102(2):322-333.
11. Kuhl D, Mieler WF. Ciliary body. In: Kuhn F, Pieramici DJ, eds. *Ocular Trauma: Principles and Practice.* New York, NY: Thieme; 2002:157-168.
12. Banta JT, Cebulla CM, Quinn CD. Closed globe injuries: anterior chamber. In: Banta JT, ed. *Ocular Trauma.* Philadelphia, PA: Saunders Elsevier; 2007:82-88.
13. Simmons, ST. *Basic and Clinical Science Course Section 10: Glaucoma.* San Francisco, CA: American Academy of Ophthalmology; 2007.
14. Mateo-Montoya A, Dreifuss S. Anterior segment optical coherence tomography as a diagnostic tool for cyclodialysis clefts. *Arch Ophthalmol.* 2009;127(1):109-110.
15. Ormerod LD, Baerveldt G, Sunalp MA, Riekhof FT. Management of the hypotonous cyclodialysis cleft. *Ophthalmology.* 1991;98(9):1384-1393.
16. Krohn J. Cryotherapy in the treatment of cyclodialysis cleft induced hypotony. *Acta Ophthalmol Scand.* 1997;75(1):96-98.
17. Ormerod LD, Baerveldt G, Green RL. Cyclodialysis clefts: natural history, assessment, and management. In: Weinstein GW, ed. *Open-Angle Glaucoma.* New York, NY: Churchill Livingstone; 1986:201-225.
18. Hwang JM, Ahn K, Kim C, Park KA, Kee C. Ultrasonic biomicroscopic evaluation of cyclodialysis before and after direct cyclopexy. *Arch Ophthalmol.* 2008;126(9):1222-1225.
19. Delgado MF, Daniels S, Pascal S, Dickens CJ. Hypotony maculopathy: improvement of visual acuity after 7 years. *Am J Ophthalmol.* 2001;132(6):931-933.

DRAINAGE OF
CHOROIDAL EFFUSIONS

Leon W. Herndon, MD

Serous choroidal detachment is characterized by exudative detachment of the retina and choroid following leakage of fluid from the choriocapillaris into the suprachoroidal space. This accumulation of fluid has been known to be a complication of various intraocular surgeries (cataract, glaucoma, and retinal detachment) where hypotony is combined with postoperative inflammation.[1] The terms *edema, effusion,* and *detachment* are often used interchangeably in describing this uveal disorder.

ANATOMICAL FEATURES

The suprachoroidal space forms a transition zone and potential space between the choroid and the sclera and is composed of thin connective tissue fibers that branch and connect melanocytes, smooth muscle cells, and ganglion cells. Because there are virtually no capillaries or lymphatic spaces to facilitate drain-off, fluid in this area must re-enter vascular channels in the choroid and exit by way of the vortex veins[2] or seep through perforations in the sclera.[3]

PATHOPHYSIOLOGY

The physiologic pressure in the suprachoroidal space is approximately 2 mm Hg less than the intraocular pressure (IOP) in the anterior and vitreous chambers.[4] Any decrease in the IOP is transmitted to the choroid, and the reduced pressure may promote vascular engorgement and transudation. Such mechanical factors partly explain the suprachoroidal edema that results when the pressure in the eye decreases substantially at the time of surgery or trauma.[4,5] An increase in the permeability of the choroidal

Kahook M.
Essentials of Glaucoma Surgery (pp 253-260).
© 2012 SLACK Incorporated.

vessels also increases the protein leakage into the suprachoroidal space. This reduces the intravascular colloid osmotic force that is responsible for fluid reabsorption. Relative hypotony accompanies choroidal effusion. In the past, this was attributed to decreased production of aqueous.[6] Experimental evidence[7] suggests that there is increased uveoscleral outflow in eyes with choroidal detachment. Less commonly, a hemorrhagic choroidal detachment can develop from rupture of the capillary membrane.[8]

CLINICAL FEATURES

In the clinical setting of ocular surgery, trauma, or inflammation, shallowing of the anterior chamber with a drop in intraocular pressure should suggest possible choroidal effusion. With forward displacement of the lens–iris diaphragm and angle closure, the IOP may be elevated.[9] Acute onset of myopia, resulting from the anterior displacement of the lens, may also be a clue.[10] Visual acuity usually is reduced, including light perception, depending on the degree of interference with the visual axis. Choroidal edema may resemble retinal detachment; however, darkness of the uvea, lack of tremulousness, and normal retinal vessels indicate a probable uveal process. Visualization of the ora serrata without scleral depression is also a reliable sign.[11] The onset of a hemorrhagic choroidal detachment is usually accompanied by pain, IOP elevation, and a shallow or flat anterior chamber. Detachment can occur after a Valsalva maneuver, straining at stools, coughing, or sneezing. Anticoagulants and aspirin may facilitate bleeding. Intraoperative hemorrhage is characterized by the development of positive pressure, visualization of an enlarging dark mass obscuring the fundus reflex, and tendency to extrude eye contents.

Choroidal effusions may have an annular, lobular (Figure 29-1), or flat ophthalmoscopic appearance. Annular detachments occur around the ciliary body and peripheral choroid. Lobular types are large hemispheric detachments that bulge toward the center of the globe. Flat effusions are most often apparent in isolated peripheral choroidal areas where local structures limit fluid extension. B-scan ultrasonography may be used to help differentiate between a retinal detachment and an effusion as well as between a hemorrhagic and a serous choroidal effusion. Retinal detachments are mobile and highly reflective, whereas choroidal detachments are smooth, dome-shaped, and thick. Virtually no movement of the detachment is seen with eye movement. When extensive, one can see multiple dome-shaped detachments, which may "kiss" in the central vitreous cavity. When choroidal detachments are hemorrhagic rather than serous, the suprachoroidal space is filled with a multitude of dots in contrast to the echolucent suprachoroidal space of a serous choroidal detachment.

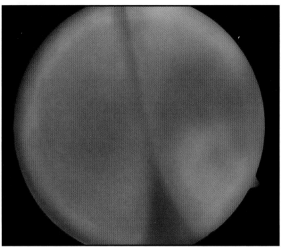

Figure 29-1. Lobular appositional choroidal effusion.

Serous choroidal detachments usually resolve spontaneously with the normal rise in IOP that occurs during the first days to weeks postoperatively. However, prolonged edema may lead to major complications. Peripheral anterior synechiae and secondary glaucoma may result from long-term flattening of the anterior chamber, especially when there is a concurrent low-grade uveitis. Secondary cataract and cyclitic membrane may develop as well. Retinal adhesions from the apposition of "kissing choroidals" and secondary retinal detachment have also been reported.[12] Persistent choroidal effusion and hypotony eventually result in phthisis bulbi.

MEDICAL THERAPY

Topical corticosteroids, cycloplegics, and mydriatics should be prescribed for patients. Oral steroids can be used and are indicated when inflammation is a factor. When the IOP is high, which can occur with hemorrhagic choroidal detachments, IOP-lowering drugs can be used. Osmotics and aqueous suppressants are recommended.

Parasympathomimetics are contraindicated. If a significant choroidal detachment persists longer than 1 week after the underlying cause has been identified and addressed, drainage of the suprachoroidal fluid should be considered. The 7-day limit is an indication only; individualized assessment is key. If an improvement is suspected, waiting longer and closely monitoring the patient may be warranted. Immediate action is indicated when lens–cornea touch or intraocular lens (IOL)–cornea touch exists. This condition causes endothelial corneal damage and acceleration of lens opacities. If the anterior chamber (AC) remains flat after the cause has been identified and addressed, injection of viscoelastics into the AC should be considered. If lens–cornea touch or IOL–cornea touch exists, the AC reformation should be performed immediately at the slit lamp, if possible, while waiting to assess the need for suprachoroidal fluid drainage. A waiting period of 7 to 10 days after suprachoroidal hemorrhage is advised before surgical intervention to allow the fibrinolytic response to liquefy the clot, which permits more effective evacuation of the suprachoroidal space, with retinal and choroidal flattening.[13]

SURGICAL THERAPY

The most definitive treatment of choroidal detachment is drainage of the fluid in the suprachoroidal space. If the eye is extremely soft, a sub-Tenon's block is favored over a retrobulbar block. If the original paracentesis cannot be found, a new beveled paracentesis is made slowly with a 15-degree knife. Care in making the incision prevents rapid entry into the anterior chamber, which could result in damage to the iris or lens. If fixation of the globe becomes difficult, it may be helpful to place a small, partial-thickness scratch incision into the cornea near the limbus with a 15-degree knife. An incision approximately 2 mm long and one-third thickness is usually adequate. This groove can then be used for fixation allowing development of a paracentesis. After the paracentesis is made, the anterior chamber is reformed with injection of balanced salt solution through a 27-gauge cannula.

A 3- to 4-mm circumferential or radial conjunctival incision is made 3 to 6 mm from the limbus in the inferonasal and inferotemporal quadrants (away from the filtering site). Small episcleral blood vessels are gently cauterized before the sclerotomy is performed. Two 2- to 3-mm radial sclerotomies are centered in the inferior quadrants 3 to 4 mm from the limbus (Figure 29-2). We prefer to use a No. 64 Beaver blade (Becton Dickinson, Franklin Lakes, New Jersey) to make the sclerotomies because it is sharp enough to incise the sclera, but not too sharp to cut through to the choroid on contact. The blade is used to make gentle "scratch-down" strokes to approach the suprachoroidal space. Xanthochromic fluid often drains spontaneously after the incision is carried into the suprachoroidal space. Egress of fluid can be enhanced by placement of an infusion cannula through the paracentesis to pressurize the globe during these maneuvers (Figure 29-3). To further facilitate drainage, forceps are used on either edge of the sclerotomy to gape the wound further by alternatively pushing down on one edge of the sclerotomy while pulling up on the other edge of the sclerotomy. After the fluid flow slows, the tip of a cyclodialysis spatula can be carefully inserted into the suprachoroidal space in a circumferential direction (Figure 29-4). This maneuver is particularly helpful with facilitating drainage of loculated fluid as is often found in patients with hemorrhagic choroidals. The spatula is then removed and reinserted in

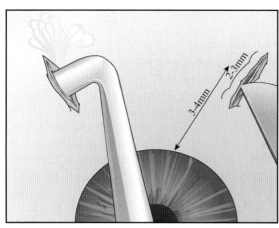

Figure 29-2. Sclerotomy sites in the inferior quadrants, 2- to 3-mm in length and centered 3 to 4 mm from the limbus. (Reprinted with permission of R. Rand Allingham, MD.)

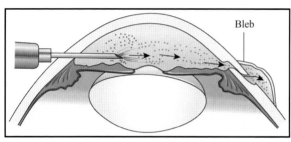

Figure 29-3. Injection of balanced salt solution deepens the anterior chamber and elevates the filtration bleb. (Reprinted with permission of R. Rand Allingham, MD.)

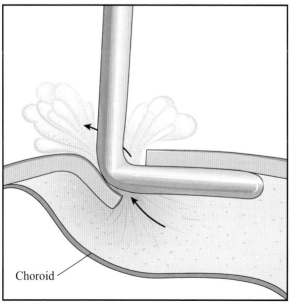

Figure 29-4. Side view of sclerotomy. The heel of the cyclodialysis spatula is used to depress the lip of the wound to aid the escape of suprachoroidal fluid. (Reprinted with permission of R. Rand Allingham, MD.)

the opposite direction. The sclerotomy is manipulated until no further fluid presents at the wound (typically, the brown color of the underlying choroid comes into view). An indirect ophthalmoscope is then used to confirm flattening of the retina before the other inferior sclerotomy is entered.

After the choroidal effusions have been drained, the edges of the sclerotomies are left unopposed to allow for continued drainage.[14] This can be accomplished by gaping the edges of the scleral wound with cautery or by excising a small piece of sclera with a punch or trephine.[15] The conjunctival wounds are closed with 8-0 Vicryl suture and atropine and antibiotic ointment are applied to the eye, followed by a patch and an eye shield. Occasionally, concurrent bleb revision is necessary and if cataract extraction needs to be performed, it may be combined with choroidal drainage.[16] The cataract surgery follows the choroidal drainage.

KEY POINTS

1. In the setting of ocular surgery, trauma, or inflammation, shallowing of the anterior chamber with a decrease in IOP suggests a possible choroidal effusion.

2. Medical therapy for choroidal effusions includes topical corticosteroids, cycloplegics, mydriatics, and occasionally oral steroids.

3. The most definitive treatment of choroidal effusions is surgical drainage of the fluid in the suprachoroidal space.

4. Surgical drainage involves creation of two 2- to 3-mm radial sclerotomies centered in the inferior quadrants 3 to 4 mm from the limbus.

5. During surgical drainage of choroidal effusions, egress of fluid can be enhanced by placement of an infusion cannula through the paracentesis to pressurize the globe.

6. The sclerotomies are manipulated with forceps and a cyclodiaylsis spatula until no further fluid presents at the wound and the brown color of the underlying choroid comes into view.

REFERENCES

1. Brubaker RF, Pederson JE. Ciliochoroidal detachment. *Surv Ophthalmol.* 1983;27(5): 281-289.

2. Weiter JJ, Ernest JT. Anatomy of the choroidal vasculature. *Am J Ophthalmol.* 1974;78(4):583-590.

3. Bill A. Intraocular pressure and blood flow through the uvea. *Arch Ophthalmol.* 1962;67:336-348.

4. Moses RA. Detachment of the ciliary body: anatomic and physical considerations. *Invest Ophthalmol.* 1965;4(5):935-941.

5. Capper SA, Leopold IH. Mechanism of serous choroidal detachment. *Arch Ophthalmol.* 1956;55(1):101-113.

6. Chandler PA, Maumenee AE. A major cause of hypotony. *Am J Ophthalmol.* 1961;52: 609-618.

7. Pederson JE, Gasterland DE, McClean HM. Experimental ciliochoroidal detachment: effect on intraocular pressure and aqueous humor flow. *Arch Ophthalmol.* 1979;97(3):536-541.

8. Bellows AR, Chylack LT, Hutchinson BT. Choroidal detachment: clinical manifestation, therapy and mechanism of formation. *Ophthalmology.* 1981;88(11):1107-1115.

9. Schepens CL, Brockhurst RJ. Uveal effusion: I. Clinical picture. *Arch Ophthalmol.* 1963;70:189-201.

10. Hyman BN, Hagler WS. Bilateral annular detachment and myopia. *Am J Ophthalmol.* 1970;70(5):853-855.

11. Hertz V. Choroidal detachment with notes on sclera depression and pigmented streaks in the retina. *Acta Ophthalmol.* 1954;41(Suppl):1-256.

12. Berrocal J. Adhesion of the retina secondary to large choroidal detachment as a cause of failure in retinal detachment surgery. *Mod Probl Ophthalmol.* 1979;20:51-52.

13. Lambrou FH, Meredith TA, Kaplan HG. Secondary surgical management of expulsive choroidal hemorrhage. *Arch Ophthalmol.* 1987;105(9):1195-1198.

14. Abrams GW, Thomas MA, Williams GA, et al. Management of postoperative suprachoroidal hemorrhage with continuous infusion air pump. *Arch Ophthalmol.* 1986;104(10):1455-1458.

15. Dellaporta A. Scleral trephination for subchoroidal effusion. *Arch Ophthalmol.* 1983;101(12):1917-1919.

16. Berke SJ, Bellows AR, Shingleton BJ, et al. Chronic and recurrent choroidal detachment after glaucoma filtering surgery. *Ophthalmology.* 1987;94(2):154-162.

30

ANGLE SURGERY
GONIOTOMY AND TRABECULOTOMY

Danielle M. Ledoux, MD; Suzanne Johnston, MD;
and David S. Walton, MD

Goniotomy and trabeculotomy are performed to improve the facility
of outflow of aqueous humor from the eye by incising abnormal trabecular
meshwork. This creates an improved conduit between the anterior chamber
and Schlemm's canal rather than creating an alternative aqueous bypass as
in filtration or tube shunt surgery.

EXAMINATION UNDER ANESTHESIA

Examination under anesthesia contributes essential information in
preparation for angle surgery and is very often necessary in caring for
pediatric patients. To minimize artificially low intraocular pressure (IOP)
measurements, which can be caused by inhaled anesthetics, IOP measurements should be taken soon after the induction of anesthesia. IOP measured
during an examination under anesthesia must be considered in conjunction
with the other findings because the pressure measured is often different
than that measured if the child were awake. A Tono-pen (Reichert Technologies, Depew, New York), Schiotz, or Perkins tonometer is used. Calipers
or a ruler is used to measure the corneal diameter for future comparison.
Axial length measurements are also helpful for future comparison and can
be used in concert with changing refractive error and corneal diameter to
identify disease progression. Careful slit-lamp examination should then
be performed. A diagnostic goniolens such as a Koeppe lens coupled with
balanced salt solution is then placed on the cornea, and a hand-held slit-
lamp device can be used to carefully examine the cornea, iris, and angle
structures. Alternatively, a mirrored lens or a Koeppe lens may be used
with the operating microscope. Both the cornea and angle structures can

Kahook M.
Essentials of Glaucoma Surgery (pp 260-272).

be examined while the goniolens is in place. The examiner should look for evidence of Haab's striae, which are horizontal breaks in Descemet's membrane. In addition, corneal stromal and/or epithelial edema may be noted. The quality of the view to the angle is crucial in deciding between the goniotomy and trabeculotomy procedures. The surgeon must evaluate the angle and become familiar with its anatomy. Careful observation will reveal abnormalities in the angle and iris structures, as well as evidence of previous angle procedures. This information is helpful not only in determining the etiology of glaucoma but also to orient the surgeon with the architecture of the angle prior to the procedure. Finally, a direct ophthalmoscope may be used to examine the optic nerve through an undilated pupil. This can also be accomplished through the pupil with the Koeppe lens in place after completing gonioscopy.

GONIOTOMY

Indications

Goniotomy is the procedure of choice for infantile primary congenital glaucoma and is also used for other types of developmental glaucoma, as well as some types of secondary glaucoma. However, angle surgery is not indicated in all types of childhood glaucoma. The decision about type of surgery has to be tailored to the individual's diagnosis and case. Goniotomy and trabeculotomy obtain similar results in experienced hands; however, individual surgeons may have a preference for one procedure over the other. Trabeculotomy is particularly helpful when the angle view is limited by opacification of the cornea. Advantages of goniotomy include a relatively short procedure time and preservation of conjunctiva for future filtration procedures. Also, anatomical landmarks for a trabeculotomy may be challenging to identify in a severely buphthalmic eye.

Preparation and Instrumentation

Glaucoma medications, such as oral acetazolamide 10 to 15mg/kg/day, may be used preoperatively to help reduce the IOP, as well as to help clear the cornea, so that a goniotomy may be performed. Other topical glaucoma medications may also be used preoperatively to help reduce pressure, including topical carbonic anhydrase inhibitors and beta-blockers. Alpha-adrenergic receptor agonists are typically avoided in infants because of possible somnolence and apnea. The exception to this is the intraoperative use of apraclonidine 0.5% (see Surgical Procedure section on page 264).

TABLE 30-1: PROPER POSITIONING FOR GONIOTOMY

Goniotomy

Instruments

- Goniotomy knife (eg, Storz SP7-62233) or 25-gauge 1.5-inch needle
- 2 locking fixation forceps (eg, Moody forceps)
- Operating gonioscopy lens (eg, Barkan or Swan-Jacob lens [both from Ocular Instruments Inc.; Bellevue, Washington])
- Operation magnification instruments (microscope and/or loupes)

Supplies

- Apraclonidine 0.5%
- 10-0 absorbable suture
- Ophthalmic viscoelastic device
- Balanced salt solution
- 70% isopropyl alcohol (if needed to débride epithelium)

Trabeculotomy

Instruments

- Right- and left-handed trabeculotomes (eg, Harms)
- Westcott scissors
- #57 blade
- Fine sharp knife
- Fine forceps
- Handheld cautery

Supplies

- 6-0 nylon suture
- 10-0 absorbable scleral suture
- Ophthalmic viscoelastic device
- 6-0 Prolene suture (for 360-degree suture trabeculotomy)

Goniotomy may be performed with an operating microscope or with loupes for magnification. The operating microscope is tilted to 45 degrees to provide an optimal view of the angle structures. During the cleaning and preparation, a few drops of dilute betadine are placed in the eye. The surgeon is seated opposite the operative angle. A trained assistant can help to stabilize and rotate the eye during the procedure. See Table 30-1 for appropriate surgical instruments and supplies.

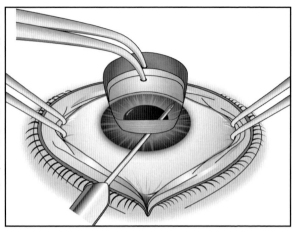

Figure 30-1. Goniotomy. The eye is fixated by the assistant with forceps grasping the superior and inferior recti muscles. The surgeon places the gonioprism on the cornea centrally, not obscuring the limbus, to facilitate entry of the knife or needle through the cornea.

Surgical Procedure

Typically, goniotomy is performed under general anesthesia. First, examination under anesthesia is performed as described above. The corneal epithelium may be removed if edematous using 70% isopropyl alcohol to improve visualization. Apraclonidine 0.5% on a spear (to limit the amount of medication absorbed systemically and avoid mydriasis) may be applied to the limbus adjacent to the planned goniotomy cleft to reduce the reflux of blood into the anterior chamber. The surgeon sits opposite the portion of the angle to be operated with the patient's head turned slightly away from the surgeon. The assistant stabilizes the eye with locking forceps secured at the insertion of the superior and inferior rectus muscles. Next, the operating goniolens is placed on the cornea.

Either a goniotomy knife or a 25-gauge needle on a viscoelastic-filled syringe is introduced into the anterior chamber through the peripheral cornea. The instrument's tip is visualized as it is advanced across the anterior chamber, parallel to the iris, to the opposite angle (Figure 30-1). It is then introduced to the mid to posterior third of the trabecular meshwork and a circumferential incision is made in one direction and then in the opposite direction, with the assistant carefully rotating the eye when requested by the surgeon (Figures 30-2 and 30-3). During the procedure, the surgeon will note the iris moving posteriorly, the release of iris processes, and the formation of a cleft. Approximately 4 clock hours can be treated with one procedure. After this incision is made, the instrument is removed from the anterior chamber and the anterior chamber is deepened with balanced salt solution or a sterile gas bubble. Normally, reflux of blood into the anterior chamber will occur concurrent with shallowing of the anterior

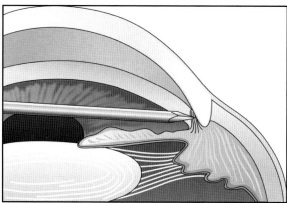

Figure 30-2. Goniotomy. The plane of entry of the cutting instrument is parallel to the iris, taking care to avoid the anterior vault of the lens.

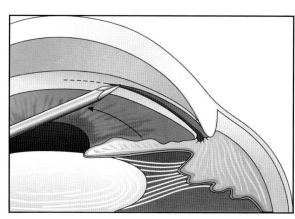

Figure 30-3. Goniotomy. The incision in the trabeculum is visualized behind the path of the cutting instrument.

chamber and hypotony. After the instrument is removed, forceps points held together are used to gently hold the incision closed. A 10-0 absorbable suture is used to secure the incision with the knot buried. The eye is then dressed with topical steroid drops and antibiotic drops. A patch and shield are then placed on the eye.

Complications and Prognosis

A small hyphema is common following goniotomy and typically clears within a few days. Observe the patient closely for progression of hyphema, which may require an anterior chamber washout. More severe trauma to the iris and angle structures, such as iridodyalysis or cyclodyalysis, can also occur, potentially leading to hypotony. Trauma to the cornea and retinal detachment can also occur. Great care should be taken to avoid trauma to the lens and subsequent cataract formation. Corneal edema can obscure the surgeon's view and increase the risk of these complications. If a tapered knife is used, it is important to be sure that the chamber does not collapse, which could lead to lens trauma. There is also a small risk of intraocular infection or inflammation. Prognosis is dependent on the etiology of glaucoma. Many children require further surgical intervention to control IOP.

Key Points of Goniotomy Surgery

1. Proper positioning of the patient, microscope, and assistant are crucial to performing a successful goniotomy. Practicing the procedure with the assistant just before the procedure can alert the team to potential difficulties that may arise during the procedure. For example, the surgeon's view may not be adequate or the assistant may be unaware of how to manipulate the eye smoothly in a given position.

2. It is easy to introduce air bubbles under the goniolens when placing it on the eye. To avoid this, the head of the patient is tilted away from the surgeon; the lens is initially placed at a 45-degree angle to the cornea as the goniolens is lowered to the surface of the cornea over a small amount of saline or viscoelastic.

3. A gonioknife typically has a tapered shaft. As a result, it is possible for the corneal wound to leak as the blade is removed from the anterior chamber. This is not true for a 25-gauge needle, which has a straight shaft. The needle is placed on a viscoelastic-filled syringe and the chamber can be deepened if it becomes shallow during the procedure.

4. If a 25-gauge needle is used for the procedure, care should be taken to enter the cornea parallel to the iris so that the flexible needle does not pivot in an anterior-posterior direction while the angle incision is being created.

TRABECULOTOMY

Indications

Trabeculotomy is a surgical procedure that can be performed when the cornea is not adequately clear to view the angle structures and perform goniotomy. Some surgeons choose trabeculotomy as their procedure of choice when angle surgery is indicated, particularly if performing a 360-degree suture trabeculotomy is preferred. A 360-degree suture trabeculotomy offers the potential to treat the entire angle with one procedure. Angle surgery is often the procedure of choice for a child with glaucoma but not for all forms of glaucoma. The decision about type of surgery has to be tailored to the individual's diagnosis and case.

Preparation and Instrumentation

Following the examination under anesthesia, the eye is prepared and positioned based on the surgeon's preferred approach. A temporal approach is often selected to avoid the nose and to preserve the superior conjunctiva if future filtration surgery is needed. During the cleaning and preparation, a few drops of dilute betadine are placed in the eye. See Table 30-1 for appropriate surgical instruments and supplies.

Surgical Procedure

Conjunctival Peritomy and Scleral Flap Creation

A fornix-based peritomy for approximately 3 clock hours is performed with Westcott scissors and fine forceps to expose sclera above Schlemm's canal for the creation of a 3-mm equilateral triangular scleral flap (Figure 30-4). Light cautery can be used to achieve hemostasis. The scleral flap is partial thickness and created with the #57 blade. Dissection of this flap is extended anteriorly until darker limbal tissue is easily seen anterior and adjacent to the sclera.

Dissection to Schlemm's Canal

A 2-mm radial incision is created with the #57 blade at the junction of the scleral and limbal tissue (see Figure 30-4). Successive deeper layers of sclera are dissected by "scratching down" with gentle downward pressure and side-to-side movements of the #57 blade. The circumferential fibers of Schlemm's canal may be appreciated on dissection to the outer wall of the canal. The use of higher magnification and a sharp pointed blade can facilitate this final dissection. Entry into Schlemm's canal is heralded by a slow egress of blood-tinged aqueous humor. Rapid egress of fluid should raise suspicion of inadvertent direct entry into the anterior chamber. If inappropriate entry into the anterior chamber has occurred, the incision should be sutured closed with 10-0 absorbable sutures and the dissection should be performed slightly posterior to the initial site. The presence and patency of Schlemm's canal may be confirmed by introducing a short segment of 6-0 Prolene or nylon suture material, which should enter with minimal difficulty. If significant resistance is encountered, consider which anatomic space has been entered (eg, the suprachoroidal space). Once Schlemm's canal has been successfully identified, a peripheral corneal paracentesis is created to allow reformation of the anterior chamber with ophthalmic viscoelastic devices if needed.

Figure 30-4. Trabeculotomy. The radial incision is made at the junction of the sclera and posterior limbus and is deepened until Schlemm's canal is entered.

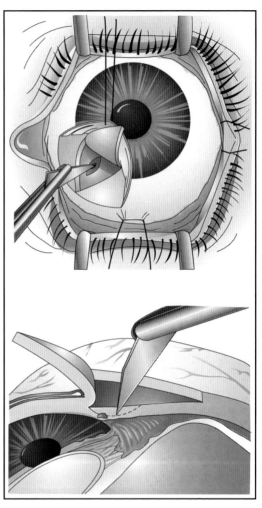

Opening of Trabecular Meshwork

Using the metal Trabeculotome, the distal arm of the Trabeculotome is placed through Schlemm's canal at the dissection site. The proximal arm is used as a guide and should track along the limbus external to the eye as the distal arm moves with minimal resistance through Schlemm's canal circumferentially for approximately 2 hours (Figure 30-5). The instrument is then rotated into the anterior chamber over the iris leaf surface until three-fourths of the length of the Trabeculotome is directly visualized in the anterior chamber (Figure 30-6). The Trabeculotome is then withdrawn.

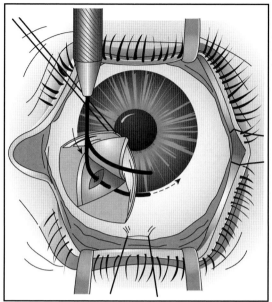

Figure 30-5. Trabeculotomy. Minimal resistance is encountered when the distal arm of the Trabeculotome is placed in Schlemm's canal.

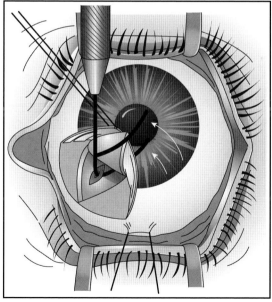

Figure 30-6. Trabeculotomy. The Trabeculotome is rotated parallel to the iris to lessen the risk of injury to the cornea and iris.

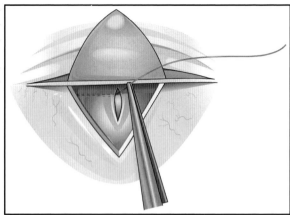

Figure 30-7. Technique of trabeculotomy. Schlemm's canal is cannulated with a suture to confirm entry into the canal and its patency.

Often the anterior chamber shallows and/or hyphema occurs. Injecting an ophthalmic viscoelastic device (OVD) through the paracentesis may be needed to partially reform the anterior chamber and move the iris posterior before initiating use of the opposite metal Trabeculotome. The opposite Trabeculotome is placed through the opposite side of the incision into Schlemm's canal for an additional 2 clock hours and rotated into the anterior chamber as previously described.

If suture trabeculotomy is chosen instead of the metal Trabeculotome, a 6-0 Prolene suture is measured along the external border of the limbus and trimmed to a few millimeters longer than this measured distance. The leading end of the suture is melted into a mushroom shape with the use of cautery held in close proximity to the suture without contact. This mushroomed leading end of the suture is thread through Schlemm's canal and recovered from the opposite side of the incision after passing 360 degrees (Figure 30-7). Resistance to passing the suture may be encountered 180 degrees from the introduction site. If this occurs and it is not easy to pass, a second flap can be created at this location to recover the suture and introduce an additional suture for the remaining 6 clock hours. The leading end is grasped external to the eye, and then both leading and trailing ends are grasped with equal force and pulled tangentially through the trabecular meshwork into the anterior chamber (Figure 30-8).

Closure

The scleral flap is closed with interrupted 10-0 absorbable sutures; typically a single suture is sufficient. If significant OVD or hyphema is in the anterior chamber, the flap can be loosely closed and serve as a temporary

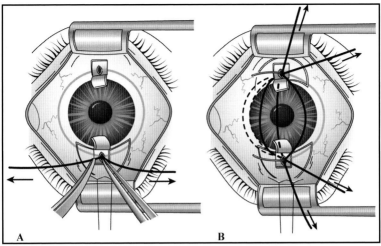

Figure 30-8. Both leading and trailing ends are grasped with equal force and pulled tangentially through the trabecular meshwork into the anterior chamber.

filter. Finally, the peritomy is closed watertight with 10-0 absorbable suture. After applying antibiotic and corticosteroid medications, the eye is patched and shielded.

Complications and Prognosis

False passages are possible, either into the anterior chamber or the suprachoroidal space. Postoperative hypotony is therefore a risk. Postoperative hyphema often occurs, but viscoelastic and apraclonidine 0.5% can help to control this. Observe the patient closely for progression of hyphema, which may require an anterior chamber washout. A small risk of postoperative infection exists. The patient needs to be followed closely for an elevation of IOP; repeat angle surgery or other procedures and medication control may be required. Prognosis is often related to the etiology of the glaucoma.

Key Points of Trabeculotomy Surgery

1. Preparing the correct location and positioning the patient prior to entry into the eye is an important first step of a successful procedure.
2. A partial-thickness scleral flap allows for easier identification and dissection to Schlemm's canal.

3. A gentle approach to Schlemm's canal is used by scratching down at the scleral–limbal junction through the scleral fibers with a knife in a side-to-side motion with slight downward pressure.

4. When Schlemm's canal is located, slow egress of blood or pigment-tinged fluid will be appreciated. Rapid egress of fluid should raise suspicion of entry into the anterior chamber.

5. Entering the suprachoroidal space with either the suture or metal Trabeculotome is possible. Significant resistance to passing the instrument should raise suspicion for the incorrect location.

6. With initial rotation of the metal Trabeculotome, if it is directed posteriorly, movement of the iris will be seen. If this position is not corrected, an iridodialysis will occur.

7. To avoid corneal or lenticular damage, OVDs may be necessary to maintain and deepen the anterior chamber partway through the procedure.

SUGGESTED READINGS

Beck AD, Lynch MD. 360-degree trabeculotomy for primary congenital glaucoma. *Arch Ophthalmol.* 1995;113(9):1200-1202.

Freedman SF. Medical and surgical treatments for childhood glaucomas. In: Allingham RR, ed. *Shields' Textbook of Glaucoma.* 5th ed. Philadelphia, PA: Lippincott Williams & Wilkins; 2005:626-643.

Mandal AK, Netland PA. *The Pediatric Glaucomas.* Philadelphia, PA: Elsevier; 2006.

Walton DS. Goniotomy, trabeculotomy, and goniosynechiolysis. In: Higginbotham EJ, Lee DA, ed. *Clinical Guide to Glaucoma Management.* Woburn, MA: Butterworth Heinemann; 2004:412-423.

Walton DS. Pediatric glaucoma: angle surgery and glaucoma brainage devices. In: Giaconi JA, Law SK, Coleman AL, Caprioli J, eds. *Pearls of Glaucoma Management.* Berlin, Germany: Springer-Verlag; 2010:403-408.

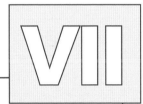

SURGICAL MANAGEMENT OF
COMPLICATED GLAUCOMAS

31

Surgical Management of Neovascular Glaucoma

Jonathan A. Eisengart, MD

It is more difficult to achieve an optimal outcome in neovascular glaucoma than in primary open-angle or other more common types of glaucoma. First, the lack of trabecular outflow tends to make a low intraocular pressure (IOP) difficult to achieve (some functional trabecular outflow remains in most eyes having undergone glaucoma surgery and likely improves final IOP control). Second, the rate of complications—bleeding and surgical failure—is higher in eyes with neovascular glaucoma (NVG) than primary open-angle glaucoma (POAG). Last, posterior segment ischemia often limits visual outcome. On the plus side, however, these eyes often do not have a primary glaucomatous optic neuropathy and often do well with an IOP in the high teens or low 20s.

The best glaucoma surgical outcome is achieved when the eye is quiet and neovascularization is regressed. Active anterior segment neovascularization can lead to blocked outflow surgery through hyphema or progressive synechiae. Eyes with active ischemia are more likely to scar or heal poorly. Active inflammation can lead to hypotony, scarring, or fibrin, complicating surgical outcomes.

When possible, it is best to delay surgery until neovascularization, ischemia, and inflammation are controlled. Typically, this means maximizing medical therapy and following the patient carefully to appropriately time surgical intervention.

Antivascular Endothelial Growth Factor Therapy

Traditionally, ischemia and neovascularization have been treated with panretinal photocoagulation (PRP). However, not only does PRP take days

Kahook M.
Essentials of Glaucoma Surgery (pp 275-278).
© 2012 SLACK Incorporated.

to weeks to produce results, it often cannot be adequately performed in eyes with NVG due to vitreous hemorrhage, corneal edema, poor papillary dilation, or dense cataract.

Recently, anti-vascular endothelial growth factor (VEGF) therapy has revolutionized initial treatment of NVG. Anti-VEGF therapy may reduce surgical complications by inducing rapid regression of neovascularization and control of ischemia,[1] and unlike PRP, it is not dependent on clarity of the eye's optical media. Additionally, anti-VEGF therapy may reduce scarring and improve the success rate of outflow surgery.[2] It is important to note, however, that because anti-VEGF agents have a limited duration of action, they do not replace PRP. PRP should be performed (or a second anti-VEGF injection given) within 4 to 6 weeks of the initial anti-VEGF injection.

Practically speaking, when an eye presents with uncontrolled NVG, I typically initiate maximum topical therapy and sometimes oral acetazolamide. I ensure that an intravitreal injection of an anti-VEGF drug is given the same day or as soon as possible. I will follow closely and choose to do surgery later if the IOP remains too high. Not uncommonly, especially if the angle is still open on presentation, IOP will respond to medical therapy and surgery may not be needed.[3] If glaucoma surgery cannot be delayed due to pain or extremely elevated IOP, I will inject anti-VEGF therapy intraoperatively.

Bevacizumab and ranibizumab are the 2 agents currently available that are useful in treating neovascular glaucoma. Although *neither one is FDA-approved* for treating NVG, Lucentis is approved for intraocular injection (for exudative age-related macular degeneration). However, cost considerations and insurance coverage issues dictate that bevacizumab is more commonly given for NVG.

The most effective route of administration for treatment of NVG is intravitreal injection. The typical dose of bevacizumab is 1.25 mg/0.05 mL (25 mg/mL). The vitreous gel acts like a depot and probably allows sustained release of the anti-VEGF agent over 4 weeks or more. Intracameral injection is an option to cause regression of anterior segment neovascularization but likely has a shorter duration of action and may not be as beneficial to posterior segment disease.

GLAUCOMA DRAINAGE DEVICE VERSUS TRABECULECTOMY VERSUS CYCLOPHOTOCOAGULATION

Three main surgical approaches can be used to lower IOP in medically uncontrolled NVG: glaucoma drainage device (GDD), trabeculectomy with antifibrotics, and cyclophotocoagulation (CPC). When choosing a surgical approach, the following questions should be considered:

- Is there active ischemia and neovascularization?
- Is there active inflammation?
- Are other surgical interventions going to be performed concomitantly or in the future?
- What is the visual potential of the eye?
- What is the target pressure?
- What is the general health of the patient?

Glaucoma Drainage Device

In many cases, GDDs provide the most robust, predictable outcome for treating NVG. They tend to maintain function relatively well through subsequent surgery and through active inflammation, ischemia, and neovascularization. I tend to use a GDD to treat NVG whenever there is any degree of useful vision or if there is any inflammation.

Implanting a GDD in an eye with NVG takes no modification of technique other than that the tube tip probably should not touch the iris, where it can cause hyphema if rubeosis is present. If anterior segment neovascularization is present and hyphema forms, this can lead to tube occlusion (see Chapter 12).

The choice of device is based on surgeon preference. One caveat is that an ischemic eye may be more prone to hypotony due to aqueous hyposecretion, and a Baerveldt 350-mm² implant probably should be used only in people who are expected to rapidly generate thick capsules. Personally, I tend to prefer the Baerveldt 250 mm² or Ahmed FP7 in most NVG eyes.

In eyes that also need vitrectomy for nonclearing vitreous hemorrhage, tractional retinal detachments, or other posterior segment problems, I prefer to place the GDD through the pars plana in conjunction with my vitreoretinal colleague. Not only does this technique save the patient from 2 separate trips to the operating room, but placement of the tube through the pars plana eliminates the chance that the tube will contact rubeotic vessels and cause hyphema.

Trabeculectomy With Mitomycin C

In acute NVG, trabeculectomy tends to work poorly due to intense scarring, marked anterior chamber hemorrhage, and fibrin formation. However, in quiet eyes with chronic or regressed NVG, trabeculectomy with mitomycin C (MMC) is the procedure preferred by some.[4] The advantages are the ability to achieve a lower IOP off medication (at least in the short term) and lack of an implanted foreign body.

Trabeculectomy is not the best choice if subsequent vitreoretinal surgery is likely because of the potential to induce scarring and failure of the filtering bleb.

Cyclophotocoagulation

CPC is, in my opinion, underutilized for the treatment of NVG. The transscleral approach is quick, effective, and has almost no bleeding risk. The drawbacks are that it is inflammatory, difficult to titrate, and irreversible. I consider transscleral CPC an excellent choice for eyes with poor visual potential, patients with advanced dementia or other health issues that make incisional surgery less safe, and patients on anticoagulation. I avoid performing CPC in patients with active or recurrent inflammation because this procedure can significantly worsen inflammation.

Ischemic eyes are more likely to develop hypotony, so initial treatment should be limited to 270 degrees (or perhaps even 180).[5] When performing transscleral CPC, I routinely use transillumination to identify the ciliary body and direct my treatment accordingly.

KEY POINTS

1. When rubeosis is present, anti-VEGF therapy should be administered at least 24 to 72 hours prior to surgery, if possible. Otherwise, it may be administered intraoperatively.

2. In eyes with rubeosis or otherwise active NVG, GDDs and transscleral cyclophotocoagulation are the most helpful treatment options.

REFERENCES

1. Saito Y, Higashide T, Takeda H, Ohkubo S, Sugiyama K. Beneficial effects of preoperative intravitreal bevacizumab on trabeculectomy outcomes in neovascular glaucoma. *Acta Ophthalmol.* 2010;88(1):96-102.

2. Horsley MB, Kahook MY. Anti-VEGF therapy for glaucoma. *Curr Opin Ophthalmol.* 2010;21(2):112-117.

3. Wakabayashi T, Oshima Y, Sakaguchi H, et al. Bevacizumab for iris neovascularization and neovascular glaucoma. *Ophthalmology.* 2008;115(9):1571-1580.

4. Alkawas AA, Shahien EA, Hussein AM. Management of neovascular glaucoma with panretinal photocoagulation, intravitreal bevacizumab, and subsequent trabeculectomy with mitomycin C. *J Glaucoma.* 2010;19(9):622-626.

5. Ramli N, Htoon HM, Ho CL, Aung T, Perera S. Risk factors for hypotony after transscleral diode cyclophotocoagulation. *J Glaucoma.* 2011;21(3):169-173.

32

Surgical Management of Uveitic Glaucoma

Jonathan A. Eisengart, MD

Surgical Assessment of Uveitic Glaucoma

Glaucoma surgery in patients with uveitis is not easy. First, uveitis reduces the success rate of glaucoma surgery. Not only are eyes with uveitis more likely to scar and fail glaucoma outflow surgery, but they are also more prone to hypotony. Second, glaucoma surgery itself can exacerbate uveitis. Not only can surgical trauma cause a flare of inflammation, but it can also lead to initiation or worsening of cystoid macular edema. Therefore, great care must be taken in planning and timing surgical intervention to minimize risks and maximize the chance of success.

Mechanisms of Glaucoma in Uveitis

- Closed Angle
    - Peripheral anterior synechiae
    - Pupillary block
    - Neovascular glaucoma
- Open Angle
    - Steroid response
    - Clogging of TM by cells, fibrin, inflammatory debris
    - Chronic TM damage and scarring of outflow channels

As mentioned above, eyes with chronic or recurrent uveitis are more prone to hypotony after glaucoma surgery. It is commonly known that actively inflamed eyes hyposecrete aqueous acutely. However, it is equally

Kahook M. *Essentials of Glaucoma Surgery* (pp 279-284). © 2012 SLACK Incorporated.

important to realize that repeated bouts of ciliary body inflammation can lead to profound atrophy of the ciliary processes[1] and chronic aqueous hyposecretion. This can lead to a dreaded "high-low" syndrome of uncontrolled high intraocular pressure (IOP) prior to glaucoma surgery, intractable hypotony after glaucoma surgery, and again uncontrolled IOP after outflow surgery is reversed.

Preoperative Considerations

When possible, surgical intervention should be delayed until inflammation is absent, or at least minimized. If necessary, oral acetazolamide can be useful to help delay surgical intervention. In some cases without severe optic nerve damage, it may be safer to observe elevated IOP for several weeks while control of acute inflammation is achieved than to intervene in an inflamed eye.

In the days leading up to surgery, it is important to maximize anti-inflammatory therapy. Topical nonsteroidal anti-inflammatory drugs (NSAIDs) may be added because they will not exacerbate IOP. If a significant steroid response component is not present, topical, and sometimes oral, corticosteroids should be maximized.

If the uveitis is related to herpes virus, prophylaxis with full-treatment dose of oral antivirals surgery (ie, acyclovir 400 mg 5 times daily for herpes simplex virus or 800 mg 5 times daily for herpes zoster) should be started 1 to 3 days prior to surgery and continued as long as the patient is on elevated steroid dosing.

Intraoperative Considerations

When operating in an eye with uveitis, it is important to minimize intraocular manipulation by operating efficiently, entering the eye as few times as possible, avoiding the iris and uvea, and taking particular care to be gentle.

Not uncommonly, the ocular tissues in uveitics are found to be friable, likely due to repeated bouts of inflammation and chronic steroid exposure. The conjunctiva is more likely to tear or bleed, and subconjunctival fibrosis can make dissection more difficult. Scleral flaps can perforate from toothed forceps, avulse, and sutures can cheese-wire through these flaps. The iris can be floppy, dilate poorly, or tear easily, and iris hooks can cheese-wire.

Postoperative inflammation can lead to posterior synechiae and iris bombe, so creation of a surgical iridectomy is often advisable. This is especially true if lysis of posterior synechiae or other iris manipulation was performed.

In uveitics, it is especially important to avoid hypotony that can lead to worsening inflammation or macular edema. Therefore, the surgeon should not leave the operating room until the eye can maintain an appropriate pressure. If necessary, additional sutures should be placed through trabeculectomy flaps; tube shunts need a reliably functioning valve or adequate occlusion. Viscoelastic may be left in the anterior chamber if self-limited postoperative hypotony is anticipated.

Postoperative Considerations

Early, aggressive steroid use can be helpful in reducing risk of complications. An intravenous bolus at the conclusion of surgery can be helpful, and consideration should be given to periocular corticosteroids or intravitreal preservative-free triamcinolone. A rapidly tapering course of oral steroids can also help minimize early postoperative inflammation. Prednisolone every 1 to 2 hours, or difluprednate every 3 to 4 hours, should be started and tapered based on the clinical examination. Topical NSAIDs and cycloplegics should be given in most cases.

Sustained-Release Steroid Implants

Eyes with steroid response glaucoma secondary to steroid implants, particularly Retisert (fluocinolone intravitreal implant), behave somewhat differently than a typical uveitic eye. These eyes with sustained-release steroid implants tend to have little, if any, inflammation and typically do not require more than routine postoperative prednisolone use. However, they may have impaired wound healing due to the steroid implant (personal experience), and late conjunctival dehiscence can occur. I recommend meticulous and tension-free conjunctival closure and securely anchoring glaucoma drainage devices (GDDs) with nonabsorbable sutures.

CHOOSING SURGICAL APPROACH

Laser Trabeculoplasty

Neither argon laser trabeculoplasty nor selective laser trabeculoplasty are appropriate for the management of uveitic glaucoma. The failure rate can approach 80%, and the chance of causing a flare of uveitis is reported to be 60%.[2]

Glaucoma Drainage Device

GDDs should be considered the mainstay of uveitic glaucoma management. Their effectiveness in the face of recurrent bouts of inflammation is their primary advantage over trabeculectomy.

Due to the potential for acute or chronic aqueous hyposecretion, valved devices such as the Ahmed provide the greatest margin of safety and are often a first choice.[3,4] However, I have seen several cases of uveitic glaucoma in which an occlusion develops within the valve mechanism, presumably from inflammatory debris.

Baerveldt tubes probably have a higher success rate[5] but also have a higher hypotony risk. With nonvalved devices, hypotony tends to manifest during acute flares of inflammation associated with aqueous hyposecretion but can also occur chronically due to ciliary atrophy. I tend to use the Baerveldt 250 mm^2 in cases with well-controlled inflammation when acute aqueous hyposecretion is a lesser risk (steroid implant recipients tend to make good candidates for nonvalved devices). The Baerveldt 350-mm^2 implant should be used with caution in uveitics, as it can lead to profound hypotony. I have personally used this device in uveitics only after the patient has proven to scar or encapsulate intensely.

Trabeculectomy With Mitomycin C

Trabeculectomy with mitomycin C (MMC) can provide good long-term IOP control in uveitic glaucoma, although the reported success rate may be lower than with tube implants.[6] The advantages include lack of implanted foreign material and saving glaucoma drainage device surgery as a backup if the bleb eventually fails. However, trabeculectomies tend to be less durable than tubes and probably are not the best choice if there is active or recurrent inflammation or if subsequent surgery (other than clear corneal phacoemulsification) is planned.

Because eyes with Retisert remain quiet for years, they probably do well with trabeculectomy. Also, eyes with very well-controlled uveitis, or uveitis in long-term remission, may do well with trabeculectomy.

Cyclophotocoagulation

For good reason, cyclophotocoagulation (CPC) is traditionally considered to be contraindicated in uveitis. Because this procedure directly injures uveal tissue, it can cause a severe uveitis reactivation. Furthermore, it may lead to irreversible hypotony. However, there are a few case series suggesting safety and efficacy of transscleral CPC for uveitic glaucoma.[7,8] Personally, I would still be highly reluctant to try any form of cyclodestruction for treatment of uveitic glaucoma if any type of outflow surgery or medical option remained.

KEY POINTS

1. Patients with uveitis need careful pre- and postoperative planning.
2. A prophylactic peripheral iridectomy should be performed if there is lysis of synechia or other manipulation of iris tissue.
3. Tube implants are generally preferred for uveitic glaucoma, although trabeculectomy may be appropriate for cases of uveitis in remission.

REFERENCES

1. da Costa DS, Lowder C, de Moraes HV Jr, Oréfice F. The relationship between the length of ciliary processes as measured by ultrasound biomicroscopy and the duration, localization, and severity of uveitis [Portuguese]. *Arq Bras Oftalmol.* 2006;69(3):383-388.
2. Foster CS. *Secondary glaucoma.* Ocular Immunology and Uveitis Foundation Web site. Retrieved from www.uveitis.org/medical/articles/clinical/clinglahtm.html.
3. Da Mata A, Burk SE, Netland PA, Baltatzis S, Christen W, Foster CS. Management of uveitic glaucoma with Ahmed glaucoma valve implantation. *Ophthalmology.* 1999;106(11):2168-2172.
4. Papadaki TG, Zacharopoulos IP, Pasquale LR, Christen WB, Netland PA, Foster CS. Long-term results of Ahmed glaucoma valve implantation for uveitic glaucoma. *Am J Ophthalmol.* 2007;144(1):62-69.
5. Ceballos EM, Parrish RK 2nd, Schiffman JC. Outcome of Baerveldt glaucoma drainage implants for the treatment of uveitic glaucoma. *Ophthalmology.* 2002;109(12):2256-2260.
6. Ceballos EM, Beck AD, Lynn MJ. Trabeculectomy with antiproliferative agents in uveitic glaucoma. *J Glaucoma.* 2002;11(3):189-196.
7. Schlote T, Derse M, Zierhut M. Transscleral diode cyclophotocoagulation for treatment of refractory glaucoma secondary to inflammatory eye disease. *Br J Ophthalmol.* 2000;84(9):999-1003._
8. Puska PM, Tarkkanen AH. Transscleral red laser cyclophotocoagulation for the treatment of therapy-resistant inflammatory glaucoma. *Eur J Ophthalmol.* 2007;17(4): 550-556.

GLAUCOMA SURGERY IN THE NANOPHTHALMIC EYE

Tiffany N. Szymarek, MD; Sayoko E. Moroi, MD, PhD; and Jonathan A. Eisengart, MD

The surgical management of glaucoma in eyes with nanophthalmos requires special consideration because these eyes are prone to serious postoperative complications, including significant inflammation, uveal effusion syndrome, retinal detachment, cystoid maculopathy, aqueous misdirection, and severe vision loss.[1] Fortunately, surgical outcomes have improved due to better recognition of the full clinical spectrum of the "small eye"[2] and advances in cataract surgery, as well as glaucoma surgeries.

DEFINITION AND CLINICAL FEATURES

Nanophthalmos is characterized by a small eye without other malformations. Clinical features include a narrow palpebral fissure, a small orbit, a short axial length, axial hyperopia, a small to normal corneal diameter, a shallow anterior chamber, thickened choroid, thickened sclera, and a high lens-eye volume ratio.[2] The angle-closure form of glaucoma occurs frequently in such eyes. The "pushing" pupillary block mechanism is caused by a relatively large lens in a small anterior segment, which leads to narrowing of the angle and peripheral anterior synechiae (PAS) formation. Another, less common mechanism occurs in the presence of an annular ciliochoroidal effusion in which the anteriorly rotated ciliary processes displace the peripheral iris to close the anterior chamber angle.[3]

Diagnostic evaluation should include refraction, gonioscopy, and biometry measurements of the axial length, keratometry readings, and anterior chamber (AC) depth. Imaging with standard B-scan ultrasound provides helpful information about the combined retinal-choroidal-scleral thickness.[2] Although there are no absolute biometric parameters for nanophthalmos, an axial length <21.0 mm and scleral thickness

Kahook M.
Essentials of Glaucoma Surgery (pp 285-292).
© 2012 SLACK Incorporated.

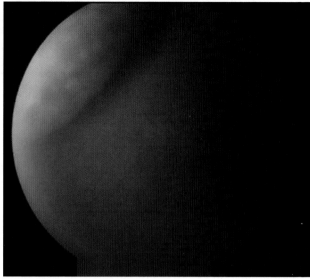

Figure 33-1. Choroidal effusion after laser iridotomy for narrow-angle glaucoma in a nanophthalmic eye with 22.18-mm axial length and 1.65-mm scleral thickness by B-scan ultrasound.

>1.7 mm support the diagnosis of nanophthalmos.[2] A variety of retinal pathology has been described in these eyes, such as macular hypoplasia, retinal cysts, macular folds, retinoschisis, pigmentary retinopathy, and disc drusen.[2]

MEDICAL AND LASER TREATMENT

Traditionally, the first-line treatment of glaucoma in nanophthalmic eyes has been medical and laser therapy due to the high rate of complications with incisional surgery. Typically, aqueous suppressants such as beta-blockers, alpha-adrenergic agonists, and carbonic anhydrase inhibitors are used. In addition, the prostaglandin outflow agents can also be used to lower intraocular pressure (IOP). Miotic agents should be used with caution, as they may worsen pupillary block by relaxing the zonules, which allows the lens to "push" forward and further crowd the anterior segment.[3,4]

Laser iridotomy can relieve the pupillary block, and iridoplasty can further open the drainage angle.[1,4] These interventions should be performed before extensive PAS develops.[4] It is important to remember that nanophthalmic eyes are more prone to significant postoperative inflammation, therefore steroids should be used judiciously. Such patients may develop uveal effusions after laser procedures (Figure 33-1), which may require oral prednisone in addition to topical prednisolone. If such effusions do not respond to aggressive steroid use, unsutured sclerotomies may be required to allow for posterior drainage of the effusions.[4]

INCISIONAL SURGERY

The decision for incisional surgery in an eye with nanophthalmos requires careful planning of anesthesia and surgical approach. In such eyes, it is advised to keep a simple approach given the increased risk of complications. As there are no clinical trial results to guide treatments in such eyes, the following considerations are based on clinical experience.

Preoperative Management

If a patient has shown increased propensity for inflammation, such as spontaneous uveal effusions or marked inflammatory reaction after laser treatments, then preoperative prednisone should be considered 2 to 3 days before surgery at a dose of 40 to 60 mg. To minimize the risk of increased posterior pressure and intraoperative aqueous misdirection, mannitol (12.5 to 25 g intravenously) or acetazolamide may be given.

Anesthesia

When planning anesthesia for these patients, it is important to consider general anesthesia. If a patient has a shallow orbit, then an anesthetic block may cause significant posterior pressure and severe chemosis to a degree that may preclude the surgery from being performed.[2] Topical anesthetic surgery is not advised due to the risk of intraoperative aqueous misdirection. If a block is performed, then only a small volume (ie, <3 cc) should be given, and one should consider applying a Honan balloon (The Lebanon Corporation, Lebanon, Indiana) for at least 10 minutes to ensure a soft eye.[5]

Phacoemulsification

Several recent case series have indicated that small-incision phacoemulsification can be safe and effective in patients with nanophthalmos for both visual improvement and IOP control.[2,5,6] In eyes with no preoperative evidence of choroidal effusion, prophylactic sclerotomies were not necessary, and no postoperative effusions were reported.[2]

Factors to keep in mind when performing phacoemulsification in nanophthalmic eyes include the following:

- Given very shallow ACs with limited working space, great care must be taken to avoid damage to the corneal endothelium. Frequent reapplication of viscoelastic against the endothelium and performing phacoemulsification in-the-bag are important.

- Poorly dilating pupils with posterior synechiae require synechialysis, pupil stretching, and iris retraction, including an iris retractor posterior to the temporal clear cornea incision. Such manipulations can cause significant postoperative inflammation.
- Hydrodissection should be performed carefully to prevent overfill in the capsular bag and iris prolapse through the corneal incision.
- Use increased height of infusion to maintain AC depth, but be aware of potential risk for diverting the infusion into the posterior segment.
- The intraocular lenses (IOLs) required are high-powered and will often need special ordering. If using a single-piece IOL, consider the use of a capsule tension ring, which will provide stable tension at the equator of the residual capsule bag with the implication of a stable planar configuration.
- Consider using a 3-piece IOL because the flexible haptics may provide more capsular tension, help stabilize the zonules, and decrease the risk of aqueous misdirection.
- We do not advise piggyback IOLs (ie, one in-the-bag and one in the sulcus) due to the limited space in the eye and to minimize the risk of the sulcus-placed IOL causing chaffing of the iris and/or ciliary body in eyes that are susceptible to inflammation.

Trabeculectomy

If the IOP is still uncontrolled after lens extraction, a good next option is trabeculectomy. In nanophthalmos, the sudden decrease in IOP on opening the globe can result in rapid uveal effusion, secondary retinal detachment, vitreous hemorrhage, and aqueous misdirection.[3,6] Several surgical modifications to trabeculectomy have been suggested to minimize the risk of these complications, including the following[3]:

- Stabilizing the anterior chamber depth with viscoelastic prior to performing the sclerostomy.
- Pre-placing the scleral flap sutures.
- Tight scleral flap closure.
- Leaving viscoelastic in the AC.
- Inferior sclerotomies or sclerectomies.

To decrease the risk of trabeculectomy failure because of the thick sclera, a deep sclerectomy should be considered. After dissecting the scleral flap just anterior to the surgical limbus, the underlying scleral tissue can be dissected off, leaving a thin layer of sclera over the uvea.

Glaucoma Drainage Devices

To our knowledge, there are no studies reporting on surgical results of glaucoma drainage devices in patients with nanophthalmos. Factors to consider are a small orbit and small globe, which may make placement of the plate challenging. Also, there may be limited space in the crowded AC for a tube.

Postoperative Management

It is important to remember that patients with nanophthalmos are prone to significant postoperative inflammation.[2] Frequent topical steroid administration should be a mainstay of postoperative treatment. Consideration should also be given to subconjunctival or oral steroids to supplement control of inflammation. Topical nonsteroidal anti-inflammatory drugs (NSAIDs) may also be helpful. Other postoperative complications should be managed as with any other case.

SPECIAL CONSIDERATIONS IN NANOPHTHALMOS

It is of utmost importance to recognize aqueous misdirection and uveal effusions in nanophthalmic eyes. The following management steps are options when these complications occur during specific procedures or during the postoperative period.

Aqueous Misdirection

When performing any type of incisional surgery on nanophthalmic eyes, there is an increased risk of intraoperative aqueous misdirection, which is characterized by elevated IOP and persistent AC shallowing, with or without accompanying iris prolapse. As noted above in the preoperative management section, mannitol or acetazolamide may help decrease the risk of aqueous misdirection by decreasing vitreous pressure and lowering IOP, respectively.

If intraoperative aqueous misdirection occurs with AC shallowing, the following steps may be taken in the given clinical setting:

During phacoemulsification:

- Administer the hyperosmotic agent, mannitol, intravenously (suggested 12.5 to 25 g single dose, infused slowly over 30 to 60 minutes, but up to 1 to 2 g/kg body weight may be given; however, in the authors' opinion this large dose is not necessary to achieve the hyperosmotic effect), and aqueous suppressant acetazolamide (500 mg intravenously).
- Raise the bottle height to increase the infusion pressure, but be cautious to avoid introducing more fluid into the vitreous cavity.

- Decrease the aspiration rate, but be cautious to recognize the risk of introducing more fluid into the vitreous cavity.
- Perform a vitrectomy with the goal to disrupt the anterior hyaloid vitreous face—either via a posterior pars plana approach or an anterior approach with iridectomy and hyaloid-zonulectomy. If the IOL has not yet been placed, then a posterior capsulectomy and anterior vitrectomy may be considered.
- Use cycloplegics and aqueous suppressants at the end of the surgery.
- Avoid miotic agents, as this drug class exacerbates aqueous misdirection.

During trabeculectomy:

- Administer the hyperosmotic agent, mannitol, intravenously (see suggested dose in the section above), and aqueous suppressant acetazolamide (500 mg intravenously).
- Perform vitrectomy either through the pars plana approach or an anterior approach through an iridectomy and hyaloid-zonulectomy.
- Use cycloplegics and aqueous suppressants at the end of the surgery.
- Avoid miotic agents, as this drug class exacerbates aqueous misdirection.

During postoperative period:

- Avoid miotic agents, as this drug class exacerbates aqueous misdirection.
- Adminster aqueous suppressants.
- Administer cycloplegics.
- Perform Nd:YAG laser anterior hyaloidotomy.
- Perform surgical pars plana vitrectomy with anterior hyaloidotomy.

Uveal Effusion

In patients with a history of choroidal effusion or an existing choroidal effusion, it may be prudent to perform an unsutured sclerotomy or sclerectomy either several weeks prior to or at the time of planned incisional surgery. This leaves a thinner scleral area open for posterior uveoscleral drainage from the choroid which helps resolve an existing choroidal effusion. Several techniques have been described. Two techniques described by Jin and Anderson,[4] which were successful in a series of patients are as follows:

- Sclerectomy: Remove a partial (two-thirds) thickness rectangle of sclera approximately 5 × 7 mm in a quadrant, then remove a 1-mm, full-thickness piece in the bed.

- Unsutured sclerotomy: Create a full-thickness V-shaped incision through the sclera into the suprachoroidal space. The site should be positioned anteriorly over the pars plana region.

The unsutured sclerotomy technique is preferred because it causes less posterior scleral weakness, which is a risk for rupture with retina and vitreous incarceration. The anterior site is protected by a thicker uveal layer and a firm vitreous base. These procedures may also be performed in the event of postoperative uveal effusion, and the effusion will likely resolve within 2 weeks.

KEY POINTS

1. Nanophthalmos is characterized by a small eye with short axial length, shallow anterior chamber, normal lens, thickened choroid and sclera, and a high risk for angle-closure glaucoma.

2. Nanophthalmic eyes are prone to significant postoperative inflammation, uveal effusions, and aqueous misdirection, even following uncomplicated laser procedures.

3. First-line management of glaucoma should be medical and laser treatment due to increased risk of intra- and postoperative complications.

4. Small incision phacoemulsification can often be performed safely and successfully without the need for prophylactic sclerotomies.

5. Trabeculectomy can be performed with several minor surgical modifications to minimize the risk of intraoperative uveal effusion and aqueous misdirection.

6. It is important to promptly recognize and treat aqueous misdirection and uveal effusion.

REFERENCES

1. Singh OS, Simmons RJ, Brockhurst RJ, Trempe CL. Nanophthalmos: a perspective on identification and therapy. *Ophthalmology.* 1982;89(9):1006-1012.
2. Wu W, Dawson DG, Sugar A, et al. Cataract surgery in patients with nanophthalmos: results and complications. *J Cataract Refract Surg.* 2004;30(3):584-590.
3. Yalvac IS, Satana B, Ozkan G, Eksioglu U, Duman S. Management of glaucoma in patients with nanophthalmos. *Eye (Lond).* 2008;22(6):838-843.
4. Jin JC, Anderson DR. Laser and unsutured sclerotomy in nanophthalmos. *Am J Ophthalmol.* 1990;109(5):575-580.
5. Faucher A, Hasanee K, Rootman DS. Phacoemulsification and intraocular lens implantation in nanophthalmic eyes: report of a medium-size series. *J Cataract Refract Surg.* 2002;28(5):837-842.
6. Yuzbasioglu E, Artunay O, Agachan A, Bilen H. Phacoemulsification in patients with nanophthalmos. *Can J Ophthalmol.* 2009;44(5):534-539.

34

GLAUCOMA SURGERY IN ANIRIDIA PATIENTS

Jeffrey M. Zink, MD

Aniridia patients present unique surgical challenges. Aniridia is a panocular disease that is associated with higher incidence of glaucoma and cataract. It is also associated with foveal hypoplasia, stem cell deficiency, nystagmus, and subluxated lenses. Approximately 50% of aniridia patients will develop aniridic glaucoma.[1] Many patients who develop aniridic glaucoma eventually require glaucoma surgery. Initially, it has been shown that some patients with aniridic glaucoma can be controlled with topical medicines.[2] When medications fail or ocular surface disease precludes adding multiple glaucoma drops, there are many different techniques that have been described in the surgical treatment of aniridic glaucoma. In addition, prophylactic goniotomy in a select group of younger aniridia patients may also be effective in preventing the development of aniridic glaucoma.[1]

GONIOTOMY

Chen and Walton[1] have described goniotomy as a prophylactic procedure in young ariridia patients (mean age 37 months) with iris adhesions to the posterior trabecular meshwork for greater than 180 degrees. This technique, in a select group of younger patients with early angle changes, may be effective in preventing aniridic glaucoma.[1] In their retrospective study that examined 50 eyes in 33 patients with aniridia, 49 (89%) had an intraocular pressure (IOP) <22 mm Hg without medications at last follow up. This was with an average of 1.65 procedures and average of 200 degrees of goniosurgery. No operative complications were noted, and no eye had a decrease in visual acuity at last follow-up. This series suggests that the incidence of glaucoma development in aniridia patients may be significantly affected by goniosurgery. Goniotomy requires an adequate gonioscopic view of the

Kahook M.
Essentials of Glaucoma Surgery (pp 293–300).
© 2012 SLACK Incorporated.

angle, which can which can become more limited if worsening aniridic keratopathy develops over time. This procedure may be a good option in some younger aniridia patients, before more severe aniridic keratopathy develops, which can limit a clear view of the angle.

TRABECULOTOMY

Trabeculotomy has also been shown to be a reasonable option in aniridia patients. The advantage of trabeculotomy is that it does not require a clear gonioscopic view and can be done in patients with corneal opacities that may limit the ability to perform goniotomy surgery. In a series of aniridia patients undergoing initial surgery for glaucoma, Adachi et al[3] found that 10 (83%) out of 12 eyes in trabeculotomy patients were controlled with 9.5 years of follow-up, compared with 3 (18%) out of 17 eyes that underwent goniotomy, trabeculectomy, traceculectomy combined with trabeculotomy, and Molteno implant.

GLAUCOMA DRAINAGE IMPLANTS

Glaucoma drainage implants are effective at controlling pressure in aniridic glaucoma. Molteno implants were effective at controlling pressure in 5 (83%) out of 6 eyes in a series by Wiggens and Tomey.[4] Similarly, Baerveldt glaucoma drainage implants have been shown to control IOP in aniridic glaucoma.[5] Success with Ahmed valves in aniridia patients with glaucoma has also been demonstrated, but some patients required needling and 5-fluorouracil.[6] Glaucoma drainage implants have been the treatment of choice in my practice for older patients with aniridia, and I have been very satisfied with the level of pressure control achieved with these techniques (Figure 34-1). The surgeon has to be prepared to manage surface-related complications such as tube erosions, which may occur at a higher rate in patients with severe surface disease and stem cell deficiency (Figure 34-2).

CYCLODESTRUCTIVE PROCEDURES

Traditionally, cyclodestructive procedures have been reserved for refractory glaucomas or glaucomas associated with a very poor visual potential. Cyclocryotherapy procedures have been described in aniridia with limited success. In a series by Wiggens and Tomey,[4] cyclocryotherapy was successful in only 25% of eyes, and complications such as phthisis bulbi and progressive cataract were observed. Wagle et al[7] reported a much higher rate of phthis using cyclocryotherapy in pediatric glaucoma patients with aniridia resistant to maximal medical and surgical interventions compared with pediatric patients with glaucoma not associated

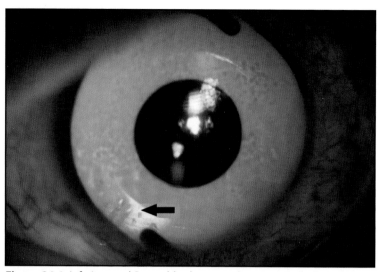

Figure 34-1. Inferior nasal Baerveldt glaucoma drainage implant in a patient with aniridia and an artificial iris. The tube is seen well positioned in the anterior chamber, in front of the Ophtec 311 artificial iris (Ophtec, Boca Raton, Florida).

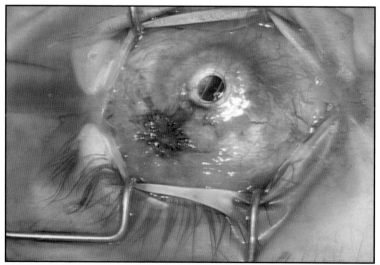

Figure 34-2. Aniridia patient with keratoprosthesis and prior pars plana Baerveldt glaucoma drainage tube insertion. A tissue patch graft (corneal patch) was required to repair a tube erosion in this patient.

with aniridia. This study cautions the use of cyclodestructive procedures in aniridia patients with glaucoma. It remains to be seen whether other cyclodestructive procedures, such as endoscopic cyclophotocoagulation or transscleral cyclophotocoagulation, which have been used to treat secondary glaucomas in childhood,[8] have a place in the treatment of glaucoma associated with aniridia.

TRABECULECTOMY

Conflicting results have been reported in the literature with regard to the success of trabeculectomy for glaucoma in patients with aniridia. In a retrospective review of aniridic glaucoma patients under the age of 40 years following trabeculectomy (17 patients) and trabeculectomy with mitomycin C (MMC) (3 patients), the mean period of postoperative success (defined as IOP below 21 mm Hg with or without medicines) after the filtering surgery was 14.6 months (range: 2 to 54 months).[9] Other studies have shown minimal benefit of trabeculectomy in aniridia. Wiggens et al[4] found that trabeculectomy controlled the IOP in only 9% of cases in which it was performed.

SPECIAL CONCERNS WITH ANIRIDIA PATIENTS

Central Corneal Thickness

Central corneal thickness has been shown to be increased in aniridia patients, which is an important consideration when measuring IOP by Goldmann applanation tonometry in these patients.[10,11] Clinicians may be overestimating IOP when using Goldmann applanation tonometry techniques in aniridia patients with increased central corneal thickness.

Surface Disease

Stem cell deficiency and ocular surface disease are special concerns that occur in patients with aniridia. In some patients with aniridia, the surface failure can be successfully treated with stem cell transplantation or keratoprosthesis surgery. In the case of stem cell transplantation, it is often desirable to have tube shunt surgery prior to surface rehabilitation surgery, such as a keratolimbal allograft, to minimize the potential deleterious effects of glaucoma drops on the transplanted tissue.

In our practice, when patients require 2 to 3 topical medicines preoperatively to control their glaucoma, we generally recommend glaucoma drainage implant surgery prior to undergoing keratolimbal allograft surgery. In general, the glaucoma worsens following the keratolimbal allograft

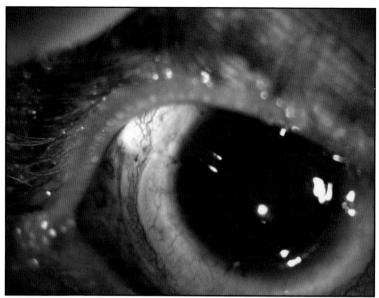

Figure 34-3. Patient that underwent combined cataract and Baerveldt glaucoma drainage implant surgery for a visually significant cataract and uncontrolled glaucoma. This patient has aniridia and prior keratolimbal allograft for stem cell deficiency. The corneal surface is clear following stem cell transplantation, and a well-positioned anterior chamber tube is present.

surgery, and it is desirable to minimize topical glaucoma medicines following the stem cell transplant. It is also possible to place a tube shunt following keratolimbal allograft surgery. Careful attention needs to be taken to preserve the keratolimbal allograft integrity during the tube shunt insertion (Figure 34-3).

Tube insertion in a keratolimbal allograft patient starts by creating a conjunctival peritomy at the posterior lip of the keratolimbal allograft for approximately 100 degrees. The glaucoma drainage implant plate is placed in a routine fashion and secured to the sclera. A dissection is carried out between the sclera and keratolimbal allograft segment. Usually, this is fairly easy because there is already a plane between the keratolimbal allograft lenticule and the sclera. The segment of the keratolimbal allograft is then elevated, a 23-gauge needle is used to make an entry into the anterior chamber 1.5 mm posterior to the limbus, and the tube is inserted into the eye. After the tube is at the desired length and positioned in the anterior chamber, the keratolimbal allograft is then placed back in its original position and secured to the sclera with interrupted 10-0 nylon sutures. A small tissue patch graft is then placed behind the

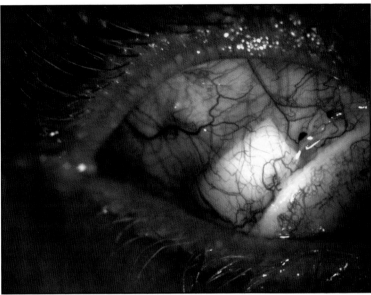

Figure 34-4. Baerveldt glaucoma drainage implant seen in an aniridia patient with prior keratolimbal allograft for stem cell deficiency. The scleral patch graft was placed just posterior to the keratolimbal allograft lenticule with some degree of patch overlap to ensure complete coverage of the tube.

keratolimbal allograft segment, and the anterior portion of the tissue patch graft is positioned against and slightly posterior to the lip of the keratolimbal allograft to allow a small amount of "patch overlap." This is done to ensure there is no gap in tube coverage by patch material (Figure 34-4). The conjunctival flap is closed by suturing the flap to the posterior lip of the keratolimbal allograft. I prefer a monofilament 9-0 Vicryl running suture on a Vas-100 needle.

Aniridia Fibrosis Syndrome

Aniridia fibrosis syndrome is described in aniridia patients that have undergone multiple surgeries in which there is progressive anterior chamber fibrosis. A retrolenticular and retrocorneal membrane forms, which can be seen clinically involving the ciliary body and anterior retina. Histopathologic evidence in this condition demonstrates extensive fibrotic tissue originated from the root of the rudimentary iris and entrapped in the intraocular lens (IOL) haptics.[12] Patients with aniridia and multiple prior surgeries (penetrating keratoplasty, tube shunts, cataract surgery) are at risk for aniridia fibrosis syndrome. Early recognition is important because early surgical intervention is recommended to prevent phthisis.[12] In our practice, pars plana vitrectomy with aggressive epiciliary membrane peeling has been successful in preventing some of these eyes from progressing to phthisis from ciliary fibrosis.

KEY POINTS

1. Aniridia patients present many unique challenges to the glaucoma surgeon.

2. Tube shunt surgery, trabeculotomy, and goniotomy have shown the most favorable results.

3. Early goniotomy should be considered in patients in whom angle changes are occurring that predispose them to developing aniridic glaucoma.

4. Cyclodestructive procedures should be used with caution given the higher rates of severe complications in aniridia patients.

REFERENCES

1. Chen TC, Walton DS. Goniosurgery for prevention of aniridic glaucoma. *Arch Ophthalmol.* 1999;117(9):1144-1148.
2. Filous A, Odehnal M, Brunova B. Results of treatment of glaucoma associated with aniridia [Czech]. *Cesk Slov Oftalmol.* 1998;54(1):18-21.
3. Adachi M, Dickens CJ, Hetherington J Jr, et al. Clinical experience of trabeculotomy for the surgical treatment of aniridic glaucoma. *Ophthalmology.* 1997;104(12):2121-2125.
4. Wiggens RE, Tomey, KF. The results of glaucoma surgery in aniridia. *Arch Ophthalmol.* 1992;110:503-505.
5. Arroyave CP, Scott IU, Gedde SJ, Parrish RK II, Feuer WJ. Use of glaucoma drainage devices in the management of glaucoma associated with aniridia. *Am J Ophthalmol.* 2003;135(2):155-159.
6. Lee H, Meyers K, Lanigan B, O'Keefe M. Complications and visual prognosis in children with aniridia. *J Pediatr Ophthalmol Strabismus.* 2010;47(4):205-210.
7. Wagle NS, Freedman SF, Buckley EG, Davis JS, Biglan AW. Long-term outcome of cyclocryotherapy for refractory pediatric glaucoma. *Ophthalmology.* 1998;105(10): 1921-1926.
8. Wallace DK, Plager DA, Snyder SK, Raiesdana A, Helveston EM, Ellis FD. Surgical results of secondary glaucomas in childhood. *Ophthalmology.* 1998;105(1):101-111.
9. Okada K, Mishima HK, Masumaoto M, Tsukamto H, Takamatsu M. Results of filtering surgery in young patients with aniridia. *Hiroshima J Med Sci.* 2000;49(3):135-138.
10. Brandt JD, Casuso LA, Budenz DL. Markedly increased central corneal thickness: an unrecognized finding in congenital aniridia. *Am J Ophthalmol.* 2004;137(2):348-350.
11. Whitson JT, Liang C, Godfrey DG, et al. Central corneal thickness in patients with congenital aniridia. *Eye Contact Lens.* 2005;31(5):221-224.
12. Tsai JH, Freeman JM, Chan CC, et al. A progressive anterior fibrosis syndrome in patients with post surgical congenital aniridia. *Am J Ophthalmol.* 2005;140(6):1075-1079.

35

GLAUCOMA SURGERY IN CORNEAL TRANSPLANT PATIENTS

Preeya K. Gupta, MD and John P. Berdahl, MD

Glaucoma is a frequent comorbid condition in corneal transplant patients. Glaucoma may develop after transplantation secondary to chronic steroid use or synechiae-induced angle closure, or it could be a pre-existing condition related to traumatic injury. Common indications for corneal transplant include Fuchs' dystrophy, aphakic or pseudophakic bullous keratopathy, corneal infections, traumatic injury, scarring, and irregular astigmatism. Penetrating keratoplasty performed for aphakic and pseudophakic bullous keratopathy, as well as inflammatory conditions, are more likely to cause postoperative glaucoma than keratoconus and Fuchs' endothelial dystrophy because the former is often associated with damage to the trabecular meshwork. Newer transplantation techniques, such as Descemet's stripping endothelial keratoplasty (DSEK), used to treat corneal edema secondary to endothelial dysfunction (ie, Fuchs' dystrophy, aphakic and pseudophakic bullous keratopathy) have allowed for faster visual recovery. However, glaucoma is still a significant comorbid condition.

In the Collaborative Corneal Transplantation Studies, a history of preoperative glaucoma increased the graft failure rate from 29% to 48%.[1] Further, in the Cornea Donor Study, the rate of graft failure was 11% without glaucoma, 20% with glaucoma treated with medications alone, 29% with glaucoma treated with surgery alone, and 58% with glaucoma treated by both medication and surgery.[2] Repeated studies have shown that the risk of graft failure is increased in patients with uncontrolled intraocular pressure (IOP), making management of glaucoma an integral component to graft survival.[3,4]

Kahook M.
Essentials of Glaucoma Surgery (pp 301-306).
© 2012 SLACK Incorporated.

Preoperative risk factors for uncontrolled IOP after corneal transplant include the following:

- Steroid-induced ocular hypertension
- Prior angle trauma
- Pre-existing glaucoma with uncontrolled IOP
- Aphakia
- Intolerance or allergy to IOP-lowering medications
- Poor compliance with medications

SURGICAL OPTIONS

Surgical intervention for glaucoma primarily includes either trabeculectomy with antimetabolite or implantation of a glaucoma drainage device. In the case of refractory glaucoma, cycloablative procedures such as cyclophotocoagulation may be considered.[5] The major factors influencing one's decision regarding these surgical options include the intended degree of IOP reduction and the risk of bleb failure due to comorbidities. Trabeculectomy may achieve a lower IOP compared with glaucoma drainage devices (GDDs). However, trabeculectomy is more sensitive to postoperative inflammation, and when performing combined lens exchange and/or vitrectomy, there may be a higher risk for bleb failure. Further, trabeculectomy surgery may not be feasible in patients who have prior conjunctival scarring secondary to trauma, chemical exposure, limbal stem cell deficiency, or other ocular surface diseases. Thus, prior to performing trabeculectomy, it is important to have any ocular surface inflammation under maximal control.

The surgical procedure of choice for glaucoma requiring moderate IOP reduction in the setting of prior corneal transplant is a GDD (Figure 35-1). Typically, these devices allow for adequate IOP control and are relatively uncomplicated to implant. Further, multiple GDDs can be placed to achieve lower IOP. Tube shunt surgery can be done at the same time as penetrating keratoplasty in a staged fashion, with the tube shunt performed 4 to 6 months prior to corneal surgery or after prior corneal transplant. Valved (Ahmed, Krupin, Molteno) and nonvalved (Baerveldt) implants can be used alone or in combination. Careful placement of the GDD within the anterior chamber is of importance, as there is a risk of endothelial damage should repeated contact occur between the tube and endothelium.

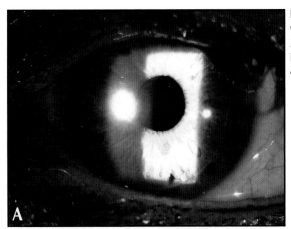

Figure 35-1. Patient with DSEK, Baerveldt 350 Tube Shunt, and inferior peripheral iridotomy.

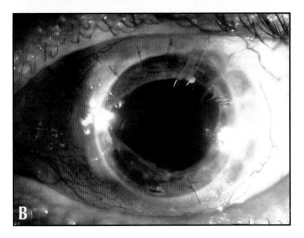

SURGICAL PLANNING

Preoperative Clinical Considerations

- Posterior capsule and hyaloid face status
- Presence or absence of vitreous into the anterior chamber
- Altered lens status: aphakia; sutured posterior chamber lens
- Ocular surface inflammation
- Conjunctival vascularity and/or scarring

A thorough preoperative examination for the presence of vitreous in the anterior chamber is essential prior to surgical intervention. The presence of vitreous in the anterior chamber increases the risk of glaucoma surgery failure. Vitreous can become incarcerated into the tube opening or sclerostomy site, causing poor outflow and elevated IOP. If vitreous is present, a thorough anterior vitrectomy is required at the time of glaucoma surgery to prevent failure.

Ocular surface inflammation and vascularity can be a source of bleb failure in patients undergoing trabeculectomy. Adequate control of inflammation with steroids or immunomodulating agents is essential prior to surgery. GDD is preferred in patients with significant ocular surface inflammation, as these patients have a tendency toward developing bleb fibrosis with subsequent bleb failure.

Anterior chamber depth is important when considering implantation of a GDD in a patient with either penetrating keratoplasty (PK) or DSEK. Eyes with a shallow anterior chamber depth are at higher risk for tube–endothelium contact, which risks failure of the transplanted tissue and corneal decompensation over time.

Intraoperative Considerations

- Location of tube placement
- Length of tube
- Placement of venting slits and/or ripcord

GDD tubes can be placed in the anterior chamber or through the pars plana. The length of the tube is of critical importance because corneal decompensation and graft failure will ensue with chronic tube–cornea touch. Placement of the tube in the pars plana prevents tube–cornea touch, but a complete vitrectomy is required prior to the placement of the tube in this location to prevent incarceration of the vitreous.

When placing a nonvalved GDD, such as the Baerveldt, the surgeon has the option to place venting slit incisions within the tube, in addition to occluding the tube with a nylon suture and Vicryl ligature to prevent postoperative hypotony. Venting incisions within the tube allow for early flow through the tube until a bleb has formed over the plate of the tube and the ripcord can be removed, typically 4 to 6 weeks after implantation.

Postoperative Considerations

- Complications: Hypotony, graft failure, suprachoroidal hemorrhage, malignant glaucoma
- Chronic topical steroid use and potential IOP elevation
- Choice of topical ocular hypotensive medications in patients with a corneal graft

Suprachoroidal hemorrhage is a dreaded complication of cornea transplant surgery. It is more common in patients who have pre-existing glaucoma, vascular disease, and preoperative elevated IOP. Suprachoroidal hemorrhage can occur during glaucoma surgery but is more common in corneal transplantation because the IOP is reduced to atmospheric pressure. If the choroidal pressure is elevated during this time, a suprachoroidal hemorrhage and/or expulsion of intraocular contents occurs secondary to the absence of IOP to counterbalance the choroidal pressure. For this reason, in patients undergoing corneal transplantation, it is advisable to use a Honan balloon or other device to decompress the vitreous and lower IOP at the time of surgery.

Patients with corneal transplant often need to be on chronic steroid therapy. Chronic steroid therapy can increase IOP, and the elevated IOP should be weighed against the increased risk of corneal graft rejection. Intensive topical steroids are often critical early in the postoperative period to avoid graft rejection and can be gradually tapered over time. However, graft rejection can occur at any point in time, therefore, careful attention should be paid to graft health during the tapering of topical steroids.

For patients who have had corneal transplantation and glaucoma surgery whose IOP is still not adequately controlled, beta-blockers (timolol) or alpha-agonists (brimonidine) are the medications of choice. Prostaglandin analogue drugs (eg, latanoprost, bimatoprost, travoprost) should be avoided because they can increase inflammation, leading to graft rejection. Similarly, carbonic anhydrase inhibitors (eg, dorzolamide, brinzolamide) can lead to graft failure by inducing decreased endothelial cell pump function, leading to corneal edema. In the end, placement of multiple glaucoma drainage devices to achieve adequate IOP control is an option if other interventions prove inadequate, as good IOP control is critical to graft survival.

CONCLUSION

Corneal graft failure is a potential complication that can occur at any point in the postoperative period. Should it occur, it is critical to identify the etiology of graft failure, which may be secondary to uncontrolled IOP or due to mechanical damage from glaucoma implant hardware. Graft failure due to mechanical trauma from intraocular hardware should prompt revision of the tube with repeat corneal transplant. The intraocular portion of the glaucoma drainage device can be trimmed to a shorter length or repositioned to a location that is directed further away from the cornea (ie, in the iris plane, behind the iris, or in the pars plana).

KEY POINTS

1. Glaucoma is common in patients with corneal transplantation.
2. Glaucoma increases the risk of graft failure.
3. Glaucoma drainage devices are usually preferred in patients with corneal transplantation.
4. Ideally, prostaglandins are avoided in the setting of corneal transplantations.

REFERENCES

1. Maguire MG, Stark WJ, Gottsch JD, et al. Risk factors for corneal graft failure and rejection in the collaborative corneal transplantation studies. Collaborative Corneal Transplantation Studies Research Group. *Ophthalmology*. 1994;101(9):1536-1547.
2. Sugar A, Tanner JP, Dontchev M, et al. Recipient risk factors for graft failure in the cornea donor study. *Ophthalmology*. 2009:116(6):1023-1028.
3. Lee RK, Fantes F. Surgical management of patients with combined glaucoma and corneal transplant surgery. *Curr Opin Ophthalmol*. 2003;14(2):95-99.
4. Aldave AJ, Rudd JC, Cohen EJ, et al. The role of glaucoma therapy in the need for repeat penetrating keratoplasty. *Cornea*. 2000;19(6):772-776.
5. Shah P, Lee GA, Kirwan JK, et al. Cyclodiode photocoagulation for refractory glaucoma after penetrating keratoplasty. *Ophthalmology*. 2001;108(11):1986-1991.

GLAUCOMA SURGERY IN THE KERATOPROSTHESIS PATIENT

Jeffrey M. Zink, MD

KERATOPROSTHESIS: THE GLAUCOMA PROBLEM

Patients with a history of keratoprosthesis present many challenges for the glaucoma specialist. An extremely high incidence of glaucoma is seen in patients who have undergone keratoprosthesis surgery. Many of these patients have pre-existing glaucoma or develop glaucoma following keratoprosthesis placement. Netland et al[1] published a retrospective case series of 55 eyes of 52 patients treated with a keratoprosthesis and found glaucoma present in the majority (64%) of eyes treated with keratoprosthesis (36% before and 28% following keratoprosthesis).

The incidence of glaucoma is already high in patients who need to undergo keratoprosthesis surgery. This includes patients with a history of severe surface disease, chemical injury, ocular cicatricial pemphigoid, status/postkeratolimbal allograft surgery, herpes keratitis, and aniridia. Glaucoma can also be exacerbated following keratoprosthesis surgery. Development of angle-closure glaucoma following keratoprosthesis surgery is common. Keratoprosthesis patients are often on chronic steroids, so this predisposes them to a steroid-induced component as well.

Currently there are 2 artificial corneas approved for use in the United States—the AlphaCor (Addition Technology, Des Plaines, Illinois) artificial cornea and the Dohlman-Doane or Boston keratoprosthesis (Massachusetts Eye & Ear Infirmary, Boston, Massachusetts). The Boston keratoprosthesis was first described in 1974 by Sayech et al[2] and was approved by the Food and Drug Administration (FDA) for use in the United States in 1992. There are 2 types, depending on the severity of ocular surface disease (Type I and Type II).

The Multicenter Boston Type 1 Keratoprosthesis Study (MBTKS), a prospective series of 141 patients from 17 centers, revealed that many of these patients do reasonably well from a visual outcome standpoint.[3] The

Kahook M.
Essentials of Glaucoma Surgery (pp 307-312).
© 2012 SLACK Incorporated.

study showed a visual acuity of greater than 20/40 in 23% of patients and better than or equal to than 20/200 in 57% of patients.

Failure of visual acuity to improve was attributed to underlying ocular disease such as advanced glaucoma, macular degeneration, or retinal detachment. This study demonstrated the importance of controlling glaucoma in this patient population.

DIAGNOSIS AND MONITORING

Intraocular pressure measurement is difficult because there is no reliable way to monitor intraocular pressure (IOP) in this patient population. Measurements taken over the prosthesis will be markedly elevated, and measurements taken over the sclera are not accurate.[4] At this time, finger palpation is felt to be the best approach to estimation of the IOP. I prefer palpating over the upper lid with an index finger from each hand while the patient is looking down to get an approximation of IOP. This is a skill that can be developed by a clinician by palpating many normal eyes and comparing the estimated IOP by palpation to the IOP measured with applanation tonometry. With practice, surgeons can learn to better estimate the IOP using palpation techniques.

In these patients, glaucoma is followed using tactile IOP, visual field testing, and optic nerve examinations. Stereoscopic optic nerve examinations can be difficult secondary to retroprosthetic membrane formation, nystagmus, and limited keratoprosthesis aperture. Anterior segment optical coherence tomography may be useful in documenting stability of the device around the stem and to better characterize angle anatomy.[5]

Eventually, an IOP sensor would be the best way to monitor IOP more accurately in keratoprosthesis patients. Techniques using laser interferometry (eg, FISO Inc, Ottawa, Canada) and Radiowave telemetry (eg, Medical Sensors Technology Inc, Germany) may hold some promise.[6] The future application of these technologies in humans is yet to be determined.

MANAGEMENT

Medications

Medications can be helpful, but many patients require surgical intervention. Typically, aqueous suppressants are a good option for first-line treatment. Prostaglandin analogues can also be helpful in these patients. Preservative-free preparations, such as preservative-free timolol maleate, can be an ideal option in keratoprosthesis patients with severe surface disease. These can minimize the toxic surface effects of preservatives, as many patients with a keratoprosthesis have severe underlying surface disease. Oral carbonic

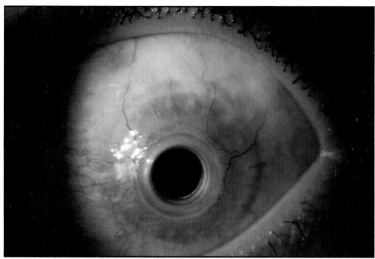

Figure 36-1. Young aniridia patient with a keratoprosthesis that required a 250 mm² Baerveldt glaucoma drainage implant for uncontrolled glaucoma.

anhydrase inhibitors, such as acetazolamide or methazolamide, can also be helpful in keratoprosthesis patients when the IOP is difficult to control.

Glaucoma Drainage Implants

Various options of glaucoma drainage implants can be used in these patients, but I prefer either an Ahmed or smaller-plate Baerveldt (250 mm²). A Molteno3 (175 mm²) would also be a good option in these patients because of the theoretical lower risk of hypotony. Tube placement should be done prior to keratoprosthesis placement when possible. Drainage implants placed in the anterior chamber prior to keratoprosthesis placement usually continue to function well following keratoprosthesis surgery. There is a risk of tube occlusion from retroprosthetic inflammatory membrane formation in tubes placed in the anterior chamber prior to keratoprosthesis placement. If the patient has already had keratoprosthesis surgery and develops glaucoma following surgery, a combined pars plana vitrectomy with pars plana tube insertion is a good option (Figures 36-1 and 36-2). I recommend doing this in conjunction with a vitreoretinal surgeon who is comfortable with endoscopic vitrectomy techniques because the view can be limited and the patient is at risk of tube occlusion by vitreous without a complete vitrectomy. Glaucoma drainage implant surgery can also be done at the time of keratoprosthesis placement but may be difficult to arrange for logistical reasons.

A recent published report described a series in which the glaucoma drainage implant plate was connected with a tube to the lacrimal sac,

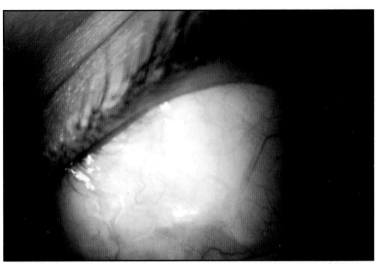

Figure 36-2. Filtration bleb seen overlying the Baervelt 250 mm² implant plate in this young aniridia patient with a keratoprosthesis.

ethmoid or maxillary sinus, or lower lid fornix to facilitate aqueous drainage in keratoprosthesis patients.[7] The authors found that the incidence of severe infection rates was very low with these techniques. Although this technique is reasonable, more conventional tube shunt surgery has been shown to be effective in keratoprosthesis patients. Vajaranant et al[8] recently published a cases series using the technique of combined vitrectomy and pars plana glaucoma shunt placement in keratoprosthesis patients.

Cyclophotocoagulation

I prefer the transscleral cyclophotocoagulation option in patients with severe conjunctival scarring who are poor candidates for tube shunt placement. Recently, Rivier and colleagues reported a series between 1993 and 2007 in which 18 eyes of 18 patients underwent diode laser transscleral cyclophotocoagulation (DLTSC), either before (n = 3), during (n = 1), or after (n = 14) keratoprosthesis surgery. Mean postoperative IOP was significantly reduced at 6, 12, 24, 36, and 48 months after DLTSC.[9] In my practice, I typically begin with 180 degrees of treatment, which is usually adequate in achieving the desired IOP lowering in most patients. Because cyclodestructive procedures are permanent, I recommend conservative treatment initially, as more treatment can always be added in the future.

Endoscopic cyclophotocoagulation is a good option in patients who have severe surface disease, conjunctival scarring, or prior keratolimbal allograft surgery. In my experience, transscleral cyclophotocoagulation may not be as effective following keratolimbal allograft surgery given the increased thickness of perilimbal tissue that needs to be penetrated to reach the ciliary processes. In patients with severe conjunctival scarring that precludes tube shunt placement, endoscopic cyclophotocoagulation can be a great option if a vitrectomy is already being performed for another indication.

KEY POINTS

1. Patients with a history of keratoprosthesis surgery have a high incidence of glaucoma and need to be followed very closely to prevent permanent visual loss.

2. Medications, aqueous drainage implants, and cyclodestructive procedures are all reasonable options, but many patients will require surgical intervention.

3. Be ready for additional challenges when caring for these patients.

4. Better ways of measuring IOP are needed in these patients to improve long-term monitoring capabilities. New technologies may eventually make this possible.

REFERENCES

1. Netland, PA, Terada H, Dohlman, CH. Glaucoma associated with keratoprosthesis. *Ophthalmology.* 1998;105(4):751-757.

2. Sayech RR, Ang LPK, Foster CS, Dohlman CH. The Boston keratoprosthesis in Steven's-Johnson syndrome. *Am J Ophthalmol.* 2008;145(3):438-444.

3. Zerbe BL, Belin MW, Ciolino JB. Results from the multicenter Boston Type 1 Keratoprosthesis Study. *Ophthalmology.* 2006;113(10):1779.e1-7.

4. Birkholz ES, Goins KM. *Boston keratoprosthesis: an option for patients with multiple failed corneal grafts.* Accessed March 9, 2009. Retrieved from www.webeye.ophth.uiowa.edu/eyeforum/cases/94-Boston-Keratoprosthesis-Failed-Corneal-Grafts.htm.

5. Garcia JP, de la Cruz J, Rosen RB, Buxton DF. Imaging implanted keratoprostheses with anterior-segment optical coherence tomography and ultrasound biomicroscopy. *Cornea.* 2008;27(2):180-188.

6. Melki S, Lopez M, Dohlman C. Intraocular pressure sensors in KPRO. *Boston Keratoprosthesis Update,* Newsletter VI: 2009. Accessed February 10, 2010. Retrieved from www.masseyeandear.org/gedownload!/2009%20KPro%20Newsletter.pdf?item_id=48224001&version_id=48224002.

7. Dohlman CH, Grosskreutz CL, Chen TC, et al. Shunts to divert aqueous humor to distant epithelialized cavities after keratoprosthesis surgery. *J Glaucoma.* 2010:19(2):111-115.

8. Vajaranant TS, Blair MP, McMahaon T, Wilensky JT, de la Cruz J. Special considerations for pars plana tube-shunt placement in Boston type 1 keratoprosthesis. *Arch Ophthalmol.* 2010;128(11):1480-1482.

9. Rivier D, Jayter P, Kim E, Dohlman, CH, Grosskreutz CL. Glaucoma and keratoprosthesis surgery: role of adjunctive cyclophotocoagulation. *J Glaucoma.* 2009;18(4):321-324.

37

CONCOMITANT GLAUCOMA DRAINAGE DEVICES AND CORNEAL TRANSPLANTATION

Preeya K. Gupta, MD and John P. Berdahl, MD

A number of conditions may necessitate combined corneal transplantation and implantation of a glaucoma drainage device. Conditions such as trauma, iridocorneal endothelial (ICE) syndrome, herpetic infection, aphakia, or neovascular glaucoma are commonly associated with elevated intraocular pressure (IOP) and corneal scar or decompensation. The anterior segment procedures can be performed in combination by a glaucoma and corneal surgeon or simultaneously by a single anterior segment surgeon. It is important for the surgeon to determine preoperatively the risk of elevated IOP after keratoplasty. The risk of glaucoma after keratoplasty depends on the indication for corneal transplant; patients with keratoconus or Fuchs' dystrophy have been found to have significantly less postoperative glaucoma than patients with corneal ulcer, herpetic disease, and aphakia.

PREOPERATIVE CONSIDERATIONS

Corneal graft survival and maximization of visual potential are intimately tied to adequate IOP control. In a patient undergoing corneal transplantation, a comprehensive evaluation prior to surgery is necessary to determine whether a combined surgery is the best option for the patient. Glaucoma surgery for uncontrolled IOP usually takes precedence over the corneal transplant because the damage that occurs with glaucoma is irreversible. Glaucoma surgery almost always can be performed first while delaying the cornea transplantation; the exception is corneal melt or perforated cornea in which the cornea transplantation becomes urgent. If the progression of glaucoma can be arrested, the surgeon can safely come back at a later time and perform corneal

Kahook M.
Essentials of Glaucoma Surgery (pp 313-318).
© 2012 SLACK Incorporated.

transplantation. This staged procedure has the potential to increase the success rate for both surgeries, as there is adequate pressure control at the time of transplantation and less overall inflammation; however, outcomes of staged vs combined surgeries have been variable in the literature. Ultimately, the decision between staged vs combined glaucoma and transplant surgery is determined by the surgeon and patient. In some situations, such as in a patient with severely uncontrolled preoperative IOP, poor medication compliance, medical contraindications to multiple surgeries, or in very controlled situations such as an ICE syndrome in which the eye is not in an inflamed state, one may prefer to perform combined glaucoma and corneal transplant surgery. In most cases, glaucoma drainage devices (GDDs) are preferable over trabeculectomy generally because of the increased inflammatory reaction present following corneal transplantation, which could lead to bleb failure.

DESCEMET'S STRIPPING ENDOTHELIAL KERATOPLASTY COMBINED WITH GLAUCOMA DRAINAGE DEVICE

Performing combined GDD implantation and Descemet's stripping endothelial keratoplasty (DSEK) is possible in patients who have endothelial dysfunction and uncontrolled glaucoma. One reason for combining this procedure is in patients with ICE syndrome who have abnormal endothelial cell function and deterioration of the angle and trabecular meshwork. Further, certain patients with Fuchs' dystrophy who have combined endothelial dysfunction and uncontrolled IOP may also be good candidates for this procedure because elevated IOP can increase corneal edema and decrease the quality of vision.

The first step in a combined DSEK and glaucoma surgery should be implantation of the GDD. The rationale for placing the glaucoma implant first is that it is easier to suture the GDD plate to the sclera on a relatively firm eye. Additionally, the insertion of the tube into the anterior chamber would likely cause a collapse of the anterior chamber or detachment of the DSEK lenticule, thus the DSEK should be performed after the GDD portion of the surgery is completed (see Chapter 8 for a complete description of the surgery). Similar to the standard GDD implantation procedure, after securing the plate, the tube is cut to the appropriate length and inserted into the eye. It is very important in the combined surgery to ensure that the tube is cut to the appropriate length and is angled in the iris plane or directed slightly posteriorly. The intraocular portion of the tube should be trimmed relatively short to prevent it from interfering with graft insertion and from chronically touching the corneal transplant, which would cause it to decompensate (Figure 37-1). A patch graft of sclera or pericardium should be secured over the tube, and the conjunctiva can be repositioned and fastened with sutures.

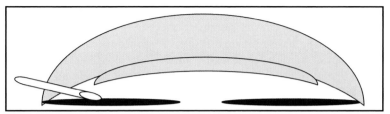

Figure 37-1. Note that the tube should be directed away from the DSEK graft and cut short to avoid contact with the graft.

Next, viscoelastic is inserted into the anterior chamber; then Descemet's membrane can be scored, stripped, and removed from the eye. An inferior peripheral iridotomy is used by some surgeons to prevent pupillary block from the air bubble that will be placed in the anterior chamber. The inferior peripheral iridotomy also allows the surgeon to leave a relatively large air bubble, which can be advantageous for increased air tamponade of the graft to the stroma or in patients in whom air escape is anticipated (aphakia, trabeculectomy, and/or patent tube shunt present preoperatively). The inferior peripheral iridotomy can be created prior to removal of the viscoelastic with microforceps and microscissors, or preoperatively with the YAG laser. A 4- to 5-mm clear corneal or scleral tunnel incision should be created approximately 90 degrees away from the insertion of the glaucoma tube. The viscoelastic is removed and the corneal transplant tissue cut to the appropriate size. Once the DSEK lenticule is separated from the rest of the corneal tissue, it can be inserted into the anterior chamber using an insertion device or tissue forceps. The graft is unfolded in the anterior chamber with balanced salt solution and an air bubble. The graft is positioned into place, and then a large air bubble is instilled into the anterior chamber. Air bubble management can be challenging in patients with a preexisting GDD, given the propensity for air to rise and escape through the tube. In a combined procedure, because the tube is typically tied off or valved, air does not go through the GDD. However, if this is a problem, viscoelastic can be inserted into the tip of the tube to help provide a temporary plug so pressure can be maintained to facilitate DSEK graft attachment. A large air bubble can either be left in place with an inferior iridotomy or can be exchanged for balanced salt solution after an appropriate period of time with a full air bubble. A full air bubble is a 100% fill of air in the anterior chamber, which is typically left in place for 8 to 10 minutes after graft insertion to facilitate adhesion of the donor lenticule to the host stroma. Then, the size of the air bubble is adjusted based on the surgical technique used (ie, only a small amount of air is exchanged with balanced salt solution if an inferior iridotomy is present and a large bubble of air is left) or about 50% of the air bubble is exchanged for balanced salt solution in the absence of an inferior peripheral iridotomy to avoid pupillary block.

Patients who have combined DSEK and glaucoma surgery often need to take topical steroids for at least 1 year. The prolonged steroid use can cause a rise in IOP, and this should be monitored closely. Additionally, as the bleb wall forms around the GDD plate, there can be a hypertensive phase between weeks 2 and 10, requiring the addition of topical medications. If glaucoma medications are needed in addition to the GDD to lower IOP, alpha-agonists or beta-blockers are typically the medications of choice. Prostaglandin analogues can increase the inflammatory response and increase the chance of corneal graft rejection, and carbonic anhydrase inhibitors can inhibit endothelial cell pump function, thereby limiting the effectiveness of the corneal graft.

GLAUCOMA DRAINAGE DEVICE IN COMBINATION WITH PENETRATING KERATOPLASTY

Diseases that affect the corneal stroma or induce severe irregular astigmatism, such as scarring after trauma, infectious corneal ulcers, or herpetic infection, are better treated with full-thickness corneal transplant than DSEK. If the patient also has progressive glaucoma that is not controllable with medications, one could consider combined full-thickness cornea transplant with GDD implantation. The most common cause of a combined full-thickness corneal transplant and glaucoma surgery is trauma (although other causes, such as inflammatory conditions or herpetic keratouveitis, are also possible).

Again, the GDD should be performed first to facilitate securing the plate to the sclera. Given the increased risk of graft failure with a GDD, it is important to ensure that the intraocular portion of the glaucoma tube is directed away from the cornea and that it is not too long inside the eye. After the GDD is placed, the typical steps of a full-thickness cornea' transplant can be performed. A vacuum trephine, the diameter of which depends on the location of the pathology present, is used to trephinate the host cornea. Similarly, a punch trephine is used to cut a corneal button of similar or slightly larger size to transplant into the host cornea. A 10-0 nylon suture is used in an interrupted and/or running fashion to secure the full-thickness corneal transplant to the host eye. Interrupted sutures are preferred in an inflammatory condition so that selective suture removal may be performed if any of the sutures become a source of inflammation. The postoperative period involves gradual visual recovery and requires topical steroids for an extended period of time. The IOP must be watched carefully during this period and treated appropriately. Again, prostaglandin and carbonic anhydrase inhibitors are ideally avoided because of the pro-inflammatory component of prostaglandin analogues and the decrease in endothelial cell pump function with carbonic anhydrase inhibitors.

POSTOPERATIVE CONSIDERATIONS

The failure rate of glaucoma surgery and cornea transplantation is variable but can be higher in combined surgeries as mentioned previously. In some cases, the benefits of providing simultaneous surgery outweigh the risks of surgical failure. Postoperatively, both the glaucoma surgery and the corneal transplant need to be monitored for signs of failure. Corneal rejection is identified by intraocular cell and flare, keratic precipitates present on the endothelium, corneal edema, epithelial irregularity, or other signs such as a Khodadoust line. Glaucoma failure is determined predominantly by the morphology of the overlying bleb and the IOP. Multiple glaucoma tubes can be placed in eyes with prior corneal transplantation should the IOP be inadequate. The risk of graft failure should be weighed against the risk of progressive glaucoma in this setting. Cycloablative procedures are also an option to achieve better IOP control without implantation of more hardware.

SPECIAL CONSIDERATIONS

In patients who have had a vitrectomy and need glaucoma surgery combined with a corneal transplant, it is advisable to place the GDD tube into the posterior segment to avoid all possibility of corneal decompensation secondary to the cornea–tube touch.

CONCLUSION

Corneal transplantation and glaucoma surgery can be performed concomitantly. Glaucoma surgery usually takes precedence over corneal transplantation because the damage caused by glaucoma is irreversible. In the setting of endothelial dysfunction, a DSEK combined with GDD is the preferred approach. If corneal scarring or irregular astigmatism is present, penetrating keratoplasty combined with GDD is typically performed. The majority of the glaucoma portion of the procedure is usually performed prior to entering the intraocular space. It is important to avoid endothelial tube touch, which can cause corneal decompensation. Managing postoperative inflammation is critical to the survival of both the corneal transplant and the glaucoma surgery.

KEY POINTS

1. Combined corneal transplantation and glaucoma surgery can be performed.
2. Usually a GDD is combined with corneal transplantation.

3. Avoiding endothelial tube touch is important to prevent corneal decompensation.

4. Aggressively managing postoperative inflammation is critical for the success of the corneal transplant and glaucoma surgery.

SUGGESTED READINGS

Ayyala RS. Penetrating keratoplasty and glaucoma. *Surv Ophthalmol.* 2000;45(2):91-105.

Lee RK, Fantes F. Surgical management of patients with combined glaucoma and corneal transplant surgery. *Curr Opin Ophthalmol.* 2003;14(2):95-99.

Price FW Jr, Price MO. Is it worthwhile to combine penetrating keratoplasty with glaucoma drainage implants? *Cornea.* 2008;27(3):261-262.

Glaucoma Drainage Device Implantation Combined With Pars Plana Vitrectomy

Jonathan A. Eisengart, MD

Typically, glaucoma drainage devices (GDDs) and pars plana vitrectomy (PPV) are combined when the drainage tube needs to be placed through the pars plana. Although there are multiple reasons why a tube would be placed through the pars plana instead of the anterior segment, there are roughly 3 broad categories: to protect compromised corneal endothelium, the anterior segment will not anatomically accept a tube, or perilimbal conjunctival thinning or scarring. Additionally, if a vitrectomy and a GDD are both required (ie, neovascular glaucoma with nonclearing vitreous hemorrhage), combining a PPV and GDD may be more convenient and lead to a better outcome than performing the surgeries separately.

Considerations for Combining Glaucoma Drainage Device and Pars Plana Vitrectomy

Effectively combining efforts requires that the vitreoretinal surgeon and the glaucoma surgeon communicate well and plan the surgery. Important points to discuss include the following:

1. *Anesthesia.* A combined PPV and tube insertion likely will be longer and more involved than either procedure separately. Although retrobulbar block is appropriate for many patients, general anesthesia may be more appropriate for some.

2. *Location of the GDD.* The planned location for GDD placement may affect placement of the PPV ports. If the vitrectomy is done with a 23- or 25-gauge system, one of the ports may be positioned so that it can be reused for tube insertion. Additionally, the vitreoretinal surgeon should be reminded to thoroughly trim the vitreous base, particularly in the planned quadrant for tube insertion.

Kahook M.
Essentials of Glaucoma Surgery (pp 319-322).
© 2012 SLACK Incorporated.

Reasons to Consider PPV and Pars Plana Tube Insertion

1. Compromised corneal endothelium.
   ◦ Fuchs' or pseudophakic bullous keratopathy.
   ◦ Corneal edema secondary to anterior chamber tube (ie, reposition tube into pars plana).
   ◦ Penetrating keratoplasty or endothelial graft.
2. Anterior segment will not accept a tube.
   ◦ Extensive high peripheral anterior synechiae.
   ◦ Vitreous prolapse anteriorly/unicameral eyes.
   ◦ Unable to visualize anterior chamber for tube placement (ie, keratoprosthesis).
   ◦ Chronic anterior segment neovascularization (ie, hyphema could block tube).
   ◦ Very shallow anterior chamber.
3. Ocular surface disorders.
   ◦ Extensive anterior/perilimbal conjunctival scarring or recession from previous surgery.
   ◦ Reposition eroded tube into pars plana.
4. Complicated disease requiring simultaneous vitreoretinal and glaucoma surgery.

3. *Opening conjunctiva.* Many glaucoma doctors are quite particular about how the conjunctiva is handled, and this issue should be discussed with their vitreoretinal colleague. If a 20-gauge PPV is going to be performed, the extent and location of the peritomy should be planned to accommodate the GDD and the PPV sclerostomies. Even for 23- or 25-gauge vitrectomies that can be done transconjunctivally, the conjunctiva should be opened in the quadrant of the tube prior to placement of the trochars to avoid conjunctival holes.

4. *Order of surgical steps.* Typically I begin the combined surgery by opening up the conjunctiva and securing the plate to the eye. The vitreoretinal specialist will then complete a PPV. Finally, I will insert the tube into the pars plana, secure the patch graft, and close the conjunctiva.

It may be more convenient or efficient for the vitreoretinal surgeon to perform the complete PPV first, thereby allowing the glaucoma specialist to follow and complete the entire tube implant surgery uninterrupted. However, the eye is often quite hypotonous immediately following the PPV, which can make placement of the plate more difficult.

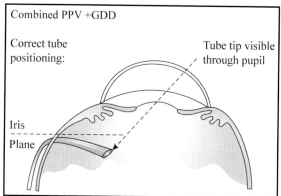

Combined PPV +GDD

Correct tube positioning:

Tube tip visible through pupil

Iris
Plane

Figure 38-1. Diagram of correct pars plana tube positioning: length, angle.

Pars Plana Tube Insertion

Placement of the tube through the pars plana is straightforward. The tube should be laid across the limbus and trimmed so that it extends approximately 2- to 3-mm past the limbus. This technique should ensure adequate length so that the tube can be visualized postoperatively at the slit lamp. The tube is then trimmed with a *posterior* bevel so that if it rotates anteriorly, it will not become obstructed by iris. If an existing PPV port is not being utilized, a 23-gauge needle is used to make a sclerostomy tract, directing the needle parallel to, or slightly posterior to, the plane of the iris; if it is pointed too posteriorly, the tube may rarely "kink" at the sclerostomy. The sclerostomy should be created 3.5 to 4mm posterior to the limbus in pseudophakes and 4mm in phakic patients. The tube is then inserted and visually inspected through the pupil in the anterior vitreous cavity; rotating the eye toward the quadrant with the tube or gently depressing in the area of the tube entry can facilitate visualization (Figure 38-1). The tube is covered with donor sclera, and the conjunctiva closed with 8-0 Vicryl suture.

An alternative to placing the bare tube directly through the pars plana is to use a dedicated pars plana "knuckle" (Model: PC, New World Medical Inc). This device fits onto an existing tube and bends it gently, avoiding a kink. I have never found this device necessary, but if used, it should be covered with graft material.

Vitreous Incarceration

Vitreous incarceration is a complication that can occur at any time intra- or postoperatively. This complication is uncommon if the vitreoretinal surgeon is able to remove the majority of the vitreous body.

Vitreous blocking the tube may be recognized intraoperatively if fluid fails to pass through the tube after insertion. After the tube is inserted into the eye, I like to pressurize the anterior chamber before closing the conjunctiva and ensure that fluid is flowing through the tube (or through the fenestration slits if the tube is tied off) and that the eye pressure comes down as expected.

If vitreous blocks the tube postoperatively, an elevated intraocular pressure (IOP) and flat bleb will be noted. If the intraocular portion of the tube was left long enough to be visualized at the slit lamp, vitreous may be seen extending into the tube. YAG laser vitreolysis can be successful in restoring tube function. If the tube cannot be visualized, or if YAG laser is unsuccessful, a repeat PPV to remove remaining vitreous or repositioning the tube into the anterior segment will be required.

KEY POINTS

1. The pars plana is an excellent location for tube insertion when the anterior chamber is not safe or available and may be the primary location whenever the eye has had a complete vitrectomy.

2. Good communication and planning between surgeons is necessary to successfully combine glaucoma drainage device insertion and pars plana vitrectomy.

3. Careful trimming of the vitreous skirt is important to prevent tube occlusion.

SUGGESTED READINGS

De Guzman MH, Valencia A, Farinelli AC. Pars plana insertion of glaucoma drainage devices for refractory glaucoma. *Clin Experiment Ophthalmol.* 2006;34(2):102-107.

Diaz-Llopis M, Salom D, García-Delpech S, Udaondo P, Millan JM, Arevalo JF. Efficacy and safety of the pars plana clip in Ahmed valve device inserted via the pars plana in patients with refractory glaucoma. *Clin Ophthalmol.* 2010;4:411-416.

Gandham SB, Costa VP, Katz LJ, et al. Aqueous tube-shunt implantation and pars plana vitrectomy in eyes with refractory glaucoma. *Am J Ophthalmol.* 1993;116(2):189-195.

Rothman RF, Sidoti PA, Gentile RC, et al. Glaucoma drainage tube kink after pars plana insertion. *Am J Ophthalmol.* 2001;132(3):413-414.

Smiddy WE, Rubsamen PE, Grajewski A. Vitrectomy for pars plana placement of a glaucoma seton. *Ophthalmic Surg.* 1994;25(8):532-535.

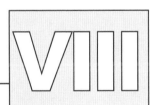

VIII

NOVEL APPROACHES

39

EX-PRESS
GLAUCOMA FILTRATION DEVICE

Mahmoud A. Khaimi, MD and Malik Y. Kahook, MD

Since its inception in the 1960s, the gold standard for surgical treatment of glaucoma has been the trabeculectomy.[1] The goal of this glaucoma filtering surgery is to create an alternative route for aqueous humor to drain out of the eye and into a subconjunctival reservoir, thus creating a bleb. More recently, incremental advancements in microsurgical device manufacturing has paved the way for the introduction of the Ex-Press glaucoma filtration device as a valuable adjunct to trabeculectomy.

OVERVIEW AND SURGICAL TECHNIQUE

The Ex-Press glaucoma filtration device is a nonvalved, MRI-compatible, stainless steel device that is inserted under a scleral flap into the anterior chamber to shunt aqueous to a subconjunctival reservoir.[2] The device is approximately 3 mm in length and has a 400-µm external lumen. Currently, the R and P models are available, with the P model being the most widely used. The P model is available with 50- or 200-µm internal lumens (Figure 39-1). The devices are preloaded on an injector device to minimize intraoperative device manipulation and for simplification of delivery (Figure 39-2).

The surgical technique for a trabeculectomy using the Ex-Press device is very similar to the standard trabeculectomy procedure. However, there are key differences that will be noted. The anesthetic used for this procedure should not vary from what the surgeon is originally accustomed to with traditional trabeculectomy. We prefer a retrobulbar block containing a half-and-half mixture of 0.4% lidocaine, 0.75% marcaine, and added wydase for a total of 5 cc. The patient is prepped and draped in the same fashion and a standard fornix or limbal-based conjunctival flap is then created to

Kahook M.
Essentials of Glaucoma Surgery (pp 325-330).
© 2012 SLACK Incorporated.

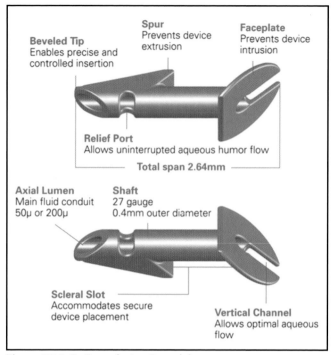

Figure 39-1. Ex-Press device, P-model.

Figure 39-2. Ex-Press injector device.

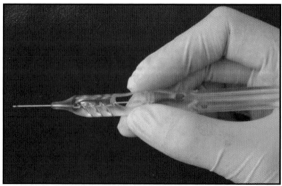

provide access to the scleral bed at the limbus. Wet-field cautery is used for homeostasis and a scleral flap is then created with the surgeon's blade of choice. The scleral flap should extend into clear cornea. **Note: Close attention should be paid to the following: (1) fashion a scleral flap that is a least half-thickness wide and, at minimum, 3- to 3.5-mm wide and long;**

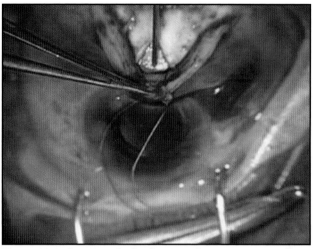

Figure 39-3. Creation of scleral ostia with a 25-gauge needle.

and (2) create a uniplanar flap dissection. Both of these critical points will ensure adequate coverage of the device face plate to avoid overfiltration and conjunctival extrusion.[3-13] As with traditional trabeculectomy, the shape of the flap (triangular, pentagonal, rectangular) does not seem to affect the outcome. Antifibrotics are then used in the usual manner for trabeculectomy. In anticipation of device placement, a clear corneal paracentesis is then created to provide access for reformation of the anterior chamber and assessment of aqueous egress.

The prefashioned scleral flap is then lifted and the "blue line" (trabecular meshwork) adjacent to clear cornea should be identified. Next, a 25-gauge needle (a 26- or 27-gauge needle may also be used) is then used to enter the anterior chamber just posterior to the blue line (Figure 39-3). The needle should be directed parallel to the iris plane, and the tip of the needle should fully enter the anterior chamber. Care should be taken to avoid needle-to-iris or -lens contact to minimize complications. However, the needle must completely enter the eye to create a patent scleral ostia for proper insertion of the implant. The Ex-Press, which is preloaded on an injector, is then threaded into the eye through the ostium (Figure 39-4) created in the previous step. **Note: Close attention should be paid to entering the anterior chamber at the same angle used with the needle. Failure to do so may result in difficulty in inserting the implant, which may potentially widen the ostia and subsequently lead to overfiltration and loose fixation of the device to the sclera.** The surgeon should also become familiarized with the injector device and specifically the central ridge,

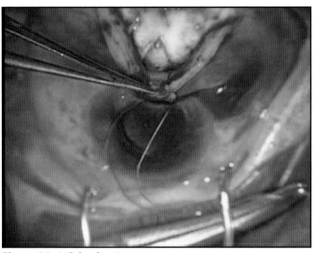

Figure 39-4. Scleral ostia.

where one must press to release the device prior to inserting it. Placement of the surgeon's finger anterior or posterior to the central ridge will result in greater effort required to release the device. Knowing the intricacies of the preloaded injector will help to promote a safer and uncomplicated insertion of the device. After the device is inserted, care is taken to make sure that it is well placed into the anterior chamber away from the corneal endothelium and iris and well situated on the scleral bed (face plate flush with the sclera). Furthermore, for the P version implants, the posterior groove on the footplate should point posteriorly toward the apex of the flap to promote posterior flow of aqueous.

As with traditional trabeculectomy, the scleral flap is then reapproximated to sclera with 10-0 nylon sutures. Two to 5 interrupted sutures are typically placed through the scleral flap. Flow can be assessed by injecting balanced salt solution through the previously created corneal paracentesis. After the amount of fluid flow is deemed appropriate and the eye pressure is adequate, the conjunctiva is closed with the surgeon's suture and technique of choice (ie, single versus double, running versus interrupted).

Our postoperative care is similar to our standard post-trabeculectomy regimen of topical steroids and antibiotics. Furthermore, postsurgical modifications, such as laser suture lysis, are similar to standard trabeculectomy parameters. Anecdotally, however, we have found that with the utilization of the Ex-Press device, earlier and more aggressive suture lysis is possible without an increased rate of hypotony.

Conclusion

The Ex-Press glaucoma filtration device has been a promising adjunct to the traditional glaucoma filtering procedure. Kanner et al[14] in a large case series, along with other studies,[15,16] have shown that use of the Ex-Press device under a scleral flap had similar intraocular pressure (IOP)-lowering efficacy compared with trabeculectomy. Thus, over the past half decade, placement of the Ex-Press device has exponentially increased. The Ex-Press has gained vast popularity worldwide for its ease of usage and for the advantages it offers both the patient and surgeon intra- and postoperatively over traditional trabeculectomy. One major difference between the traditional trabeculectomy and Ex-Press implantation is there is less intraocular manipulation of tissue when using the Ex-Press device. Unlike traditional trabeculectomy, a surgical iridectomy is not performed when using an Ex-Press device. This avoids the complication that can potentially arise when performing a surgical iridectomy (ie, hyphema and inflammation) and has led to less of an inflammatory response in the immediate postoperative period.[15,17,18] Furthermore, because the scleral ostia is much smaller than a typical sclerotomy created by a Kelley punch, intraopertively, the eye tends to be much more stable with less incidence of hypotony leading to shallow or flat chambers.[14-16] Less intraocular instability and complications have led many to believe that the postoperative visual recovery is faster in patients in whom an Ex-Press filtering procedure has been performed. In fact, a recent study conducted by Good and Kahook[16] has shown that patients who received an Ex-Press device had quicker visual recovery, fewer postoperative visits, and experienced fewer episodes of postoperative hypotony and hyphema compared with patients who had traditional trabeculectomy. The Ex-Press glaucoma filtration device procedure has thus emerged as a safe and effective alternative to the traditional trabeculectomy procedure.

References

1. Cairns JE. Trabeculectomy: preliminary report of a new method. *Am J Ophthalmol.* 1968;66(4):673-679.
2. Seibold LK, Rorrer RA, Kahook MY. MRI of the Ex-Press stainless steel glaucoma drainage device. *Br J Ophthalmol.* 2011;95(2):251-254.
3. Kaplan-Messas A, Traverso CE, Sellem E, Zagorsky ZF, Belkin M. The Ex-Press miniature glaucoma implant in combined surgery with cataract extraction: prospective study. *Invest Ophthalmol Vis Sci.* 2002;43:E-abstract 3348.
4. Gandolfi S, Traverso CF, Bron A, et al. Short-term results of a miniature drainage implant for glaucoma in combined surgery with phacoemulsification. *Acta Ophthalmol Scand Suppl.* 2002;236:66.
5. Traverso CE, De Feo F, Messas-Kaplan A, et al. Long term effect on IOP of a stainless steel glaucoma drainage implant (Ex-Press) in combined surgery with phacoemulsification. *Br J Ophthalmol.* 2005;89:425-429.

6. Wamsley S, Moster MR, Rai S, et al. Results of the use of the Ex-Press miniature glaucoma implant in technically challenging, advanced glaucoma cases: a clinical pilot study. *Am J Ophthalmol.* 2004;138:1049-1051.

7. Wamsley S, Moster MR, Rai S, et al. Optonol Ex-Press miniature tube shunt in advanced glaucoma. *Invest Ophthalmol Vis Sci.* 2004;45:E-abstract 994.

8. Stewart RM, Diamond JG, Ashmore ED, et al. Complications following Ex-Press glaucoma shunt implantation. *Am J Ophthalmol.* 2005;140:340-341.

9. Rivier D, Roy S, Mermoud A. Ex-Press R-50 miniature glaucoma implant insertion under the conjunctiva combined with cataract extraction. *J Cataract Refract Surg.* 2007;33:1946-1952.

10. Tavolato M, Babighian S, Galan A. Spontaneous extrusion of a stainless steel glaucoma drainage implant (Ex-Press). *Eur J Ophthalmol.* 2006;16:753-755.

11. Garg SJ, Kanitkar K, Weichel E, et al. Trauma-induced extrusion of an Ex-Press glaucoma shunt presenting as an intraocular foreign body. *Arch Ophthalmol.* 2005;123:1270-1272.

12. Filippopoulos T, Rhee DJ. Novel surgical procedures in glaucoma: advances in penetrating glaucoma surgery. *Curr Opin Ophthalmol.* 2008;19:149–154.

13. Stein JD, Herndon LW, Bond JB, Challa P. Exposure of Ex-Press miniature glaucoma devices: case series and technique for tube shunt removal. *J Glaucoma.* 2007;16:704-706.

14. Kanner E, Netland PA, Sarkisian SR, Du H. Ex-Press miniature glaucoma device implanted under a scleral flap alone or in combination with phacoemulsification cataract surgery. *J Glaucoma.* 2009;18(6):488-491.

15. Maris PJ Jr, Ishida K, Netland PA. Comparison of trabeculectomy with Ex-Press miniature glaucoma device implanted under scleral flap. *J Glaucoma.* 2007;16:14-19.

16. Good TJ, Kahook MY. Assessment of bleb morphologic features and postoperative outcomes after Ex-Press drainage device implantation versus trabeculectomy. *Am J Ophthalmol.* 2011;151(3):507-513.

17. Nyska A, Glovinsky Y, Belkin M, et al. Biocompatibility of the Ex-Press miniature glaucoma drainage implant. *J Glaucoma.* 2003;12:275-280.

18. Mermoud A. Ex-Press implant. *Br J Ophthalmol.* 2005;89:396-397.

CANALOPLASTY

Mahmoud A. Khaimi, MD

Traditionally, the gold standard for surgical treatment of open-angle glaucoma (OAG) has been trabeculectomy with the use of antifibrotic therapy. The goal of the trabeculectomy procedure is to create an alternative route for aqueous humor to drain out of the eye and into a subconjunctival reservoir, thus creating a bleb. Despite the fact that the trabeculectomy surgery has proven to be effective in both lowering intraocular pressure (IOP) and halting the progression of the disease process, it is not without the risk of immediate or delayed postsurgical complications.[1-6] Therefore, there has been a growing interest amongst surgeons to seek out and develop IOP-lowering procedures that do not rely on the creation of a bleb and avoid the utilization of antifibrotics. One such procedure that has successfully fulfilled these requirements is canaloplasty with circumferential dilation and suture tensioning of Schlemm's canal. Canaloplasty has gained increasing popularity as a surgical procedure that promotes the rejuvenation of the natural convential outflow pathway without the formation of a bleb. Studies have shown that canaloplasty has proven to be similar to trabeculectomy in effectively lowering IOP and appears to have a safer postoperative profile.[7-8]

SURGICAL PROCEDURE

Canaloplasty is accomplished by exposing Schlemm's canal via non-penetrating dissection and using the iTrack 250 flexible microcatheter (Figure 40-1) to circumferentially viscodilate and intubate Schlemm's canal with a tensioning suture. Furthermore, the microcatheter is also unique in that it has a beacon tip to allow for transscleral illumination during catheterization.

Typically, anesthesia and akinesia are achieved with a retrobulbar block. A corneal traction suture is placed superiorly next to the limbus. Next, a fornix-based conjunctival incision is created, followed by careful dissection

Kahook M.
Essentials of Glaucoma Surgery (pp 331–336).
© 2012 SLACK Incorporated.

Figure 40-1. iTrack 250 flexible microcatheter.

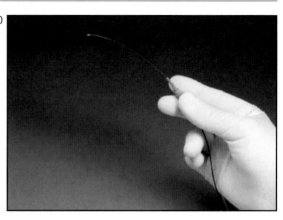

Figure 40-2. Fornix-based conjunctival peritomy.

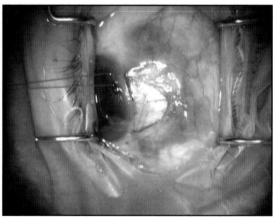

of conjunctiva and Tenon's capsule down to bare sclera (Figure 40-2). I favor a superonasal approach during this step, as it leaves the superior and superotemporal conjunctiva undisturbed should future incisional surgeries be necessary. Hemostasis is achieved with wetfield cautery. No antifibrotics, such as mitomycin C (MMC), are necessary.

Once bare sclera is exposed, a superficial one-third- to one-half-thickness scleral flap is created at the limbus. A 5- x 5-mm parabolic shape may be used; however, I predominantly use a triangular scleral flap. Within the base of the superficial scleral flap, a deep scleral flap is created with a dissection plane just superficial to the choroid. A 4- x 4-mm parabolic deep scleral flap may suffice, or a triangular deep scleral flap smaller than the superficial flap may be preferred. The choroid may be slightly visible beneath the deep scleral flap. The deep scleral flap is dissected anteriorly to unroof Schlemm's canal.

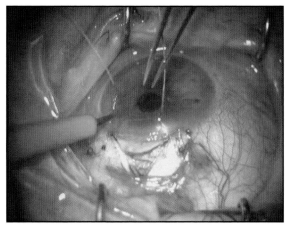

Figure 40-3. Paracentesis.

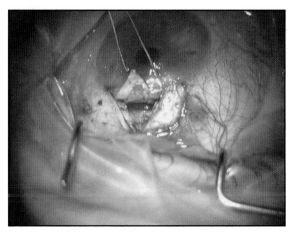

Figure 40-4. Descemet's window.

While dissecting forward, pay close attention to identifying the cross striations of the scleral spur. This assures that the surgeon has reached the correct depth and plane while fashioning the deep flap. Identifying the cross striations of the scleral spur also anatomically orients the surgeon to the location of Schlemm's canal, which is immediately anterior.

At this point, a paracentesis is performed to lower the IOP to the mid- to high-single digits (Figure 40-3). This serves to decompress the eye and decrease the risk of perforating into the anterior chamber while isolating Schlemm's canal and creating Descemet's window. After the canal is identified, the deep flap is carefully dissected further anteriorly to detach Schwalbe's line and to create an appropriately sized Descemet's window, which should, at minimum, be 500 μm (Figure 40-4). Aqueous usually, but not always, percolates through

Figure 40-5. Advancing microcatheter through Schlemm's canal.

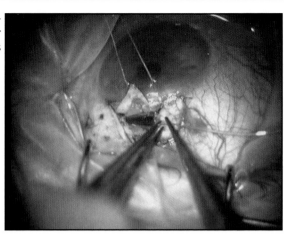

the Descemet's window. The iTrack microcatheter is then inserted through one of the canal ostia. The lights are dimmed to allow visualization of the lighted tip of the microcatheter as it is advanced through Schlemm's canal (Figure 40-5). If an obstruction is encountered during canulation, the microcatheter may be retracted, inserted into the opposite ostia, and cannulated in the other direction to achieve successful passage. After circumferential cannulation is completed, a 10-0 polypropylene suture is tied to the distal end of the catheter, which is retracted, introducing the suture into Schlemm's canal. As the suture is pulled through, ophthalmic viscosurgical device is injected at a rate of 0.5 µL/2 hours (1/8 turn of the OVD injector every 2 clock hours). The suture is tied, allowing appropriate tension to be placed on the canal without inadvertently performing a trabeculotomy. Suture tensioning is critically important because this allows for tension to be transmitted 360 degrees on Schlemm's canal and the trabecular meshwork, thereby restoring natural aqueous outflow.

Creation of a scleral lake is accomplished by excisioning the deep scleral flap followed by watertight closure of the superficial scleral flap with interrupted 10-0 nylon sutures. The conjunctiva and Tenon's capsule is reapproximated with 8-0 Vicryl at the limbus, and finally subconjunctival antibiotics are given along with topical antiobiotic-steroid ointment.

CONCLUSION

Canaloplasty offers a newer approach to surgically treating open-angle glaucoma without the formation of a bleb and the complications associated with trabeculectomy.[1-6,9-13] Ideal patient selection is key when considering canaloplasty. Patients with mild to moderate OAG with IOP desired in the mid- to low-teens are perfect candidates for canaloplasty. Furthermore, for patients with very thin conjunctiva in whom trabeculectomy with antifibrotics or glaucoma drainage device surgery would be much less desirable, canaloplasty has offered a surgical option for treating such difficult cases. Canaloplasty also appears to be an option for patients with uncontrolled ocular hypertension on maximum-tolerated medical therapy for whom laser trabeculoplasty could pose unsafe IOP spikes after laser.

Despite the increased popularity and rising acceptance of canaloplasty, like all other glaucoma surgical procedures, it has its limitations. Canaloplasty may be contraindicated in patients with chronic angle closure, narrow angles, angle recession, neovascular glaucoma, and in eyes that have undergone previous glaucoma procedures that preclude adequate cannulation of Schlemm's canal.[14] Canaloplasty outcomes will be limited in eyes in which the distal aqueous outflow network is permanently scarred down or collapsed. A learning curve for successful catheterization of Schlemm's canal and certain anatomical variations may prohibit successful catheterization, such as the microcatheter tip entering a large collector channel or meeting unknown resistance.[8] Perhaps, the biggest limitation of canaloplasty with suture tensioning is the lack of long-term data. However, because of current promising data,[7-8] and the aforementioned advantages of canaloplasty, this procedure has made its way into the surgical armamentarium of the glaucoma specialist.

KEY POINTS

1. Ideal patient selection includes the following:

   - Mild to moderate open-angle glaucoma with IOP desired in the mid- to low-teens.
   - Patients with very thin conjunctiva in which trabeculectomy with antifibrotics or glaucoma drainage devices (GDDs) would be less desirable.
   - Uncontrolled ocular hypertension with impending optic nerve damage on maximum tolerated medication.

2. Contraindications for canaloplasty include the following:

   - Chronic angle closure.
   - Narrow angles.
   - Angle recession.
   - Neovascular glaucoma.
   - Eyes that have undergone previous glaucoma procedures that preclude adequate cannulation of Schlemm's canal.

3. Surgical technique—2 points that will promote maximal pressure-lowering response are the following:

- Appropriately sized Descemet's window (≥500 μm).
- Adequate suture tensioning.

REFERENCES

1. Jones E, Clarke J, Khaw PT. Recent advances in trabeculectomy technique. *Curr Opin Ophthalmol.* 2005;16:107-113.
2. Borisuth NSC, Phillips B, Krupin T. The risk profile of glaucoma filtration surgery. *Curr Opin Ophthalmol.* 1999;10:112-116.
3. Gedde SJ, Herndon LW, Brandt JD, Budenz DL, Feuer WJ, Schiffman JC. Surgical complications in the Tube Versus Trabeculectomy Study during the first year of follow-up; the Tube Versus Trabeculectomy Study Group. *Am J Ophthalmol.* 2007;143:23-31.
4. Scott IU, Greenfield DS, Schiffman J, et al. Outcomes of primary trabeculectomy with the use of adjunctive mitomycin. *Arch Ophthalmol.* 1998;116:286-291.
5. Jampel HD, Musch DC, Gillespie BW, Lichter PR, Wright MW, Guire KE. Perioperative complications of trabeculectomy in the Collaborative Initial Glaucoma Treatment Study (CIGTS); the Collaborative Initial Glaucoma Treatment Study Group. *Am J Ophthalmol.* 2005;140:16-22.
6. Edmunds B, Thompson JR, Salmon JF, Wormald RP. The National Survey of Trabeculectomy. III. Early and late complications. *Eye.* 2002;16:297-303.
7. Lewis RA, von Wolff K, Tetz M, et al. Canaloplasty: circumferential viscodilation and tensioning of Schlemm's canal using a flexible microcatheter for the treatment of open-angle glaucoma in adults. Two-year interim clinical study results. *J Cataract Refract Surg.* 2009;35:814-824.
8. Shingleton B, Tetz M, Korber N. Circumferential viscodilation and tensioning of Schlemm canal (canaloplasty) with temporal clear corneal phacoemulsification cataract surgery for open-angle glaucoma and visually significant cataract; one-year results. *J Cataract Refract Surg.* 2008;34:433-440.
9. Mac I, Soltau JB. Glaucoma-filtering bleb infections. *Curr Opin Ophthalmol.* 2003;14:91-94.
10. Ophir A. Encapsulated filtering bleb; a selective review–new deductions. *Eye.* 1992;6: 348-352.
11. Bindlish R, Condon GP, Schlosser JD, D'Antonio J, Lauer KB, Lehrer R. Efficacy and safety of mitomycin-C in primary trabeculectomy; five-year follow-up. *Ophthalmology.* 2002;109:1336-1341.
12. Anand N, Arora S, Clowes M. Mitomycin C augmented glaucoma surgery: evolution of filtering bleb avascularity, transconjunctival oozing, and leaks. *Br J Ophthalmol.* 2006;90:175-180.
13. King AJ, Rotchford AP, Alwitry A, Moodie J. Frequency of bleb manipulations after trabeculectomy surgery. *Br J Ophthalmol.* 2007;91:873-877.
14. Khaimi MA. Canaloplasty using iTrack 250 microcatheter with suture tensioning on Schlemm's canal. *Middle East Afr J Opthalmol.* 2009;19:127-129.

41

TRABECTOME

Mina Pantcheva, MD and Malik Y. Kahook, MD

Ab interno trabeculectomy with the Trabectome has emerged as a novel surgical approach to control intraocular pressure (IOP) by effectively and selectively removing and ablating the trabecular meshwork and the inner wall of Schlemm's canal in an attempt to avoid anterior synechiae formation or other forms of wound healing with resultant closure of the cleft. This procedure seems to have an appealing safety profile with respect to early hypotony or infection if compared with trabeculectomy or glaucoma drainage device implantation. Success has been noted when combining Trabectome with cataract extraction. Long-term success of this device is still not known, and more data are needed to understand the full role of this technique in the surgical management of glaucoma. Chapter 16 should be read in combination with this chapter to fully understand how Trabectome is utilized in surgical practice today.

ANATOMICAL CONSIDERATIONS

In the human eye, the main outflow route is the trabecular or conventional outflow pathway. On this route, aqueous humor exits the eye through a well-structured tissue called the trabecular meshwork (TM). After crossing the TM, aqueous humor reaches Schlemm's canal, which drains directly to the aqueous veins. The TM tissue contains 3 differentiated layers. The layer of tissue closest to the anterior chamber is the uveal meshwork, formed by prolongations of connective tissue arising from the iris and ciliary body stromas. This layer does not offer much resistance to aqueous humor outflow because intercellular spaces are large. The next layer, known as the corneoscleral meshwork, is characterized by the presence of lamellae covered by endothelium-like cells standing on a basal membrane. The lamellae are formed by glycoproteins, collagen, hyaluronic

Kahook M.
Essentials of Glaucoma Surgery (pp 337-342).
© 2012 SLACK Incorporated.

acid, and elastic fibers. The third layer, which is in direct contact with the inner wall of endothelial cells from Schlemm's canal, is the juxtacanalicular meshwork. It is formed by cells embedded in a dense extracellular matrix, and the majority of the tissue resistance to flow is thought to be in this layer due to its narrow intercellular spaces. The layer of endothelial cells from Schlemm's canal is the last barrier that aqueous humor has to cross before exiting the eye.[1,2] Ab interno trabeculectomy using the Trabectome aims to selectively remove the TM and the inner wall of Schlemm's canal (SCIW) while leaving the rest of the outflow system (outer wall of Schlemm's canal, collector channels, and aqueous veins) relatively intact.

INSTRUMENTATION

The Trabectome device consists of a disposable handpiece tip (19.5 gauge) that will fit through a 1.6-mm corneal incision. The handpiece is connected to a console with irrigation and aspiration and also to a simple electrocautery generator. The foot pedal controls the irrigation, aspiration, and electrocautery ablation via a stepwise foot control similar to a phaco-emulsification system. The tip of the handpiece is specially designed with an insulated footplate and is pointed for ease of insertion through the TM into Schlemm's canal. The role of the footplate is critical in that it allows for the lifting of TM tissue while putting it on slight tension. It also allows for positioning the tissue for maximal discharge effect during electrocautery ablation while protecting the underlying tissues for preserving normal aqueous outflow. The footplate is coated with proprietary, multilayered polymer, which provides exceptional thermal stability, mechanical strength, biocompatibility, and chemical resistance in laboratory testing. The aspiration port is in close proximity (approximately 0.3 mm) to the cautery electrode and serves to remove debris during ablation. The irrigation is 3 mm from the surgical site and serves the dual purpose of keeping the eye pressurized and further dissipating heat energy. Although the irrigation and aspiration system role is important, the high-frequency electrocautery generator system is the pivotal point of this technology. The generator is a modified 800 EU unit from Aaron/Bovie (St. Petersburg, Florida), and operates at a frequency of 550 kHz with adjustable power setting in 0.1-W increments up to 10 W (recommended range: 0.5 to 1.5 W). The target tissue is disrupted and disintegrated by applying heat energy in bursts with a high-peak power and low-duty cycle. This ablation approach equates to high-energy bursts, which are combined into small increments with comparably long-time intervals in between. As a result, disruption and disintegration of tissue are achieved rather than a thermal-cooking effect such as that seen in traditional cautery of blood vessels.[3,4]

SETTING UP THE TRABECTOME SYSTEM

To power the system, plug in the power cords of the irrigation/aspiration console and the high-frequency generator. Turn it on, and set the power to the physician's preferred setting, typically 0.8. Turn the flow control to "Flow 1" (10 o'clock position). Toggle the black button on the foot pedal until the pinch valve indicator light is off, then turn the flow control to "Standby" (9 o'clock position). Next, fully extend the tray arm of the roller stand to drape the tray. Push the drape down into the opening of the tray holder frame to form a pocket. To set up the fluidics, close the roller clamp on the irrigation line, open the drip chamber air vent, and spike a bottle of balanced salt solution. Fill the drip chamber at least half full. Hang the bottle of balanced salt solution on the IV hook of the roller stand and raise it high. Open the pump cover and with the tubing to the left side, place the collection bag onto the pins and lay the silicone tubing across the center of the pump rollers. The silicone tubing needs to be held at the location of the fitting and without stretching, to be placed onto the left side of the V-block. Next, the cover should be closed. The Trabectome is primed by turning the flow control to "Prime" (8 o'clock position) and grasping the ends of the irrigation silicone tubing at the location of the fittings, sliding it up and down, and forcefully working it fully into the pinch valve slot. Finally, pull down to rest the upper fitting into the slot to prevent the tubing from kinking. Turn the flow control to "Standby" (9 o'clock position). Insert the handpiece bipolar plugs into the bipolar outputs of the high-frequency generator. The irrigation line needs to be lightly connected to the irrigation pigtail of the handpiece (both have color strip). With the cap in place, hold the handpiece tip up and turn the flow control to "Prime" (8 o'clock position). Then partially open the roller clamp, allowing balanced salt solution to fill the irrigation line. After balanced salt solution emerges from the tip of the handpiece, open the roller clamp completely. After the cap is filled to the height of the tip or balanced salt solution emerges from the aspiration pigtail of the handpiece, reposition the handpiece tip down (with cap in place). Lightly connect the aspiration line and continue to fill it until balanced salt solution begins to appear in the collection bag and all lines are free of air bubbles. Turn the flow control to "Standby" until the foot pedal is positioned for surgery, then turn the flow control to the physician's preferred surgical flow setting, typically "Flow 3" (12 o'clock position). Cover and secure the small drape over the irrigation/aspiration console and the high-frequency generator and check that the irrigation tubing is not kinked.

To switch to the irrigation/aspiration cannula (I/A cannula), disconnect the handpiece pigtails from the irrigation and aspiration lines and split the paratubing about 1 foot. Connect both lines to the I/A cannula using the adapter on the long line of the I/A cannula. Straighten the long line of the I/A cannula. The I/A cannula needs to be handed to the surgeon with the long line on the left side to have the suction port on the top.

TECHNIQUE

The patient's head is rotated opposite the eye receiving treatment. Various anesthetic methods can be utilized, including retrobulbar, peribulbar, and sub-Tenon's injection of 0.75% bupivacaine/2% lidocaine mixture and/or use of intracameral 1% preservative-free lidocaine. A near limbal 1.6-mm temporal corneal incision is made parallel to the iris, and viscoelastic (usually Ocucoat, Bausch + Lomb, Rochester, New York) is injected to inflate and stabilize the anterior chamber. Care is taken to avoid bubbles that can obscure the view of the angle. The Trabectome handpiece is advanced nasally across the anterior chamber with the infusion on. A modified Swan-Jacobs gonioscopy lens is used to visualize the target TM nasally as the instrument tip is advanced across the anterior chamber. The tip of the footplate is inserted through the TM into Schlemm's canal. A foot switch activates the aspiration and electrosurgical elements that ablate and remove the strip of TM and SCIW as the surgeon slowly advances the instrument along the meshwork in a clockwise and then counterclockwise direction using the insertion site as a fulcrum. A strip of TM and SCIW spanning 80 to 100 degrees is ablated and removed under direct gonioscopic visualization. Intraoperative reflux of blood through the resulting cleft is desirable in this procedure and confirms appropriate ab interno unroofing of Schlemm's canal. Switch to the I/A cannula to remove the viscoelastic. A 10-0 nylon suture is usually used to close the corneal incision.

CONCLUSION

Ab interno trabeculectomy seems to be a promising alternative surgical approach to lowering IOP when attempting to halt or slow down progression of IOP-induced glaucomatous optic neuropathy. It appears to be easy to perform, reproducible, with a low incidence of early postoperative hypotony (0% to 1%), and short-term adequate IOP control. Furthermore, the conjunctiva remains undisturbed during this procedure, allowing conventional glaucoma surgery, such as trabeculectomy or drainage implant, to remain available to the patient who is in need of better IOP control. The main disadvantage of this procedure is that it is not as effective when not combined with cataract surgery, and long-term success results are yet unknown.

KEY POINTS

1. Trabectome surgery removes trabecular meshwork and the inner wall of Schlemm's canal from an ab interno approach.

2. Trabectome is often combined with cataract surgery where it is thought to be more effective than stand-alone Trabectome surgery.

3. The main advantage of Trabectome surgery is the minimally invasive nature of the approach that does not alter the conjunctival anatomy if future filtration surgery is needed.

REFERENCES

1. Johnson DH, Tschumper RC. Human trabecular meshwork organ culture: a new method. *Invest Ophthalmol Vis Sci.* 1987;28(6):945-953.
2. Grant WM. Clinical measurements of aqueous outflow. *Arch Ophthalmol.* 1951;46(2): 113-131.
3. Francis BA, See RF, Rao NA, Minckler DS, Baerveldt G. Ab interno trabeculectomy: Development of a novel device (Trabectome) and surgery for open-angle glaucoma. *J Glaucoma.* 2006;15(1):68-73.
4. Pantcheva MB, Kahook MY. Ab interno trabeculectomy. *Middle East Afr J Ophthalmol.* 2010;17(4):287-289.

SUPRACHOROIDAL DEVICES

Sarwat Salim, MD, FACS

The 2 most commonly performed surgeries for medically uncontrolled glaucoma, at present, are trabeculectomy and glaucoma drainage devices. Although proven effective in many cases, both use a nonphysiologic pathway to direct aqueous humor from the anterior chamber to the subconjunctival space and form a filtration bleb to lower intraocular pressure (IOP). A variety of postoperative complications related to the filtration bleb are encountered with both procedures, including bleb fibrosis and failure.[1-5] Bleb formation after trabeculectomy carries a life-long risk of bleb leak, hypotony, blebitis, endophthalmitis, etc. In addition to these, the glaucoma drainage devices are associated with a unique set of tube-related complications, such as occlusion, migration, erosion, and corneal decompensation.

Because our conventional surgical procedures are far from optimal, there is significant interest in exploring newer surgical approaches that may enhance the existing physiologic outflow pathways, the trabecular outflow system, or the uveoscleral outflow system. Newer surgical approaches targeting the former pathway include Trabectome, iCath Canaloplasty (iScience Interventional, Menlo Park, California), and iStent. This chapter will discuss the uveoscleral outflow pathway system and suprachoroidal devices currently being investigated to enhance aqueous outflow.

UVEOSCLERAL OUTFLOW SYSTEM

The uveoscleral pathway consists of ciliary body, suprachoroidal space, choroid, and sclera. The aqueous humor flows from the anterior chamber, through the uveal portion (the longitudinal muscle of the ciliary body), to the suprachoroidal space. The fluid then exits the suprachoroidal space through the scleral portion, either the episcleral tissues (or the actual substance of sclera) or the choroidal vascular system. Animal studies have revealed a hydrostatic pressure differential of approximately 3.7 mm Hg

Kahook M.
Essentials of Glaucoma Surgery (pp 343–348).
© 2012 SLACK Incorporated.

between the anterior chamber and the suprachoroidal space that facilitates aqueous outflow through the uveoscleral system.[6] Although initial studies reported a total aqueous outflow of 5% to 15%, subsequent and more recent studies have reported a much greater percentage, 20% to 54%, of outflow through the uveoscleral pathway.[7,8]

The uveoscleral pathway is medically augmented by the prostaglandin analogues, which are the most potent IOP-lowering medications currently available. Although the exact mechanism by which this class of drugs improves uveoscleral outflow remains poorly understood, the two potential mechanisms are relaxation of the ciliary body and, more importantly, remodeling of extracellular matrix of the ciliary muscle.[9-11] Historically, this pathway was used in the cyclodialysis procedure, which is an operation for glaucoma first described by Heine in 1905.[12] Cyclodialysis involves separating the ciliary body from the scleral spur, creating a direct conduit between the anterior chamber and suprachoroidal space. This procedure was later abandoned because of unpredictable results and frequent complications of hypotony, hemorrhage, or failure resulting from the closure of the cyclodialysis cleft.[13-15] Various types of implants and materials have been investigated to keep the cyclodialysis cleft patent, including Teflon tube implant, hydroxyethyl methacrylate capillary strip, scleral strip, air, and sodium hyaluronate, but with limited success.[16-19] Ozdamar et al[20] implanted a modified Krupin valve into the suprachoroidal space in 4 blind eyes with a reported surgical success of 75%, defined as final IOP lower than 21 mm Hg without the use of adjunctive glaucoma medications at about 8 months' follow-up. Recently, Jordan et al[21] reported a high failure rate of 75% in 28 eyes with intractable glaucoma after a viscoelastic-assisted cyclodialysis ab interno procedure.

SUPRACHOROIDAL DEVICES

Recently, surgical interest in the uveoscleral pathway has been re-ignited using stents or shunts to allow a more controlled outflow of aqueous humor from the anterior chamber to the suprachoroidal space by using either an ab interno or ab externo approach. Three competing suprachoroidal devices under development include the Gold Shunt (SOLX Corp), Aquashunt (Opko Health Inc., Miami, FL), and CyPass Micro-Stent (Transcend Medical, Menlo Park, California).

SOLX Gold Shunt

The SOLX Gold Shunt is a 24-karat miniature gold implant that connects the anterior chamber to the suprachoroidal space through an ab externo approach. This device is the most researched of various suprachoroidal devices currently available and has evolved over 3 generations. The first-generation models are the GMS and GMS Plus. These implants are 5.2-mm long by 3.2-mm wide but have different thicknesses of 44 and 68 μm in the GMS and GMS Plus models, respectively. The GMS weighs 6.2 mg and the GMS Plus weighs 9.2 mg. All devices are composed of 2 leaflets fused together and consist of 9 channels in the body to divert aqueous humor from the anterior chamber to the suprachoroidal space. The GMS Plus has larger channels designed to increase uveoscleral outflow. The second-generation model, sGMS Plus, is 80 μm thick with one open window on the distal end of the device with flow resistance being 5 times that of the first-generation implants. Additional windows can be opened with a 790-nm titanium:sapphire pulsed laser, as needed, to reach target IOP gonioscopically postoperatively. The third-generation model, mGMS Plus, has all 9 posterior windows open with flow resistance that is 25 times that of the first-generation implants. The biocompatibility and inertness of gold have previously been reported.[22,23]

The Gold Shunt can be implanted in any quadrant as long as the integrity of the conjunctiva and sclera is well established. Preoperative gonioscopy should be performed to avoid areas of peripheral anterior synechiae. After a fornix-based conjunctival peritomy, a scleral incision approximately 3-mm long is created approximately 2 mm from the limbus at 90% depth. In eyes with high myopia, the scleral incision should be farther away from the limbus. A paracentesis is made, and viscoelastic is inserted into the anterior chamber to keep the eye pressurized or, alternatively, an anterior chamber maintainer may be used. A crescent blade or keratome is used to make a scleral tunnel into the cornea. The scleral incision is then deepened into a full-thickness incision in the suprachoroidal space. A cyclodialysis spatula may be used to correctly locate the suprachoroidal space. Attention is then diverted anteriorly, an entry is made into the anterior chamber at the level of the scleral spur, and the proximal end of the shunt is placed in the anterior chamber. The shape of the proximal end is concave to minimize contact with the iris or corneal endothelium. The distal end is then tucked into the suprachoroidal space. A small amount of balanced salt solution or viscoelastic may be injected into the suprachoroidal space to ease the shunt insertion. A Sinskey hook (Katena Products, Denville, New Jersey) or 27-gauge needle may be used to align the shunt properly at either end. All posterior drainage openings of the implant should be covered by the posterior scleral lip, and the anterior channels of the "head" of the device should be visible anteriorly; the correct position may be confirmed with intraoperative gonioscopy. The scleral wound is closed with nylon sutures, and the conjunctiva is closed with Vicryl sutures. A sterile inserter is supplied with each device to facilitate handling and insertion of the implant.

Melamed et al[24] reported the efficacy and safety of the Gold Shunt in 38 patients with uncontrolled glaucoma. They reported an IOP reduction of 32.6% from baseline and a surgical success of 79% (13% complete and

66% qualified), which was defined as IOP >5 mm Hg and <22 mm Hg. Eight patients had mild to moderate hyphema, which was the most commonly encountered complication of the surgery. In 2010, Mastropasqua and colleagues[25] described the conjunctival features with in vivo confocal microscopy (IVCM) after Gold Shunt implantation in the suprachoroidal space. No bleb formation was noted clinically. A significantly increased conjunctival microcyst density and area were observed by IVCM at the site of successful Gold Shunt implantation compared with unsuccessful Gold Shunt implantation. The authors concluded that these features suggest that aqueous filtration across the sclera may be one of the mechanisms for IOP reduction with this device.

Aquashunt

The Aquashunt is made of biocompatible polypropylene material that conforms to the shape of the globe. The device is 10-mm long, 4-mm wide, and 0.75-mm thick. The body of the device has 250-μm openings. Unlike other ab externo suprachoroidal devices, this shunt is implanted through a full-thickness incision of the sclera to the level of the suprachoroidal space. The shunt is advanced through the suprachoroidal space toward the anterior chamber with its shearing leading edge separating the attachments between the ciliary body and the scleral spur and creating an opening into the anterior chamber, allowing aqueous outflow through the shunt lumen. The device comes with an insertion tool that serves as an obturator during placement and keeps tissue from blocking the lumen of the device. The shunt and tool essentially replace a cyclodialysis spatula. After the proximal end is properly positioned in the anterior chamber, the insertion tool is removed, and the device is secured to the sclera with a single biodegradable suture. The distal end of the device is tucked beneath the posterior lip of the scleral incision, followed by closure of the conjunctiva.

A small clinical trial of Aquashunt was recently completed in Mexico and the Dominican Republic. Only 15 patients were in the clinical trial, and IOP reduction of 30% to 40% was noted in 13 patients at 12-month follow-up, although 6 required adjunctive medications. The main problem identified in the trial was fibrosis in the suprachoroidal space, suggesting the need for highly biocompatible materials and possibly antifibrotic agents, which are currently under investigation.

Ab Interno Approach

The CyPass shunt and the iStent SUPRA are a biocompatible tubular device with microholes on the surface. Unlike the previously mentioned suprachoroidal devices, the CyPass shunt uses an ab interno approach to direct fluid into the suprachoroidal space. The procedure is performed through a clear corneal incision alone or in combination with cataract extraction. A goniolens is used to visualize the angle for proper insertion of the shunt. The device and the inserter are advanced across the anterior chamber until the scleral spur and iris root are identified. The iris is gently pushed away, and a small cyclodialysis is created, placing the distal end of the device into the suprachoroidal space and the proximal collar in the anterior chamber. Clinical trials are currently under way.

CONCLUSION

Suprachoroidal devices offer promise in the surgical treatment of glaucoma by targeting the uveoscleral outflow system (ie, a physiologic pathway) to lower IOP. These devices and procedures appear appealing and potentially safer than existing options by avoiding bleb formation and its related sequelae. However, long-term efficacy of these devices remains to be determined. Large, prospective, randomized, multicenter trials are warranted to further elucidate the devices' role in glaucoma surgery.

KEY POINTS

1. Suprachoroidal devices have been in existence for several decades and in various forms.
2. These devices allow for avoidance of a bleb and thus might lead to safer long-term IOP lowering with lower risks of endophthalmitis.
3. No long-term data are available showing efficacy of these devices in various types of glaucoma.
4. The potential for fibrosis with early or late failure remains an issue, and future techniques to lessen fibrosis will likely be needed to improve the long-term performance of these devices.

REFERENCES

1. Greenfield DS, Suner IJ, Miller MP, et al. Endophthalmitis after filtering surgery with mitomycin. *Arch Ophthalmol*. 1996;114:943-949.
2. Parrish RK II, Schiffman JC, Feurer WJ, et al. Fluorouracil Filtering Surgery Study Group. Prognosis and risk factors for early postoperative wound leaks after trabeculectomy with and without 5-fluorouracil. *Am J Ophthalmol*. 2001;132:633-640.
3. Sherwood MB, Smith MF, Driebe WT Jr, et al. Drainage tube implants in the treatment of glaucoma following penetrating keratoplasty. *Ophthalmic Surg*. 1993;24(3):185-189.
4. Tessler Z, Jluchoded S, Rosenthal G. Nd:YAG laser for Ahmed tube shunt occlusion by the posterior capsule. *Ophthalmic Surg Lasers*. 1997;28:69-70.
5. Tarbak AAA, Shahwan SA, Jadaan IA, et al. Endophthalmitis associated with the Ahmed glaucoma valve implant. *Br J Ophthalmol*. 2005;89:454-458.
6. Emi K, Pederson JE, Toris CB. Hydrostatic pressure of the suprachoroidal space. *Invest Ophthalmol Vis Sci*. 1989;30:233-238.
7. Bill A, Phillips CI. Uveoscleral drainage of aqueous humor dynamics in the aging human eyes. *Exp Eye Res*. 1971;12:275-281.

8. Toris CB, Yablonski ME, Wang YL, et al. Aqueous humor dynamics in the aging human eye. *Am J Ophthalmol.* 1999;127:407-412.

9. Crawford KS, Kaufman PL. Dose-related effects of prostaglandin F2 alpha isopropylester on intraocular pressure, refraction, and pupil diameter in monkeys. *Invest Ophthalmol Vis Sci.* 1991;32(3):510-519.

10. Weinreb RN, Toris CB, Gabelt BT, et al. Effects of prostaglandins on the aqueous humor outflow pathways. *Surv Ophthalmol.* 2002;47(Suppl 1):S53-S64.

11. Nilsson SF, Sperber GO, Bill A. The effect of prostaglandin F2 alpha-1-isopropylester (PGF2 alpha-IE) on uveoscleral outflow. *Prog Clin Biol Res.* 1989;312:429-436.

12. Heine L. Die Cyklodialyse, eine neue Glaucomoperation. *Deutsche Med Wehnschr.* 1905;31:824-826.

13. Galin MA, Baras I. Combined cyclodialysis cataract extraction: a review. *Ann Ophthalmol.* 1975;7(2):271-275.

14. Shields MB, Simmons RJ. Combined cyclodialysis and cataract extraction. *Ophthalmic Surg.* 1976;7(2):62-73.

15. Seguro K, Toris CB, Pedrson JE. Uveoscleral outflow following cyclodialysis in the monkey eye using a fluorescent tracer. *Invest Ophthalmol Vis Sci.* 1985;26:810-813.

16. Portney GL. Silicone elastomer implantation cyclodialysis: a negative report. *Arch Ophthalmol.* 1973;89:10-12.

17. Miller RD, Nisbet RM. Cyclodialysis with air injection in black patients. *Ophthalmic Surg.* 1981;12:92-94.

18. Alpar JJ. Sodium hyaluronate (Healon) in cyclodialysis. *CLAO J.* 1985;11:201-204.

19. Klemm M, Balazs A, Draeger J, et al. Experimental use of space-retaining substances with extended duration: functional and morphological results. *Graefes Arch Clin Exp Ophthalmol.* 1995;233(9):592-597.

20. Ozdamar A, Aras C, Karacorlu M. Suprachoroidal seton implantation in refractory glaucoma: a novel surgical technique. *J Glaucoma.* 2003;12(4):354-359.

21. Jordan JF, Deitlein TS, Dinslage S, et al. Cyclodialysis ab interno as a surgical approach to intractable glaucoma. *Graefes Arch Clin Exp Ophthalmol.* 2007;245:1071-1076.

22. Eisler R. Mammalian sensitivity to elemental gold (Au degrees). *Biol Tr Elem Res.* 2004;100(1):1-18.

23. Sen SC, Ghosh A. Gold as an intraocular foreign body. *Br J Ophthalmol.* 1983;67(6):398-399.

24. Melamed S, Simon GJB, Goldenfeld M, et al. Efficacy and safety of gold microshunt implantation to the supraciliary space in patients with glaucoma. *Arch Ophthalmol.* 2009;127(3):264-269.

25. Mastropasqua L, Agnifili L, Ciancaglini M, et al. In vivo analysis of conjunctiva in gold micro shunt implantation for glaucoma. *Br J Ophthalmol.* 2010;94(12):1592-1596.

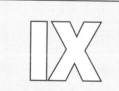

SURGICAL TRIALS AND REGULATORY INSIGHTS

REVIEW OF GLAUCOMA SURGERY CLINICAL TRIALS

Travis C. Rumery, DO; David C. Musch, PhD, MPH;
and Joshua D. Stein, MD, MS

There have been several landmark randomized clinical trials that have generated important insights into the safety and efficacy of medical therapy, laser therapy, and surgical therapy for the treatment of glaucoma. In this chapter, we will highlight several of these key randomized clinical trials by describing the rationale for the study, types of patients recruited to participate, interventions that the enrollees were randomized to receive, important primary and secondary outcomes, and implications of the trials' results. The following randomized clinical trials will be summarized in this chapter:

A. Medical therapy versus laser surgery
  a. Moorfields Primary Treatment Trial (MPTT)
  b. Glaucoma Laser Trial (GLT)
  c. Glaucoma Laser Trial Follow-Up Study (GLTFU)

B. Medical therapy versus incisional surgery
  a. Scottish Glaucoma Trial (SGT)
  b. Moorfields Primary Treatment Trial (MPTT)
  c. Collaborative initial Glaucoma Treatment Study (CIGTS)

C. Laser surgery versus incisional surgery
  a. Advanced Glaucoma Intervention Study (AGIS)
  b. Moorfields Primary Treatment Trial (MPTT)

D. Incisional surgery trials
  a. Ahmed versus Baerveldt Comparison Trial (ABC)
  b. Fluorouracil Filtering Surgery Study (FFSS)
  c. Tube versus Trabeculectomy Study (TVT)
  d. Primary Tube versus Trabeculectomy Study (PTVT)

Kahook M.
Essentials of Glaucoma Surgery (pp 351-372).
© 2012 SLACK Incorporated.

SCOTTISH GLAUCOMA TRIAL

Main Study Purpose

To test whether it was justifiable to continue with the conventional practice of using medical therapy as the initial treatment compared with using trabeculectomy as the initial treatment of patients with open-angle glaucoma.[1]

Location

Glasgow, Scotland, United Kingdom.[2]

Study Population

Patients with newly diagnosed primary open-angle glaucoma (OAG), as well as those with exfoliation syndrome glaucoma.[2]

Interventions the Participants Were Randomized to Receive

a. Medical therapy (up to a maximum of 3 different topical or systemic drugs) followed by trabeculectomy (without antimetabolites) if medical therapy failed.[2]

b. Trabeculectomy (without antimetabolites) followed by medical therapy, if trabeculotomy failed.[2]

Study Design

- Multicenter, randomized clinical trial.[1]
- 116 patients enrolled between 1980 and 1985.[1]
- 99 patients (53 in the medical therapy group and 46 in the trabeculectomy group) completed at least 1 year in the trial.[1]

Inclusion Criteria

- Untreated intraocular pressure (IOP) ≥ 26 mm Hg (Goldmann applanation tonometry) on 2 occasions.[1]
- Visual field (VF) defects characteristic of glaucoma.[1]

Length of Follow-Up

Maximum follow-up of 7 years (mean: 4.6 years).[3]

Results

Trabeculectomy group had a greater decrease in IOP than the medically treated group at 1 year.[4]

At a mean follow-up of 4.6 years, the trabeculectomy group had:
- Less VF loss than the medical group.[4,5]
- No difference in final visual acuity (VA) versus the medically treated group.[3,4]

Implications

Showed benefit to early trabeculectomy in the management of newly diagnosed OAG patients.

Notes

This trial preceded the use of many commonly used topical glaucoma medications including prostaglandin analogues, alpha agonists, and topical carbonic anhydrase inhibitors (CAI).[5]

References

1. Jay JL, Murray SB. Early trabeculectomy versus conventional management in primary open angle glaucoma. *Br J Ophthalmol.* 1988;72(12):881-889.
2. Jay JL. Earlier trabeculectomy. *Trans Ophthalmol Soc UK.* 1983;103(Pt1):35-38.
3. Jay JL, Allan D. The benefit of early trabeculectomy versus conventional management in primary open angle glaucoma relative to severity of disease. *Eye.* 1989;3(Pt5):528-535.
4. Wilson MR, Gaasterland D. Translating research into practice: Controlled clinical trials and their influence on glaucoma management. *J Glaucoma.* 1996;5(2):139-146.
5. Imami NR, Allingham RR. Initial medical treatment. In: Netland P, ed. *Glaucoma Medical Therapy: Principles and Management.* 2nd ed. New York, NY: Oxford University Press; 2008:181-190.

Moorfields Primary Treatment Trial

Main Study Purpose

To compare the efficacy of medical therapy, laser trabeculoplasty, and trabeculectomy without antimetabolites as primary treatment for patients with OAG.[1]

Location

London, England.[1]

Study Population

Patients with chronic, untreated OAG.[1]

Interventions the Participants Were Randomized to Receive

a. Initial medical therapy: pilocarpine and/or a sympathomimetic and/or timolol, as the initial therapy; increasing to maximum tolerated medical therapy, which could, in individual cases, require all 3 of these topical medications and an oral CAI.[1]

b. Initial laser trabeculoplasty: 2 treatments, each consisting of 50 burns over 180 degrees of the anterior trabecular meshwork, separated by an interval of 2 weeks (treated with pilocarpine for 2 weeks after therapy, which was tapered if IOP allowed, but continued as adjuvant therapy if IOP was not controlled by laser alone).[1]

c. Initial trabeculectomy: trabeculectomy without antimetabolites using either a fornix- or limbal-based conjunctival flap.[1]

Study Design

- Single center, randomized, clinical trial.[1]
- 168 patients (56: medical therapy group, 55: laser therapy group, and 57: trabeculectomy group) were enrolled starting in 1983.[1]

Inclusion Criteria

- IOP ≥24 mm Hg on 2 occasions.[1]
- Cup-to-disc ratio (C/D) >0.6, and/or notching, and/or pallor of the neuroretinal rim.[1]
- Glaucomatous field loss on automated perimetry.[1]
- Open drainage angle.[1]

Length of Follow-Up

Minimum of 5 years.[1]

Results

- Trabeculectomy group had the greatest IOP decrease (from 34 to 14.1 mm Hg for the trabeculectomy group, 35 to 18.5 mm Hg for the laser group, and 35 to 18.5 mm Hg for the medical therapy group) at 5 years.[1-3]
- Equal IOP decrease in the medical and trabeculectomy groups at 5 years (see above).[1]
- No difference in final VA among all groups at 5 years.[1]
- Medical and trabeculoplasty groups had greater VF loss as compared with the trabeculectomy group at 5 years.[1-3]

Implications

- Showed benefit of early trabeculectomy in the management of newly diagnosed OAG.
- Suggested a relationship between progression of VF loss and the degree of IOP lowering in OAG patients.[1]

Notes

- This trial preceded the use of many commonly used topical glaucoma medications, including prostaglandin analogues, alpha agonists, and topical CAIs.[2]
- Antimetabolites were not used in this study.
- Humphrey visual field (HVF) testing was not available for the entire follow-up period to allow for adequate data to determine progression with the HVF.[1]
- Success = IOP had been reduced to 22 mm Hg or less by 3 months and maintained below that level.[1]
- Failure = IOP was greater than 22 mm Hg on 2 repeated occasions.[1]

REFERENCES

1. Migdal C, Gregory W, Hitchings R. Long-term functional outcome after early surgery compared with laser and medicine in open-angle glaucoma. *Ophthalmology.* 1994;101(10):1651-1656.
2. Imami NR, Allingham RR. Initial medical treatment. In: Netland P, ed. *Glaucoma Medical Therapy: Principles and Management.* 2nd ed. New York, NY: Oxford University Press; 2008:181-190.
3. Wilson MR, Gaasterland D. Translating research into practice: controlled clinical trials and their influence on glaucoma management. *J Glaucoma.* 1996;5(2):139-146.

GLAUCOMA LASER TRIAL AND GLAUCOMA LASER TRIAL FOLLOW-UP STUDY

Main Study Purpose

To compare the safety and efficacy of argon laser trabeculoplasty (ALT) and topical glaucoma medications for controlling IOP in patients with newly diagnosed primary open-angle glaucoma (POAG).[1]

Location

United States.[1]

Study Population

Individuals with newly diagnosed bilateral POAG.[1]

Interventions the Participants Were Randomized to Receive

a. ALT followed by topical glaucoma medications if needed. ALT treatment consisted of 2 treatments, each consisting of 48 burns (45 to 50 allowed) over 180 degrees of the trabecular meshwork (360 degrees covered between the 2 treatments).[2]

b. Stepwise medical regimen: timolol 0.5% twice daily (step 1) → dipivefrin (step 2) → low-dose pilocarpine* (step 3) → high-dose pilocarpine◆ (step 4) → timolol with high-dose pilocarpine (step 5) → dipivefrin with high-dose pilocarpine (step 6) → ophthalmologist's discretion (step 7).[2]

*2% if brown iris, 1% otherwise.
◆4% if brown iris, 2% otherwise.

Study Design

- Multicenter, randomized, clinical trial.[1]
- Glaucoma Laser Trial (GLT): 271 patients, 542 eyes (271 eyes in each group, 1 eye randomized to each group) were enrolled between 1984 and 1987 with follow-up ending in November 1989.[3]
- Glaucoma Laser Trial Follow-Up Study (GLTFU): 203 patients (406 eyes) from the original GLT were followed between December 1990 and August 1993.[3]

Inclusion Criteria

- Age ≥35 years.[1]
- IOP ≥22 mm Hg, bilaterally, on 2 successive visits.[1]
- Glaucomatous VF loss in at least one eye or marked (C/D ≥ 0.8) disc changes in the presence of marked (≥31 mm Hg) IOP elevation.[1]
- Intereye ratio of IOP ≤ 1.50.[1]
- Best corrected visual acuity (BCVA) ≥ 20/70 in each eye.[1]
- No signs of pigmentary or exfoliation syndrome glaucoma.[1]
- No history of regular treatment with glaucoma medications within 6 months.[1]

Exclusion Criteria

Evidence of secondary glaucomas, including pigmentary or exfoliative glaucoma.[1]

Length of Follow-Up

GLT: 5 years. GLTFU: mean follow-up of 7 years (maximum: 9 years).[3]

Funding

National Eye Institute, National Institutes of Health.[1]

Results

- Initial treatment with ALT was at least as effective as initial treatment with timolol. ALT group had 1.2 mm Hg greater reduction in IOP on average over all study times. ALT group showed a small benefit in VF preservation averaged over all study times. ALT group showed less optic nerve deterioration averaged over all study times.[3-5]

- Both groups had a similar decrease in VA by approximately 0.2 to 1 line over the mean follow-up period of 7 years.[3]

- ALT group required less antiglaucoma medication (62% of the total number of medication days for the medical therapy group) compared with the medical therapy group through the mean follow-up period of 7 years.[3]

- Transient increase in IOP and formation of peripheral anterior synechiae (PAS) were 2 side effects from ALT. Patients who developed PAS had similar or better IOP reduction, similar VF status, and similar medical and surgical history as those patients who did not develop PAS throughout follow-up.[3]

Implications

Provided evidence that ALT is a reasonable alternative to topical glaucoma medications as initial treatment for POAG.[3,4,6]

Notes

- Over half of patients initially treated with ALT required medical treatment of glaucoma at 2 years.[3,4]

- This trial preceded the use of many commonly used topical glaucoma medication including prostaglandin analogues, alpha agonists, and topical CAIs.[4]

- There might have been crossover of medication effects as treatment randomization was by eyes, not patients.[5]

REFERENCES

1. The Glaucoma Laser Trial Research Group. The Glaucoma Laser Trial (GLT): 1. Acute effects of argon laser trabeculoplasty on intraocular pressure. *Arch Ophthalmol.* 1989;107(8):1135-1142.
2. Glaucoma Laser Trial Research Group. The Glaucoma Laser Trial (GLT): 3. Design and methods. *Control Clin Trials.* 1991;12(4):504-524.
3. Glaucoma Laser Trial Research Group. The Glaucoma Laser Trial (GLT) and Glaucoma Laser Trial Follow-Up Study: 7. Results. *Am J Ophthalmol.* 1995;120(6):718-731.

4. Imami NR, Allingham RR. Initial medical treatment. In: Netland P, ed. *Glaucoma Medical Therapy: Principles and Management.* 2nd ed. New York, NY: Oxford University Press; 2008:181-190.

5. Wilson MR, Gaasterland D. Translating research into practice: controlled clinical trials and their influence on glaucoma management. *J Glaucoma.* 1996;5(2):139-146.

6. The Glaucoma Laser Trial Research Group. The Glaucoma Laser Trial (GLT): 2. Results of argon laser trabeculoplasty versus topical medications. Ophthalmology. 1990;97(11):1403-1413.

FLUOROURACIL FILTERING SURGERY STUDY

Main Study Purpose

To determine the success of using postoperative subconjunctival injections of 5-fluorouracil (5-FU) in patients undergoing filtering surgery.[1]

Location

United States.[1]

Study Population

Patients with uncontrolled glaucoma and guarded prognosis for filtering surgery (aphakic and pseudophakic eyes, and phakic eyes after failed filtering surgery).[1]

Interventions the Participants Were Randomized to Receive

a. Trabeculectomy without postoperative 5-FU.[1]

b. Trabeculectomy augmented with a postoperative regimen of subconjunctival 5-FU.[1]

Study Design

- Multicenter, randomized, clinical trial.[1]
- 213 (108 in the trabeculectomy without 5-FU group, 105 in the trabeculectomy with 5-FU group) were enrolled between 1985 and 1988.[1,2]

Inclusion Criteria

- Uncontrolled glaucoma (IOP > 21 mm Hg).[1]
- Patients who had undergone prior cataract extraction or had undergone at least one unsuccessful filtering procedure in a phakic eye.[1]

Exclusion Criteria

Age <18 years, patients who had previously received 5-FU systemically or in the study eye, anterior segment neovascularization (NV) and dislocated lenses.[1]

Length of Follow-Up

Up to 8 years.[1]

Funding

- National Eye Institute, National Institutes of Health.
- Several institutional grants from participating centers.[1]

Results

- The 5-FU group was more likely to attain IOP control and to avoid reoperation through 5 years.[3]
- 5-FU reduced the 5-year failure rate following trabeculectomy: 51% of patients who received 5-FU failed compared with 74% in the trabeculectomy without 5-FU group.[3,4]
- Risk factors for surgical failure included high preoperative IOP, short time interval since last surgery involving conjunctival manipulation, number of previous surgeries with conjunctival manipulation, and Hispanic ancestry.[3,4]
- The 5-FU group had a higher incidence of late bleb leaks (9% versus 2%) through 5 years.[3,4]

Implications

- This study supported the benefits of adjunctive antifibrotic use in improving the success of trabeculectomy surgery.[4]
- Further investigations of other antifibrotic medications such as mitomycin C (MMC) were undertaken as a result of this study.[2]

Notes

- Failure = reoperation for control of IOP or an IOP >21 mm Hg at or after the first-year examination.[1]
- None of these patients had intraoperative antimetabolites.
- Eyes in the 5-FU group received a complex regimen consisting of 5.0 mg (0.5 mL) injections of 10-mg/ml 5-FU solution twice daily on postoperative days 1 to 7 and once daily on postoperative days 8 to 14.[1]

REFERENCES

1. The Fluorouracil Filtering Surgery Study Group: Fluorouracil Filtering Surgery Study one-year follow-up. *Am J Ophthalmol.* 1989;108(6):625-635.
2. Wilson MR, Gaasterland D. Translating research into practice: controlled clinical trials and their influence on glaucoma management. *J Glaucoma.* 1996;5(2):139-146.

3. The Fluorouracil Filtering Surgery Study Group: Five-year follow-up of the Fluorouracil Filtering Surgery Study. *Am J Ophthalmol.* 1996;121(4):349-366.

4. Imami NR, Allingham RR. Initial medical treatment. In: Netland P, ed. *Glaucoma Medical Therapy: Principles and Management.* 2nd ed. New York, NY: Oxford University Press; 2008:181-190.

ADVANCED GLAUCOMA INTERVENTION STUDY

Main Study Purpose

To determine the most effective way to manage patients with advanced OAG.[1]

Location

United States.[1]

Study Population

Patients with medically uncontrolled OAG.[1]

Interventions the Participants Were Randomized to Receive

a. Argon laser trabeculoplasty was given as first-line treatment. If ineffective, this was followed by trabeculectomy and, when necessary, a second trabeculectomy (ATT).[1]

b. Trabeculectomy*, was given as first-line treatment. If ineffective, this was followed by ALT, and when necessary, followed by a second trabeculectomy (TAT).[1]

   *Antimetabolites were used very sparingly in initial trabeculectomies and with greater frequency in subsequent trabeculectomies.

Study Design

- Multicenter, randomized, clinical trial.[2]
- 591 patients (789 eyes; 404 in the ATT group and 385 in the TAT group) were enrolled between 1988 and 1992.[2]

Inclusion Criteria

- Age 35 to 80 years.[1]
- Eyes had to be phakic and have advanced OAG.[1]
- On maximal medical therapy, at least 1 medication from each of 3 groups—(a) miotic; (b) beta-blocker, epinephrine derivative, or both; and (c) systemic CAIs, if not contraindicated—must have been tested and continued unless found not to be effective, not accepted, or not tolerated by the patient.[1]

- Patients met 1 of 9 specified combinations of criteria involving elevated IOP, VF loss, and damage to the optic nerve.[1]
- BCVA of 20/80 or better.[1]

Exclusion Criteria

Discernable congenital anomaly of the anterior chamber angle, eyes with secondary glaucoma, eyes with pigment dispersion, patients with exfoliative glaucoma, concurrent active disease in the study eye that may affect IOP or its measurement, patients on kidney dialysis, history of laser or incisional surgery in the eye considered for study (except laser iridotomy), laser retinal treatment anterior to the vortex vein ampullae, local retinal cryotherapy involving less than 2 quadrants for retinal holes anterior to the vortex vein ampullae, eyes that had undergone gonioplasty in more than 180 degrees of the anterior chamber angle circumference, eyes with proliferative or severe nonproliferative retinopathy, eyes with (dilated) pupil diameter of <2 mm, eyes with field loss attributed to a nonglaucoma condition, and the fellow eye previously enrolled in the Advanced Glaucoma Intervention Study.[1]

Length of Follow-Up

8 to 13 years.[3]

Funding

- Research to Prevent Blindness, Inc, New York, NY.[1]
- National Eye Institute, National Institutes of Health.[1]

Results

- IOP reduction was greatest in both Whites and Blacks with the TAT protocol.[3,4]
- Visual function was better preserved in Blacks with the ATT protocol than the TAT sequence through 7 years of follow-up.[2-5]
- Visual function was better preserved in Whites with the TAT protocol than the ATT sequence through 7 years of follow-up.[2-5]
- IOP fluctuation was associated with VF progression at a follow-up of 7 years.[6]
- Consistently low IOP is associated with reduced progression of VF (eyes that had IOP <18 mm Hg at 100% of visits had a mean IOP of 12.3 mm Hg).[7]

Trabeculectomy increases the relative risk of cataract formation by 78%.[4]

Implications

- ALT is preferable to trabeculectomy without antimetabolites in Blacks whose glaucoma is uncontrolled with medical therapy.[2]
- Identifies the importance of IOP control in reducing the risk of glaucoma progression and the significance of IOP fluctuation as a risk factor for VF progression in patients with advanced open-angle glaucoma.[4]

Notes

- Very few initial trabeculectomies used antimetabolites.[4]
- The study findings may have been very different if antimetabolites had been routinely used in trabeculectomies.[3,4]
- Prostaglandin analogues, topical CAIs, and topical selective alpha-2-adrenergic agonists were not commercially available early in the study.[4]
- The increased risk of cataract after trabeculectomy likely contributed to the greater VA loss in the TAT sequence relative to the ATT sequence, especially in the early follow-up years.[3]
- The race–treatment interactions are likely due to more scar tissue formation in Blacks after incisional glaucoma surgery without adjunctive antimetabolites, causing failure of their trabeculectomies, whereas Whites were less prone to this.

REFERENCES

1. The Advanced Glaucoma Intervention Study (AGIS): 1. Study design and methods and baseline characteristics of study patients. *Control Clin Trials.* 1994;15(4):299-325.
2. The AGIS Investigators. The Advanced Glaucoma Intervention Study (AGIS): 9. Comparison of glaucoma outcomes in black and white patients within treatment groups. *Am J Ophthalmol.* 2001;132(3):311-320.
3. Ederer F, Gaasterland DA, Dally LG, et al. The Advanced Glaucoma Intervention Study (AGIS): 13. Comparison of treatment outcomes within race: 10-year results. *Ophthalmology.* 2004;111(9):651-664.
4. Imami NR, Allingham RR. Initial medical treatment. In: Netland P, ed. *Glaucoma Medical Therapy: Principles and Management.* 2nd ed. New York, NY: Oxford University Press; 2008:181-190.
5. Beck AD. Review of recent publications of the Advanced Glaucoma Intervention Study. *Curr Opin Ophthalmol.* 2003;14(2):83-85.
6. Nouri-Mahdavi K, Hoffman D, Coleman AL, et al. Predictive factors for glaucomatous visual field progression in the Advanced Glaucoma Intervention Study. *Ophthalmology.* 2004;111:1627-1635.
7. The AGIS Investigators. The Advanced Glaucoma Intervention Study (AGIS): 7. The relationship between control of intraocular pressure and visual field deterioration. *Am J Ophthalmol.* 2000;130(4):429-440.

COLLABORATIVE INITIAL GLAUCOMA TREATMENT STUDY

Main Study Purpose

To compare the outcomes of initial management of OAG by using medical therapy versus trabeculectomy.[1]

Location

United States.[1]

Study Population

Newly diagnosed OAG (POAG, exfoliation syndrome glaucoma, and pigmentary glaucoma) patients.[1]

Interventions the Participants Were Randomized to Receive

a. Initial medical therapy: When initial treatment failed, the following protocol was followed: ALT → trabeculectomy (with or without 5-FU) → medication → trabeculectomy with antimetabolite → medication → ophthalmologist's discretion.[1]

b. Initial trabeculectomy (with or without 5-FU): When initial treatment failed, the following protocol was followed: ALT → medication → trabeculectomy with antimetabolite → medication → ophthalmologist's discretion.[1]

Study Design

- Multicenter, randomized clinical trial.[1]
- 607 patients (307 assigned to initial medical therapy and 300 assigned to initial trabeculectomy) were enrolled between 1993 and 1997.[1]

Inclusion Criteria

- Age 25 to 75 years.[1]
- Early Treatment Diabetic Retinopathy Study (ETDRS) VA better than or equal to 20/40 and 1 of the following:
  - IOP ≥ 20 mm Hg, HVF 24-2 result with ≥3 contiguous points on the total deviation plot at the <5% level and glaucoma hemifield test result that is "outside normal limits," and optic disc compatible with glaucoma.[1]
  - IOP between 20 to 26 mm Hg, HVF 24-2 result with ≥2 contiguous points on the total deviation plot at the <2% level and glaucomatous optic disc damage.[1]

· IOP ≥27 mm Hg and glaucomatous optic disc damage.[1]

Exclusion Criteria

Prior use of any glaucoma medications for more than 14 days, use of glaucoma medications within 3 weeks of baseline visit, advanced VF loss at initial presentation, ocular disease that might affect measurement of IOP, VA or VF testing, diabetic retinopathy with >10 microaneurysms, previous ocular surgery, significant cataract, and use of corticosteroids (oral or ophthalmic).[1]

Length of Follow-Up

7 to 10 years.

Funding

National Eye Institute, National Institutes of Health.[1]

Results

- Both treatment arms showed significant reduction in IOP.[2]
- Lower IOP in the trabeculectomy group as compared with the group assigned to pressure-lowering medications through 9 years of follow-up.[2]
- No substantial difference in VF progression between the groups.[3,4]
- Greater rate of cataract development in the trabeculectomy group.[4]
- Quality-of-life indicators were similar except for increased local eye symptoms in the trabeculectomy group.[5]
- Patients with more advanced VF loss at baseline fared better with initial trabeculectomy.[6]
- Less optic disc progression in the surgery group.[7]
- IOP reduction of 35% seems to stabilize glaucoma.[3]
- Patients with diabetes experienced more VF loss over time if treated with initial trabeculectomy.[6]
- There was no evidence of a substantial effect of trabeculectomy on the IOP of the untreated fellow eye during follow-up.[8]
- Patients with an early post-trabeculectomy IOP spike had significantly higher mean IOP at years 3 and 5 of follow-up, but this was not associated with subsequent VF loss.[9]
- IOP variation during treatment was associated with an increased risk of VF progression.[6]

Implications

Suggests that trabeculectomy is a reasonable alternative to initial treatment with pressure-lowering medications in patients with newly diagnosed OAG.

Notes

No MMC was used (at least in the initial trabeculectomy).

REFERENCES

1. Musch DC, Lichter PR, Guire KE, Standardi CL. The Collaborative Initial Glaucoma Treatment Study: study design, methods, and baseline characteristics of enrolled patients. *Ophthalmology.* 1999;106(4):653-662.
2. Musch DC, Gillespie BW, Niziol LM, et al. Factors associated with intraocular pressure before and during 9 years of treatment in the Collaborative Initial Glaucoma Treatment Study. *Ophthalmology.* 2008;115(6):927-933.
3. Lichter PR, Musch DC, Gillespie BW, et al. Interim clinical outcomes in the Collaborative Initial Glaucoma Treatment Study comparing initial treatment randomized to medications or surgery. *Ophthalmology.* 2001;108(11):1943-1953.
4. Feiner L, Piltz-Seymour JR. Collaborative Initial Glaucoma Treatment Study: a summary of results to date. *Curr Opin Ophthalmol.* 2003;14(2):106-111.
5. Janz NK, Wren PA, Lichter PR, et al. The Collaborative Initial Glaucoma Treatment Study: interim quality of life findings after initial medical or surgical treatment of glaucoma. *Ophthalmology.* 2001;108(11):1954-1965.
6. Musch DC, Gillespie BW, Lichter PR, et al. Visual field progression in the Collaborative Initial Glaucoma Treatment Study: the impact of treatment and other baseline characteristics. *Ophthalmology.* 2009;116(2):200-207.
7. Parrish RK II, Feuer WJ, Schiffman JC, et al. Five-year follow-up optic disc findings of the Collaborative Initial Glaucoma Treatment Study. *Am J Ophthalmol.* 2009;147(4):717-724.
8. Radcliffe NM, Musch DC, Niziol LM, et al. The effect of trabeculectomy on intraocular pressure of the untreated fellow eye in the Collaborative Glaucoma Treatment Study. *Ophthalmology.* 2010;117(11):2055-2060.
9. Chen PP, Musch DC, Niziol LM. The effect of early posttrabeculectomy intraocular pressure spike in the Collaborative Initial Glaucoma Treatment Study. *J Glaucoma.* 2011;20(4):211-214.

TUBE VERSUS TRABECULECTOMY STUDY

Purpose

To prospectively compare the safety and efficacy of trabeculectomy with adjunctive MMC as compared with implantation of a glaucoma drainage device (GDD; Baerveldt 350-mm^2) in eyes that had previously undergone filtering surgery, cataract surgery with intraocular lens (IOL implantation, or both.[1]

Location

United States and United Kingdom.[1]

Study Population

Patients with uncontrolled glaucoma who had undergone previous trabeculectomy, cataract extraction with IOL, or both.[1]

Interventions the Participants Were Randomized to Receive

a. Baerveldt 350-mm² glaucoma implant.[1]
b. Trabeculectomy with MMC (0.4 mg/mL for 4 minutes).[1]

Study Design

- Multicenter, randomized, clinical trial.[1]
- 212 patients (107 assigned to the GDD group and 105 assigned to the trabeculectomy with MMC group) were enrolled between 1999 and 2004.[1]

Inclusion Criteria

- Age 18 to 85 years.[1]
- Inadequately controlled glaucoma with IOP ≥18 and ≤40 mm Hg on tolerated medical therapy.[1]
- Previous trabeculectomy, cataract extraction with IOL implantation, or both.[1]

Exclusion Criteria

Active iris neovascularization or active proliferative retinopathy, iridocorneal endothelial syndrome, aphakia, vitreous in the anterior chamber for which a vitrectomy is anticipated, chronic or recurrent uveitis, severe posterior blepharitis, unwilling to discontinue contact lens use after surgery, previous cyclodestructive procedure, scleral buckling procedure, silicone oil present, conjunctival scarring precluding a trabeculectomy superiorly, and need for glaucoma surgery combined with other ocular procedures (ie, cataract surgery, penetrating keratoplasty, or retinal surgery), or anticipated need for additional ocular surgery.[1]

Length of Follow-Up

5 years.[2]

Funding

- Pfizer, Inc, New York, New York.[1]
- Abbott Medical Optics, Santa Ana, California (manufacturer of Baerveldt GDD).[1]
- National Eye Institute, National Institutes of Health.[1]
- Research to Prevent Blindness, Inc, New York, New York.[1]

Results

- Both treatment groups had similar IOP reduction at 3 years of follow-up.[2,3]
- Both treatment groups had similar use of supplemental medical therapy at 3 years of follow-up.[2,3]
- Trabeculectomy group had a significantly higher failure rate* compared with the GDD group at 3 years of follow-up.[2]
- Trabeculectomy group had significantly more postoperative complications than the GDD group (60% in the trabeculectomy group compared with 39% in the GDD group); however, the rate of serious complications** was similar in both groups.[2]
- Reoperation rate for glaucoma was higher in the trabeculectomy group but this did not reach statistical significance.[2]
- The GDD group was more likely to maintain IOP control and avoid persistent hypotony, loss of light perception, and reoperation for glaucoma than the trabeculectomy with MMC group during the first 3 years of follow-up.[2] (*See definitions in notes section following.)

Implications

- Prior to the TVT Study, GDD surgery was often reserved for patients who had a high risk of failure from trabeculectomy (eg, patients with neovascular glaucoma) or who had multiple past trabeculectomies.
- This study supports use of GDDs as an alternative to trabeculectomy with MMC in glaucoma patients who have had prior incisional intraocular surgery.[2]

Notes

- Fornix-based conjunctival flaps with a more diffuse application of MMC at a lower dosage has developed since the TVT study was initiated, which may affect outcomes and rates of complications.[2]
- This study is sponsored, in part, by the company that makes the Baerveldt GDD.

* Failure = IOP >21 mm Hg or not reduced by 20% below baseline on 2 consecutive follow-up visits after 3 months, IOP ≤5 mm Hg on 2 consecutive follow-up visits after 3 months, reoperation for glaucoma (additional intervention that required a return to the operating room, cyclodestruction, vitreous biopsy with injection of intravitreal antibiotics), or loss of LP (light perception) vision.[2]

** Serious complications = surgical complications that were associated with loss of 2 or more lines of Snellen VA and/or reoperation to manage the complication.[2]

REFERENCES

1. Gedde SJ, Schiffman JC, Feuer WJ, et al. The Tube Versus Trabeculectomy Study: design and baseline characteristics of study patients. *Am J Ophthalmol.* 2005;140(2):275-287.
2. Gedde SJ, Heuer DK, Parrish RK II. Review of results from The Tube Versus Trabecuectomy Study. *Curr Opin Ophthalmol.* 2010;21(2):123-128.
3. Gedde SJ, Schiffman JC, Feuer WJ, et al. Three-year follow-up of The Tube Versus Trabeculectomy Study. *Am J Ophthalmol.* 2009;148(5):670-684.

AHMED BAERVELDT COMPARISON STUDY

Main Study Purpose

To compare the outcomes and complications of the Ahmed glaucoma valve (AGV) and the Baerveldt glaucoma implant (BGI) for surgical management of refractory glaucoma.[1]

Location

- United States.[1]
- London, England (Moorfields Eye Hospital).[1]

Study Population

Refractory glaucomas (primary glaucomas with previous intraocular surgery, neovacular glaucoma, uveitic glaucoma, and other secondary glaucomas).[1]

Interventions the Participants Were Randomized to Receive

a. Ahmed glaucoma valve model FP7.[1]
b. Baerveldt glaucoma implant model 101-350.[1]

Study Design

- Multicenter, randomized clinical trial.[1]

- 276 patients (143 in the AGV group and 133 in the BGI group) were enrolled between 2006 and 2008.[1]

Inclusion Criteria

- Patients 18 to 85 years of age with inadequately controlled glaucoma despite receiving maximum tolerated medical therapy, with IOP ≥18 mm Hg.[1]
- Patients with refractory glaucoma and history of previously failed trabeculectomy or other intraocular surgery in the study eye were eligible.[1]
- Patients without previous intraocular surgery were eligible if they had secondary glaucomas known to have a high failure rate with trabeculectomy such as neovascular, uveitic, or iridocorneal endothelial syndrome-associated glaucoma.[1]

Exclusion Criteria

Patients who lacked light perception vision, patients who underwent a previous cyclodestructive procedure or previous aqueous shunt implanted in the same eye, patients who underwent a prior scleral buckling procedure or other external impediment to supratemporal drainage device implantation, patients who had presence of silicone oil, patients who had vitreous in the anterior chamber sufficient to require a vitrectomy, patients who had uveitis associated with a systemic condition, such as juvenile rheumatoid arthritis, patients who had nanophthalmos, and patients who had Sturge-Weber syndrome, other conditions associated with elevated episcleral venous pressure, or needed aqueous shunt surgery combined with other ocular procedures.[1]

Length of Follow-Up

- Ongoing study: 1 year follow-up data on 92% of the AGV group and 88% of the BGI group.[2]
- Study intends to continue following patients up to 1 year after surgery.[2]

Funding

- National Eye Institute, National Institutes of Health.[1]
- New World Medical, Rancho Cucamonga, California (company that manufactures the Ahmed GDD).[1]
- Research to Prevent Blindness, Inc, New York, New York.[1]

Results

Both surgical procedures produced a significant reduction in IOP (AVG group 31.2 ± 11.2 mm Hg preoperatively → 15.4 ± 5.5 mm Hg postoperatively; BGI group 31.8 ± 12.5 mm Hg preoperatively → 13.2 ± 6.8 mm Hg postoperatively) at 1 year.[2]

- Average IOP in the BGI group was 2.2 mm Hg lower at 1 year compared with the AVG group.[2]
- Both surgical procedures produced a significant reduction (AVG group 3.4 ± 1.1 glaucoma medications → 1.8 ± 1.3; BGI group 3.5 ± 1.1 glaucoma medications → 1.5 ± 1.4) in the need for medical therapy at 1 year.[2]
- Similar failure rates* between both treatment groups at 1 year.[2]
- BGI group had more complete successes*.[2]
- Higher rate of reoperation in the AGV group (8%) compared with the BGI group (1%) at 1 year.[2]
- Decrease of 2 or more lines of Snellen VA in 32% of patients overall at 1 year, no difference between the 2 groups.[2]
- More early (≤3 months) postoperative complications in the BGI group.[2]
- Both groups had a similar rate of late postoperative complications at 1 year♦.[2]

  *See definitions in notes section below.
  ♦See implications section below.

Implications

- BGI may be a better option for patients with advanced glaucoma who require a very low postoperative IOP.[2]
- For patients with little or no glaucomatous damage (just very elevated preoperative IOP), the Ahmed GDD is a reasonable option for stabilizing IOP.[2]
- The BGI provided slightly better IOP lowering at 1 year and less need for reoperation for elevated IOP, but patients in the BGI group had more serious complications associated with reoperation, vision loss, or both.[2]

Notes

- Failure = IOP >21 mm Hg or not reduced by 20% less than baseline or IOP ≤5 mm Hg (on 2 consecutive follow-up visits after 3 months), requiring additional glaucoma surgery, removal of the implant, or loss of light perception vision.[2]
- Complete success = eyes that had not failed and were not receiving supplemental medical therapy.[2]

References

1. Barton K, Gedde SJ, Budenz DL, Feuer WJ, Schiffman J; Ahmed Baerveldt Comparison Study Group. The Ahmed Baerveldt Comparison Study: methodology, baseline patient characteristics, and intraoperative complications. *Ophthalmology*. 2011;118(3):435-442.
2. Budenz DL, Barton K, Feuer WJ, et al. Treatment outcomes in the Ahmed Baerveldt Comparison Study after 1 year of follow-up. *Ophthalmology*. 2011;118(3):443-452.

Primary Tube Versus Trabeculectomy Study

Main Study Purpose

To compare the long-term safety and efficacy of the Baerveldt glaucoma implant versus trabeculectomy with MMC in patients who have not had prior intraocular surgery.[1]

Location

United States.[1]

Study Population

Patients with glaucoma.[1]

Interventions the Participants Were Randomized to Receive

a. Trabeculectomy with MMC.[1]
b. Baerveldt (350-mm^2) glaucoma implant.[1]

Study Design

- Multicenter, randomized, clinical trial.[1]
- Aiming to enroll 88 patients to each arm (176 patients total).[1]
- Ongoing study—plan to enroll patients from May 2008 through May 2012.[1]

Inclusion Criteria

- Age 18 to 85 years.[1]
- Glaucoma that is inadequately controlled on tolerated medical therapy with IOP ≥18 mm Hg and ≤40 mm Hg.[1]
- No previous incisional ocular surgery (including keratorefractive surgery).[1]

Exclusion Criteria

Active iris neovascularization or active proliferative retinopathy, iridocorneal endothelial syndrome, epithelial or fibrous ingrowth, chronic or recurrent uveitis, steroid-induced glaucoma, severe posterior blepharitis, unwilling to discontinue contact lens use after surgery, previous cyclodestructive procedure, conjunctival scarring from prior ocular trauma or cicatrizing disease precluding a superior trabeculectomy, functionally significant cataract, and need for glaucoma surgery combined with other ocular procedures or anticipated need for additional ocular surgery.[1]

Length of Follow-Up

Ongoing study—plan to follow patients for 5 years.[1]

Funding

- Abbott Medical Optics, Inc, Anta Ana, California.[1]
- National Eye Institute, National Institutes of Health.[1]
- Research to Prevent Blindness, Inc, New York, New York.[1]

Results

Ongoing trial.[1]

REFERENCE

1. Primary tube versus trabeculectomy (PTVT) study. Manual of procedures: version 7.0. 2010 May. 55 p. Personal communication with Dr. Steven Gedde on 12/27/10.

44

UNITED STATES FOOD AND DRUG ADMINISTRATION REGULATION OF OPHTHALMIC DEVICES

R. Lee Kramm, MD and Malvina B. Eydelman, MD

The Food and Drug Administration (FDA) is responsible for protecting the public health by assuring the safety, efficacy, and security of human and veterinary drugs, biological products, medical devices, our nation's food supply, cosmetics, and products that emit radiation, and by regulating the manufacture, marketing, and distribution of tobacco products.

An instrument or machine is considered a device if it is intended for use in the diagnosis of disease or in the cure, mitigation, treatment, or prevention of disease, or if it affects the structure or any function of the body and does not achieve its primary intended purposes through chemical action and is not dependent upon being metabolized for the achievement of its intended purposes. This definition provides a clear distinction between a device and other FDA-regulated products.

The Center for Devices and Radiological Health (CDRH), 1 of 7 FDA centers, is responsible for regulating firms that manufacture, repackage, relabel, and/or import medical devices sold in the United States.

CLASSIFICATION OF DEVICES

The Medical Device Amendments to the Food, Drug, and Cosmetic Act were enacted in 1976. These amendments categorized device types into 1 of 3 classes (Class I, II, or III) based on risks posed by the device. The class to which a specific device is assigned determines, among other things, the type of premarketing submission required for the device to be legally marketed.

Classification of medical devices identifies additional regulatory control, if any, that is necessary to assure the safety and effectiveness of a specific device. Medical devices are classified into Class I, II, and III such that the risk that a device poses to the patient and/or the user is a major

Kahook M.
Essentials of Glaucoma Surgery (pp 373-376).
© 2012 SLACK Incorporated.

factor in the class to which it is assigned. Regulatory control increases from Class I to Class III.

Class I devices are those for which general controls alone are sufficient to assure the safety and effectiveness of the device. They are generally low-risk devices and need only conform to general controls to provide reasonable assurance of safety and effectiveness. The provisions of general controls include prohibition of adulterated/misbranded devices, manufacturer registration and listing requirements, good manufacturing practices, and record keeping. Most Class I devices are exempt (subject to limitations defined in the regulations) from premarket notification (510[k]). Class I devices are subject to the least regulatory control. Ophthalmic examples of Class I devices include most visual acuity charts, perimeters, manual surgical tools, and topographers.

Class II devices are those for which general controls alone are insufficient to assure safety and effectiveness, and for which existing methods are available to provide such assurances. In addition to complying with general controls, Class II devices are also subject to special controls. Special controls may include special labeling requirements, mandatory performance standards, and postmarket surveillance. Ophthalmic examples of Class II devices include most vitrectomy and phacoemulsification instruments, tonometers, slit-lamp microscopes, glaucoma lasers, and implantable glaucoma devices for the refractory patient population.

Class III is the most stringent regulatory category for devices. Class III devices are those for which insufficient information exists to assure safety and effectiveness solely through general or special controls. Class III devices are usually those that support or sustain human life, are of substantial importance in preventing impairment of human health, or that present a potential, unreasonable risk of illness or injury. Ophthalmic examples of Class III devices include IOLs, excimer lasers, endotamponades, viscoelastics, and implantable glaucoma devices for the nonrefractory patient population.

MARKETING SUBMISSIONS

Most Class I devices and a few Class II devices are exempt from the 510(k) requirements of the Act, subject to the limitations to exemption found in each classification chapter (eg, 21 CFR 886.9). If a manufacturer's device falls into a generic category of exempted type devices and meets the exemption criteria (same intended use and same scientific fundamental technology as legally marketed devices of this type), a 510(k) and FDA clearance is not required before marketing the device in the US. (If the device exceeds the limitations to exemption, a 510(k) submission and clearance is required prior to marketing.) These devices are not, however, exempt from other general controls. All medical devices must be manufactured under a quality assurance program, be suitable for the intended use, be adequately packaged and properly labeled, and have establishment registration and device listing forms on file with the FDA. The manufacturers can confirm the exempt status and any limitations that apply to their devices at the FDA Web site for medical devices: www.fda.gov/MedicalDevices/

For most Class II devices and some not exempt Class I devices, a 510(k) submission and clearance is required for marketing. A 510(k) is a premarket submission to the FDA that compares the subject device to one or more similar devices currently legally marketed in the US, to support their "substantial equivalence." A legally marketed device(s) to which equivalence is drawn is known as a "predicate" device (see 21 CFR 807.92(a)(3)).

Due to the high risk associated with Class III devices, the FDA determined that general and special controls alone are insufficient to ensure the safety and effectiveness of Class III devices. Therefore, these devices require a PMA (premarket approval) application to obtain marketing approval. PMA is the most stringent type of device marketing application required by the FDA. PMA approval is based on a determination by the FDA that the PMA application contains sufficient valid scientific evidence to provide reasonable assurance that the device is safe and effective for its intended use(s). An applicant must receive FDA approval of its PMA application prior to marketing the device. An approved PMA is, in effect, a license granting the applicant (or owner) permission to market the device.

INVESTIGATION DEVICE EXEMPTION

For all Class III devices and some Class II devices, clinical performance data are required to be included in the regulatory marketing submissions. An investigational device exemption (IDE) allows the investigational device to be shipped and used in a clinical study to collect safety and effectiveness data required to support an application to the FDA requesting clearance to market. The purpose of an IDE is to encourage, to the extent consistent with the protection of public health and safety and with ethical standards, the discovery and development of useful devices intended for human use, and, to that end, to maintain optimum freedom for scientific investigators in their pursuit of this purpose.

All clinical evaluations of investigational devices, unless exempt (eg, certain studies of lawfully marketed devices), must have an approved IDE before the study is initiated. Investigations covered under the IDE regulation are subject to differing levels of regulatory control, depending on the level of risk. The IDE regulation distinguishes between significant and nonsignificant risk device studies. The procedures for obtaining approval to begin the study differ accordingly.

An approved IDE permits a device to be shipped lawfully for the purpose of conducting investigations of the device without complying with the requirements that apply to devices in commercial distribution. In addition, while the device is under investigation, IDE sponsors are exempt from several other regulations.

SUGGESTED READINGS

US Food and Drug Administration. *Device classification.* FDA Web site. Retrieved from www.fda.gov/MedicalDevices/DeviceRegulationandGuidance/Overview/ClassifyYour-Device/default.htm.

US Food and Drug Administration. *Medical device innovation initiative white paper.* FDA Web site. Retrieved from www.fda.gov/AboutFDA/CentersOffices/OfficeofMedical-ProductsandTobacco/CDRH/CDRHInnovation/ucm242067.htm.

US Food and Drug Administration. *Overview of device regulation.* FDA Web site. Retrieved from www.fda.gov/MedicalDevices/DeviceRegulationandGuidance/Overview/default.htm.

45

GLAUCOMA SURGERY IN RESOURCE-POOR SETTINGS

Nathan Congdon, MD, MPH

Glaucoma is the world's leading cause of irreversible blindness, affecting an estimated 60.5 million persons and responsible for vision loss among 8.4 million in 2010.[1] This chapter deals with case identification and management of this condition in areas of limited resources.

CASE IDENTIFICATION

Traditional screening tests—Goldmann tonometry, automated visual fields, and evaluation of the disc—are limited in their ability to detect glaucoma,[2,3] and there is little to suggest that newer devices[4-7] will improve screening performance soon. No trial evidence currently supports the benefit of screening for open-angle glaucoma (OAG)[8] or angle-closure glaucoma (ACG)[9], which may not be cost-effective in the developed[10-13] or developing[14,15] world. Case finding in the clinic is the best current strategy to detect glaucoma in areas of limited resources.[16]

Expense and poor accuracy among inexperienced patients[13,17] render field machines impractical in resource-poor areas. Examination of the optic nerve is better-suited to these settings and will likely identify patients at risk for blindness, the key target for case identification.

Primary angle-closure glaucoma has a greater risk of blindness compared with OAG[18] and definitely benefits from early treatment with peripheral iridectomy (PI).[19] Thus, routine assessment of the anterior chamber angle is important, particularly in areas with high angle-closure prevalence. Simpler tests, such as oblique illumination of the eye, lack diagnostic accuracy,[20,21] whereas slit-beam assessment of the peripheral angle[22] requires a slit lamp and is as resource-demanding as gonioscopy, although it may be quicker and require less training. Poor specificity limits newer imaging

Kahook M.
Essentials of Glaucoma Surgery (pp 377-380).
© 2012 SLACK Incorporated.

technologies,[9,23] which are not suited for use in poor areas. Gonioscopy appears to provide the best accuracy for modest resources in characterizing the angle.

Examination of the optic nerve and angle both presuppose significant training efforts in areas of limited resources. Few studies have examined the impact of training on accuracy in optic nerve assessment[24,25] or gonioscopy.[26]

TREATMENT

Medical therapy for glaucoma involves long-term use of therapies that may be expensive, difficult to obtain, and poorly tolerated, and is thus not well-suited for use in resource-poor areas. Glaucoma surgery may cause lens opacity[27] and vision loss[28] and is thus most appropriate for persons with vision-threatening disease.

Many patients at risk for glaucoma may also have concurrent cataract, and cataract extraction may be definitive therapy for those with narrow angles, angle closure, and possibly ACG. Trabeculectomy could be utilized for those with OAG and potentially advanced cases of ACG in which cataract extraction alone might not provide safe levels of pressure control. Few trials of glaucoma surgery have been carried out in the developing world,[29] but randomized trials in richer areas suggest generally equivalent safety and efficacy for strategies involving trabeculectomy, laser trabeculoplasty, and tube shunts.[28,30] Although laser devices are too expensive for resource-poor areas, the manufacture of high-quality, low-cost intraocular lenses (IOLs) in India and elsewhere provides a model for cheap seton devices. The recent Tube Versus Trabeculectomy Study (TVT)[28] and clinical experience suggest that tubes are at least as effective and safer than trabeculectomy, and may be more appropriate for less-experienced surgeons and more tolerant of limited follow-up and compliance with postoperative medications in poor settings.

KEY POINTS

- A combination of clinic-based case detection and surgery for severely-affected cases may be the most appropriate and sustainable approach to combatting glaucoma blindness in resource-poor settings
- While trabeculectomy and/or cataract surgery may be appropriate for many patients, as inexpensive, locally-produced tube shunts and potentially new devices for implantation into Schlemm's canal become available, these may play an increasing role in surgical treatment.

REFERENCES

1. Quigley HA, Broman AT. The number of people with glaucoma worldwide in 2010 and 2020. *Br J Ophthalmol.* 2006;90:262-267.

2. Stoutenbeek R, de Voogd S, Wolfs RC, et al. The additional yield of a periodic screening programme for open-angle glaucoma: a population-based comparison of incident glaucoma cases detected in regular ophthalmic care with cases detected during screening. *Br J Ophthalmol.* 2008;92:1222-1226.

3. Tielsch JM, Katz J, Singh K, et al. A population-based evaluation of glaucoma screening: the Baltimore Eye Survey. *Am J Epidemiol.* 1991;134:1102-1110.

4. Healey PR, Lee AJ, Aung T, et al. Diagnostic accuracy of the Heidelberg Retina Tomograph for Glaucoma: a population-based assessment. *Ophthalmology.* 2010;117: 1667-1673.

5. Zheng Y, Wong TY, Lamoureux E, et al. Diagnostic ability of Heidelberg Retina Tomography in detecting glaucoma in a population setting: the Singapore Malay Eye Study. *Ophthalmology.* 2010;117:290-297.

6. Iwase A, Tomidokoro A, Araie M, et al. Performance of frequency-doubling technology perimetry in a population-based prevalence survey of glaucoma. The Tajimi Study. *Ophthalmology.* 2007;114:27-32.

7. Wang YX, Xu L, Zhang RX, et al. Frequency-doubling threshold perimetry in predicting glaucoma in a population-based study: the Beijing Eye Study. *Arch Ophthalmol.* 2007;125:1402-1406.

8. Hatt S, Wormald R, Burr J. Screening for prevention of optic nerve damage due to chronic open angle glaucoma. *Cochrane Database Syst Rev.* 2006:CD006129.

9. Yip JL, Foster PJ, Uranchimeg D, et al. Randomised controlled trial of screening and prophylactic treatment to prevent primary angle closure glaucoma. *Br J Ophthalmol.* 2010;94:1472-1477.

10. Blanco A, Zangwill LM. Is there an appropriate, acceptable and reasonably accurate screening test? In: Weinreb R, Healey P, Topouzis F, eds. *Glaucoma Screening: 5th Consensus Report World Glaucoma Association.* Amsterdam, The Netherlands: Kugler; 2008:33-50.

11. Burr JM, Mowatt G, Hernandez R, et al. The clinical effectiveness and cost-effectiveness of screening for open angle glaucoma: a systematic review and economic evaluation. *Health Technol Assess.* 2007;11:iii-iv, ix-x, 1-190.

12. Mowatt G, Burr JM, Cook JA, et al. Screening tests for detecting open-angle glaucoma: systematic review and meta-analysis. *Invest Ophthalmol Vis Sci.* 2008;49:5373-5385.

13. Hirneiss C, Niedermaier A, Kernt M, et al. Health-economic aspects of glaucoma screening. *Ophthalmologe.* 2010;107:143-149.

14. Thomas R, Sekhar GC, Parikh R. Primary angle closure glaucoma: a developing world perspective. *Clin Exp Ophthalmol.* 2007;35:374-378.

15. Thomas R, Sekhar GC, Kumar RS. Glaucoma management in developing countries: medical, laser, and surgical options for glaucoma management in countries with limited resources. *Curr Opin Ophthalmol.* 2004;15:127-131.

16. Maul EA, Jampel HD. Glaucoma screening in the real world. *Ophthalmology.* 2010;117:1665-1666.

17. Iwase A, Tomidokoro A, Araie M, et al. Performance of frequency-doubling technology perimetry in a population-based prevalence survey of glaucoma. The Tajimi Study. *Ophthalmology.* 2007;114:27-32.

18. Foster PJ, Johnson GJ. Glaucoma in China: how big is the problem? *Br J Ophthalmol.* 2001;85:1277-1282.

19. Lam D, Tham C, Congdon N. Peripheral iridectomy for angle-closure glaucoma. In: Shaarawy TM, Hitchings RA, Crowston JG, eds. *Glaucoma: Medical Diagnosis & Therapy.* Vol 2. Philadelphia, PA: Saunders/Elsevier; 2009:61-70.

20. He M, Huang W, Friedman DS, et al. Slit lamp-simulated oblique flashlight test in the detection of narrow angles in Chinese eyes: the Liwan eye study. *Invest Ophthalmol Vis Sci.* 2007;48:5459-5463.

21. Thomas R, George T, Braganza A, et al. The flashlight test and van Herick's test are poor predictors for occludable angles. *Aust N Z J Ophthalmol.* 1996;24:251-256.

22. Nolan WP, Aung T, Machin D, et al. Detection of narrow angles and established angle closure in Chinese residents of Singapore: potential screening tests. *Am J Ophthalmol.* 2006;141:896-901.

23. Lavanya R, Foster PJ, Sakata LM, et al. Screening for narrow angles in the Singapore population: evaluation of new noncontact screening methods. *Ophthalmology.* 2008;115:1720-1727.

24. Abrams LS, Scott IU, Spaeth GL, et al. Agreement among optometrists, ophthalmologists, and residents in evaluating the optic disc for glaucoma. *Ophthalmology.* 1994;101:1662-1667.

25. Quigley HA, West SK, Munoz B, et al. Examination methods for glaucoma prevalence surveys. *Arch Ophthalmol.* 1993;111:1409-1415.

26. Congdon NG, Spaeth GL, Augsburger J, et al. A proposed simple method for measurement in the anterior chamber angle: biometric gonioscopy. *Ophthalmology.* 1999;106:2161-2167.

27. AGIS Investigators. The Advanced Glaucoma Intervention Study: 6. Effect of cataract on visual field and visual acuity. *Arch Ophthalmol.* 2000;118:1639-1652.

28. Gedde SJ, Schiffman JC, Feuer WJ, et al. Treatment outcomes in the tube versus trabeculectomy study after one year of follow-up. *Am J Ophthalmol.* 2007;143:9-22.

29. Robin AL, Ramakrishnan R, Krishnadas R, et al. A long-term dose-response study of mitomycin in glaucoma filtration surgery. *Arch Ophthalmol.* 1997;115:969-974.

30. AGIS Investigators. The Advanced Glaucoma Intervention Study: 7. The relationship between control of intra-ocular pressure and visual field deterioration. *Am J Ophthalmol.* 2000;130:429-440.

PERSPECTIVES ON SURGERY
FROM THE EXPERTS

Are You Still Withholding the "Trabeculectomy Cure"?

David L. Epstein, MD, MMM

When I was a resident, glaucoma fellow, and then junior faculty at Massachusetts Eye and Ear Infirmary (MEEI), we had a glaucoma surgical conference in which the residents would have to present their cases for filtration surgery to a large group of seasoned glaucoma experts, and they were expected to justify the need for surgical intervention. This evolved from the era of full-thickness filtration surgery, which actually was remarkably successful in achieving low intraocular pressures (IOPs) but had a significant complication rate, mostly due to postoperative flat chambers, choroidal detachments, inevitable cataract formation, etc; it took only one expulsive hemorrhage to give one a new perspective.

As I continued to advance in time on the faculty at MEEI, the more modern operation of trabeculectomy came into fashion, and I remember several of my own fellows questioning me why I was hesitant to offer the "trabeculectomy cure" more aggressively to my patients at earlier stages of their primary open-angle glaucoma (POAG) disease (without the need to document progression of their glaucoma). This was especially true after the introduction of antiproliferative eye therapy,[1] first by Richard Parrish, MD, from the Bascom Palmer Eye Institute, where we seemed to enter a somewhat naïve "golden period" of 5 to 10 years of believing in a surgical cure for glaucoma. So, indeed, how could we withhold this cure?

Of course, "glaucoma is the curse of long-term follow-up," and with further time and observation we noted some serious complications from trabeculectomy, and many glaucoma doctors became joyless "bleb doctors," dealing with thin, leaking, and occasionally infected blebs, and we soon accumulated a cadre of unhappy bleb patients despite good IOP control. Plus, sometimes the "cure" failed with time, and glaucoma control was lost. Such was the long-term cure of POAG.

Kahook M.
Essentials of Glaucoma Surgery (pp 383–386).
© 2012 SLACK Incorporated.

To me, it is amazing that now, with the further passage of time, some glaucoma experts have almost given up on trabeculectomy for POAG. I think this is an overreaction, as many patients still achieve good IOP control, but we apparently have now entered a new "curative" era of tubes and valves and external hardware that basically still just shunts fluid from the inside of the eye to the outside. Thus, "tube cures" are now replacing "trabeculectomy cures" for POAG in many places, although others are observing longer-term failures of certain tubes with their own complications, etc.

And so to me, it really is important to take a more comprehensive long-term view of our "surgical cures" for POAG. One should start at the beginning of the 20th century (that is, around 1900), when glaucoma was actually the most advanced of ophthalmology disciplines. At a time when cataracts were being couched, retinal detachments were inoperable, and corneal transplants were unknown, ophthalmologists knew that if the eye was firm, one applied the "herb" pilocarpine, and if the eye remained somewhat firm (they did not understand the difference between open-angle and angle-closure glaucoma), then one put a "hole" in the eye and externalized the anterior chamber to the subconjunctival space. Hence, this was the birth of full-thickness filtration surgery. The great advance of trabeculectomy perhaps 70 years later really consisted of still just "putting a hole in the eye," but now under a guarded scleral flap. (It is also noteworthy that trabeculectomy was not designed to produce filtration; rather to "-ectomize" the site of Grant's outflow resistance.[2]) Likewise, with modern-era "tubes," we now are once again simply externalizing the inside of the eye (through a tube) to the outside of the eye (and its accompanying hardware). How far, then, has glaucoma surgery come compared with the other advances in ophthalmology? Glaucoma physicians are still surgically "curing" POAG with some type of smaller hole into the eye.

I also continue to be amazed that, although the IOP rises in glaucoma due to abnormalities in the outflow pathway tissue, we have no targeted drugs for this tissue (which is a subject for another day and has been my life-long quest). I still think the future of surgical "cures" for POAG will some-day involve an "intra-outflow pathway" surgical procedure. There seems to be beginning efforts for this today with various Schlemm's canal surgical procedures, and I am growing optimistic, although I think we are not yet there. I think we are missing something that we do not understand, and I hope that inquisitive and observant clinicians and surgeons in the future may discover the clue to a successful Schlemm's canal surgical procedure. But I am also disappointed that many surgeons do not understand the fundamental observations of Morton Grant, MD,[2] which are the sine que non to develop such a successful intra-outflow pathway surgical procedure. Grant clearly showed that the outflow pathway functions segmentally, there is no circumferential flow in Schlemm's canal, and there is some distal scleral resistance from the outer wall of Schlemm's canal outward[2,3] that results in postoperative IOPs not being as low as when one places a true "hole" that bypasses the full outflow pathway.

Grant eliminated 75% of the resistance to aqueous outflow only by cutting into the inner wall of Schlemm's canal throughout the entire 360-degree circumference.[2,3] Therefore, segmental surgical procedures involving only 1 or even 2 hours of the circumference will eliminate only the resistance in that segment, and hence the typically resulting postoperative IOPs are in the mid- to upper-teens. Further, although we have moved along towards more circumferential surgical procedures with various suture techniques for treatments of 360 degrees of Schlemm's canal, the potential flaw here is that it has not been believed that collapse of Schlemm's canal is responsible primarily for the increased resistance to outflow (at least initially) in many glaucomas. How then is the suture technique addressing the fundamental cause of the glaucoma (except perhaps by disrupting the inner wall of Schlemm's canal)? What is the exact rationale? Further, there is a biological wound healing process inherent in trabecular meshwork outflow pathway cellular processes that can provide benefit (eg, in various laser procedures[4]) or can cause healing and scarring of the intended outcome.

So, I don't think we are quite there yet, and it is poignant to me that with the passage of time, my former fellows have themselves become seasoned glaucoma experts, and it is now their fellows who are puzzled about their hesitancy to vigorously offer a "surgical cure" for POAG.

Someday, hopefully, this will all change, but so far to me it is remarkable and disappointing how little things, in truth, are different. I worry what Drs. Chandler and Grant would say about our progress. We will all continue to carry the burdens of our glaucoma patients home with us each night until there really are both therapeutic and surgical true cures for the various glaucomas. Hopefully, the breadth of wisdom of sometimes reflective, if wizened, senior glaucoma surgeons can be combined with the inquisitive spirit of the new glaucoma generation to discover the clues necessary to accomplish this. We desperately do need new surgical "cures."

References

1. The Fluorouracil Filtering Surgery Study Group. Three-year follow-up of the Fluorouracil Filtering Surgery Study. *Am J Ophthalmol.* 1993;115(1):82-92.
2. Grant WM. Experimental aqueous perfusion in enucleated human eyes. *Arch Ophthalmol.* 1963;69:783-801.
3. Rosenquist RC, Epstein DL, Melamed S, Johnson M, Grant WM. Outflow resistance of enucleated human eyes with two different perfusion pressures and different extents of trabeculotomy. *Curr Eye Res.* 1989;8(12):1233-1240.
4. Melamed S, Epstein DL. Alterations of aqueous humor outflow following argon laser trabeculoplasty in monkeys. *Br J Ophthalmol.* 1987;71(10):776-781.

47

GLAUCOMA SURGICAL INNOVATION NEARING THE TIPPING POINT

Thomas W. Samuelson, MD

We are at a tipping point in the surgical management of glaucoma. Although most agree that trabeculectomy (guarded filtration surgery) has many imperfections, the irreversible nature of glaucoma requires a conservative approach to surgical innovation. Indeed, given the pernicious nature of some forms of glaucoma, trepidation toward surgical innovation is understandable. However, until recently, technological advancement in surgical glaucoma has been virtually nonexistent. This, despite the fact that it has been clear to many in the field that trabeculectomy, an operation for advanced and particularly high-risk glaucoma, is not a procedure for early disease. The heterogeneous nature of glaucoma, ranging from relentlessly progressive to easily controllable, mandates a more nuanced approach than the "one surgical procedure for all patients" (ie, trabeculectomy) approach that has been utilized for the past several decades. The simple fact that a filtration bleb renders a patient at risk for infection for life is unacceptable for patients with early disease or those with a more benign prognosis. It is unacceptable to subject patients at low risk for severe functional vision loss to bleb-related complications, including devastating late infections. Few procedures in medicine subject the patient to such lifelong iatrogenic risk. Further, the "therapeutic index" for trabeculectomy is unacceptably narrow to be widely used in patients with early to moderate disease. For example, a conservative filtration procedure performed with little or no antimetabolite may function well for several years but has a significant risk of failure over time. Although the bleb-related risks with this more conservative approach are diminished, this approach subjects the trabecular meshwork to several years of reduced perfusion. Subsequently, should the bleb fail, the meshwork is likely to function more poorly than prior to the procedure, owing to disuse atrophy of the distal collector system. On the other hand, antimetabolites

Kahook M.
Essentials of Glaucoma Surgery (pp 387–390).
© 2012 SLACK Incorporated.

may ensure long-term bleb stability and function. However, such measures subject the patient to the risks inherent to a weakened conjunctival barrier. Thus, the bleb that functions transiently but is prone to failure is suboptimal, and the bleb that becomes ischemic and well-established is suboptimal due to the risk of late leaks and infection. Aqueous drainage devices are a reasonable alternative to trabeculectomy with less risk of infection or conjunctiva-related complications, yet tube shunts also subject patients to significant risk, including diplopia, hypotony, corneal decompensation, and tube exposure.

Although traditional transscleral procedures, such as trabeculectomy and tube shunts, remain excellent options for advanced glaucoma, there is great need for safer surgical options for use in early glaucoma, preferably procedures that augment physiological outflow rather than bypassing it. Fortunately, the glaucoma surgical space is in the crosshairs of several well-capitalized new companies. Moreover, the purchase of the Ex-Press device by Alcon during the last year has brought new attention and ample resources to glaucoma surgical innovation as well as a safer and more precise procedure in the Ex-Press-assisted trabeculectomy.

Statistics confirm that the number of trabeculectomies performed by United States surgeons has declined considerably in recent years, despite a more aged population. Improvements in medical therapy and increased utilization of laser trabeculoplasty are important factors contributing to this decline. Another explanation for the diminishing role of external filtration surgery is the recent evidence that cataract surgery lowers intraocular pressure (IOP) more than previously appreciated. Cataract and glaucoma are common conditions and each is more prevalent with advancing age. The natural history of cataract and glaucoma is often parallel, thus it is a tempting strategy to manage both conditions with a single operation. Traditionally, a significant percentage of trabeculectomy procedures have been performed in conjunction with cataract surgery. However, this trend has decreased in recent years. The collective influence of improved glaucoma medications, the knowledge that cataract surgery often enhances physiologic outflow, and the development of less invasive surgical methods to enhance conventional outflow have made many surgeons reluctant to bypass trabecular outflow via trabeculectomy until later in the disease process or at least until after cataract surgery has been performed.

Although the mechanism of IOP reduction following cataract surgery is unclear, most believe it is due to improved physiological outflow facility. In theory, the IOP-lowering effect of cataract surgery and trabeculectomy are mutually exclusive, one negating the effect of the other. Therefore, for mild to moderate glaucoma occurring in conjunction with cataract, it seems prudent to perform either phacoemulsification alone or phacoemulsification combined with a minimally invasive glaucoma procedure, preferably one that enhances or preserves conventional outflow facility. Although a transscleral bypass procedure, such as trabeculectomy, might be the best option for patients with advanced glaucoma, eg, when fixation is threatened, patients with mild or moderate disease may be better served with a procedure that enhances physiological outflow.

Canaloplasty is an *ab externo* approach to Schlemm's canal during which the canal is intubated with a microsurgical catheter allowing 360-degree viscodilation and subsequent suture tensioning of the trabecular meshwork. The procedure has been shown to provide a reasonable balance between safety and efficacy. Published data show fewer complications than with trabeculectomy with slightly less efficacy. Although the procedure has gained gradual acceptance, its adoption rate has been less than universal due to its technical difficulty, the length of the procedure, and the fact that it expends valuable conjunctiva and scleral tissue, rendering the superior limbus suboptimal for subsequent filtration surgery if needed. My own experience with canaloplasty has been favorable for patients in the intermediate range of glaucoma severity. If a canaloplasty fails in my hands, I generally will follow it with an aqueous drainage device such as a Baerveldt implant. The Tube Versus Trabeculectomy (TVT) Study results provide reasonable validation for the use of tubes without prior trabeculectomy.

Ab interno trabeculotomy (Trabectome) is another approach to Schlemm's canal. It is appealing due to the fact that it utilizes a clear corneal conjunctival-sparing approach. It is generally performed in conjunction with cataract surgery. Published data suggest that it adds additional IOP reduction as compared to phacoemulsification alone. Yet, a controlled study has not been done to compare the effect of Trabectome alone versus Trabectome with cataract removal. Finally, the iStent, another ab interno approach to Schlemm's canal, is currently under review by the Food and Drug Administration (FDA). A panel convened by the FDA in July 2010 provided a favorable review of the iStent United States Investigational Device Exemption (IDE) trial. However, as of the time of the writing of this chapter, the FDA has not yet approved the iStent. Although the IOP-lowering effect of a single iStent was modest, patients receiving iStent required significantly less postoperative medications, and there was no measurable increased risk of phacoemulsification combined with iStent as compared with cataract surgery alone. Moreover, data from outside the United States suggest that additional efficacy is achieved when more than one stent is placed.

In summary, I currently reserve trabeculectomy for advanced glaucoma. I prefer safer, minimally invasive surgery, such as cataract extraction alone, Trabectome, canaloplasty, and when available, the iStent for patients with early to moderate glaucoma. We have made tremendous strides in our quest for a better surgery for use in early to moderate glaucoma. Given the momentum currently in place and the considerable attention dedicated to glaucoma surgery by our industry partners, I strongly believe that the best is yet to come for the surgical glaucoma patient.

48

GLAUCOMA SURGERY
A PARADOX

Richard A. Lewis, MD

I recently examined a patient with a long history of glaucoma. A number of years ago, I had performed a trabeculectomy in each eye. The surgery was uncomplicated and successfully controlled her intraocular pressure (IOP) in the 8- to 12-mm Hg range without drops. A few years later, a bleb infection developed in one eye; endophthalmitis ensued and she lost functional vision. The other eye served her well until recently. Despite low IOP, her glaucomatous cupping and visual field loss progressed. She was encouraged to discontinue driving and curtail her activities; she was declared legally blind. Unfortunately, this is not an atypical story.

Filtering procedures, in its various iterations, have been the mainstay of glaucoma surgery for over a century. Interestingly, trabeculectomy has changed little from what I learned during my fellowship in 1982. Efficacy of trabeculectomy has always been very good. However, despite various advancements in surgical technique and our enhanced understanding of wound healing, troubling short- and long-term side effects jeopardize the outcome. To a great extent, this limitation is due to the problems of directing intra-aqueous flow through the sclera to the subconjunctival space. It is not a natural space or reservoir; and despite all of our attempts with modulating use of anti-fibrotics and refined surgical technique, problems ensue.

Although directing flow to the subconjunctival space has been the primary target in glaucoma surgery, innovative and more physiologic approaches to lowering IOP utilizing the canal of Schlemm and the suprachoroidal space are actively being investigated. This recent period of innovation is not by coincidence. Various factors (including enhanced technology, funding, and broad international interest) have converged to develop a safer yet equally efficacious glaucoma operation.

Of the new procedures, the space in and around the canal is the most physiologic. The new devices are well tolerated and safe. The extent of the IOP reduction is, however, not quite to the level achieved by the

Kahook M.
Essentials of Glaucoma Surgery (pp 391–392).
© 2012 SLACK Incorporated.

subconjunctival approach but perhaps close enough. Working in the suprachoroidal space offers the chance of greater IOP reduction but raises more concern about long-term scarring and efficacy. The various devices and procedures are currently entering into phase 3 international randomized trials, and results are pending. In all likelihood, the current scope of new devices will broaden the indications for a safer surgical means of lowering IOP for glaucoma. They will also usher in the day for surgically placed drug delivery systems. Not only will this help stem the problem of patient's medication adherence but it will also open the door to posterior segment glaucoma treatment.

However, the big therapeutic advance will come in conjunction with a better understanding of the pathophysiology of the disease. We remain poorly informed of why IOP increases in selected individuals and why glaucoma patients (with and without high IOP) lose vision. Along the way, we need a better, more definitive way of classifying glaucoma. Getting away from the phenotypic or gonioscopic-defined angle classification (ie, open- versus closed-angle) in favor of a genotypic-specific diagnosis would greatly help our understanding of the disease as well as help direct customized therapy for specific glaucomas. We need a means of preventing nerve damage in susceptible patients. We need a way to protect and regenerate the optic nerve.

To say we have not made progress in the last 30 years is a misstatement. To say we have not made the progress noted in other ophthalmic specialties, such as cornea, retina, and cataract, is unmistakable. Yet, the door has begun to open for treating the complications of glaucoma, and innovation is on its way. The next few years will be like no other in the diagnosis and management of this frustrating disease.

FUTURE OF GLAUCOMA

Ramesh S. Ayyala, MD, FRCS, FRCOphth

When I look into the future of glaucoma treatment, 3 things come to mind:

1. Slow-release drug delivery systems that will avoid daily application of topical medications.

2. Development of an ideal glaucoma surgery, which should be able to lower intraocular pressure (IOP) to mid- to low-teens via a small incision and should not take more than 10 minutes to perform, with complication rates less than 0.5% and quick visual recovery.

3. Ganglion cell rehabilitation/regeneration with stem cell or similar technology.

This is easier said than done. So, I will detail those things that I think are achievable within the next 5 to 10 years.

Full-thickness filtration procedures, flat chambers, choroidal effusions, and cataract formations characterized glaucoma surgery in the first half of this century. Guarded filtration surgery and nonvalved and valved glaucoma drainage devices improved the surgical outcomes and decreased the complication rates in the second half of the 20th century. An explosion of new technology and techniques have taken glaucoma surgery to new heights in the first 10 years of the 21st century. Chances are that these changes will continue, with the ultimate goal of designing a glaucoma surgery that can be performed in 10 minutes via a 2- to 3-mm incision and have success rates similar to cataract and refractive surgery.

Traditional glaucoma surgeries divert the aqueous humor into the subconjunctival space. Failure from postoperative fibrosis and problems related to the bleb (pain and discomfort, leaky cystic blebs, bleb-related infections) are the bane of every glaucoma surgeon. The use of antifibrotic agents (eg, 5-fluorouracil [5-FU] and mitomycin C [MMC]) have increased

Kahook M.
Essentials of Glaucoma Surgery (pp 393–394).
© 2012 SLACK Incorporated.

the success of trabeculectomy operation while increasing the incidence of thin cystic blebs and bleb-related infections. The lack of standardization in the delivery of these drugs is one of the many problems that exist in the current trabeculectomy techniques. *Future research should focus on standardizing the delivery techniques of these antifibrotic agents so as to achieve the maximum benefit while minimizing the side effects. New drugs and technologies are needed that help in modulating the bleb morphology while maintaining the overall health of the bleb.* The use of antiangiogenesis drugs, such as Avastin (bevacizumab), and the new generation of collagen implants show early promise but await long-term results.

Glaucoma drainage devices (GDDs) have many advantages compared with traditional trabeculectomy such as fewer immediate postoperative complications, posterior location of the bleb, and significantly less incidence of bleb-related infections. However, they result in significantly higher-end IOP and failure rate secondary to bleb fibrosis. One-time use of anti-fibrotic agents does not appear to alter the success rate of GDDs. *The development of antifibrotic, drug-coated GDDs or GDDs attached to slow-release drug (MMC) delivery systems might decrease the postoperative fibrosis and enhance the long-term success rate of current GDDs.* If the creation of drug-coated GDDs results in IOPs comparable to trabeculectomy, then GDDs might displace trabeculectomy as the new gold standard in the foreseeable future. Animal studies using these GDDs attached to slow-release drug (MMC) delivery systems has demonstrated a significant decrease in the degree of postoperative bleb fibrosis. However, human clinical trails are still awaited.

The modification of surgeries that divert the aqueous humor into alternative pathways such as the Schlemm's canal (canaloplasty, trabeculotomy *ab interno* with the Trabectome, and iStent) and suprachoroidal space (Gold Shunt) have introduced more options to the glaucoma surgeon. Although long-term success rate of these new surgeries is not known, early results are encouraging. As more surgeons master these surgical techniques, these techniques may offer predictable results (lower IOP) with minimal complications, thus setting the stage for surgical intervention at an earlier stage in glaucoma patients who are burdened with multiple, expensive, topical glaucoma medications with numerous side effects. Although this kind of surgery might benefit the majority of patients with moderate glaucoma, there still will be a need for traditional surgery such as trabeculectomy or GDD implantation. Therefore, it is important that future research should also focus on further refinements of these age-old techniques to cater to patients with advanced glaucoma.

GLAUCOMA SURGERY
WHERE WE STARTED AND WHERE WE ARE GOING

Marlene R. Moster, MD

The world of glaucoma is vastly different now than when I first trained as a fellow from 1983 to 1984. Although the indications to perform glaucoma surgery have remained similar, the procedures available have advanced considerably. In fact, the scenario of the surgical arena in 1983 is no longer recognizable, with amazing changes occurring since then.

Let me paint the surgical picture during my fellowship with George Spaeth and Rick Wilson at Wills Eye Insitute in Philadelphia, Pennsylvania. The standard of care included large wound extracapsular cataract surgery combined with trabeculectomy (no antimetabolites), limbal-based trabeculectomies, cyclodialysis cleft formation, and bedside cryotherapy in aphakes. Patients received a retrobulbar and facial nerve block, and everyone was admitted as an inpatient. All the eyelashes were clipped and the head was draped with towels and towel clips. As a fellow, it was not uncommon to round twice a day on 20 inpatients at Wills Eye Hospital, as patients typically remained in the hospital for 4 to 5 days.

Phacoemulsification was coming of age and early on, large polymethylmethacrylate (PMMA) lenses placed in-the-bag were the first to become available. Can opener capsulorrhexis with a 25-gauge needle was routine, retained cortical remnants were no surprise, and foldable lenses were not yet invented. The combined extracapsular cataract and glaucoma surgery, as I first learned it, took easily over an hour. When 10 cases were scheduled, we would start in the morning and operate till evening. Everyone was patched, and because all eyes were blocked, the "occasional" retrobulbar hemorrhage was not really uncommon. Because antimetabolites were not

Kahook M.
Essentials of Glaucoma Surgery (pp 395–398).
© 2012 SLACK Incorporated.

yet available, scarring was almost routine. Postoperative modification of large amounts of cylinder via suture manipulation was commonplace after combined surgery when at least 6 to 8 nylon sutures closed the superior wound. Needling the bleb was unheard of, and our only option then to increase flow was laser suture lysis or subsequent tube shunt surgery (first Schockett, then Molteno, and the other shunts followed).

Having watched all these changes evolve, the real advantage that has advanced the field of glaucoma surgery is *surgeon control*. We are no longer filleting the eye open to remove large phacomorphic lenses, thus the risk of expulsive hemorrhage is way down. I recall assisting George Spaeth in managing 2 expulsives on 1 day during combined procedures.

We now have releasable sutures that can meticulously control the amount of aqueous flow in the postoperative period. Using a combination of topical, intracameral, and subconjunctival/Tenon's lidocaine, all glaucoma surgeries can be performed without either a peribulbar or retrobulbar block, allowing for immediate vision postoperatively. This is most helpful in monocular patients. Trabeculectomies or guarded filtration procedures can be done with either a fornix or the traditional limbal-based flaps. Antimetabolites like mitomycin C (MMC) placed with sponges or injected at the time of surgery improve the success. Failing trabeculectomies can be brought back to life with a combination of lidocaine and MMC injected at the time of needling. In addition, user-friendly viscoelastics can manage the chamber depth at the slit lamp should too much aqueous escape early on. Stronger topical and intracameral nonpreserved steroids, such as Triesence (triamcinolone acetonide), are now available to eradicate postoperative inflammation. We now have choices regarding lens implants and can correct large amounts of pre-existing astigmatism with toric implants, either simultaneously with cataract and glaucoma surgery or following trabeculectomy. Tube shunt options are now plentiful, and adopting techniques that modify flow early on improve the quality of the patient's vision by avoiding profound hypotony. Additionally, covering the tubes with either pericardium, sclera, amniotic membrane, or partial-thickness cornea gives the surgeon many options to better treat the individual. One advance has been the Ex-Press shunt. Unfortunately, it is still bleb-dependent, but the whole idea of standardizing glaucoma surgery so it is done efficiently with predicted flow, recognized outcomes, and fewer complications will form the new template for the future. If better control of aqueous inflow is desired, excellent visualization of the ciliary body with an endoscopic illuminator allows for limited ciliary body destruction, making cyclocryotherapy a thing of the past.

Where are we going from here? I do believe that despite the amazing advances noted above, glaucoma surgery is still in its infancy. Efforts are being made to change the morphology of the blebs by making them lower and more diffuse, with less of a tendency toward perforation or infection. A new product, Ologen (Aeon Astron, Leiden, The Netherlands), which is a collagen matrix and space maintainer, is one such idea to replace the use of MMC. I look forward to other products that will truly prevent scarring while allowing the ophthalmologist to manipulate trabeculectomy flap sutures if needed. In the future, closure with nylon sutures may be drastically reduced with affordable tissue glue products. Canaloplasty is still evolving, and I envision the surgical delivery of new drugs directly into Schlemm's canal. This may drastically modify the trabecular outflow mechanism, allowing for meticulous intraocular pressure (IOP) control while forgoing the use of topical medications and eliminating the need for blebs entirely. In addition, genetic manipulation, either intracamerally or via Schlemm's canal, may consistently lower the IOP so the optic nerve can thrive. Exploring the suprachoroidal space with an implant that allows for controlled drainage of aqueous is likely to become available, perhaps with sensors attached that will be able to constantly monitor the IOP. These are just a few of the many advances I envision that will help make glaucoma surgery safer and predictable so as to finally limit glaucomatous blindness that threatens so many throughout the world.

51

PROGRESS IN SURGERY FOR GLAUCOMA

Robert D. Fechtner, MD

Progress lies not in enhancing what is, but in advancing toward what will be.
— Khalil Gibran

WHAT WAS

My first thought when I reflect upon the state of glaucoma surgery is that not much has changed. I performed my first incisional glaucoma surgery 25 years ago. I created a partial-thickness defect in the eye wall under a scleral flap. Although it is true that we have benefited from numerous incremental refinements, the fundamental technique of trabeculectomy is quite recognizable when I refer back to the glaucoma textbooks in my library from the 1980s. We have enhanced what is. Glaucoma surgery remains a "trade" practiced by skilled craftsmen. Where are we? How did we get here? Where should we be headed? Are we advancing toward what will be?

Glaucoma was historically regarded as a disease of elevated intraocular pressure (IOP). Experimental evidence indentified that resistance to outflow resides largely in the inner wall of Schlemm's canal. It seemed logical under that model to "normalize" IOP by removing a portion of the wall to provide aqueous humor direct access to Schlemm's canal. This was the primary objective of trabeculectomy (not the diversion of aqueous to the subconjunctival space). Eventually, we abandoned this notion of using trabeculectomy to restore aqueous access to Schlemm's canal and refined the procedure as an aqueous diversion. The study of glaucoma contains a wonderful history of observation, experimentation, and refinement of hypotheses. A lifetime devoted to trying to understand glaucoma is humbling as we continue to provide care in the face of fundamental uncertainties.

Kahook M.
Essentials of Glaucoma Surgery (pp 399–402).
© 2012 SLACK Incorporated.

WHAT IS

We do not understand well the nature of the optic neuropathies that are pressure-sensitive and deserve to be included as such in our current schema of glaucomas. And we have only one proven effective surgical strategy: lower the IOP. I have the chance to repeat in print a lesson I learned from my grandfather: "If all you have is a hammer, everything looks like a nail." We continue to hammer away at IOP with surgery that provides, at best, a nonphysiologic solution to a poorly understood problem.

Modern cataract surgery might serve as our model for surgery that continues to progress toward what will be. When I was a resident, we still had some attending surgeons who performed elegant and artful intracapsular cataract surgery. Aphakic refraction was a required fundamental skill. The task of cataract surgery was clearly defined—we sought to remove the clouded crystalline lens and replace it with a lens implant without damaging the cornea or inducing astigmatism. In pursuit of this goal, we had the evolution of the intraocular lens (IOL). Extracapsular techniques invited a variety of innovative posterior chamber lens designs. Ultrasonic phacoemulsification allowed incisions smaller than the diameter of the rigid Polymethylmethacrylate (PMMA) lenses. Continuous curvilinear capsulorrhexis improved success. Lens materials advanced to allow smaller incisions. Lasers can perform some steps of the procedure. Each advance opens the door for the next one. As the techniques and technology improve, we add rapid visual rehabilitation and excellent uncorrected visual function to our goals.

Contrast this with trabeculectomy. The first trabeculectomies I performed were during my residency, following publication of the Fluorouracil Filtering Surgery Study. My attending physician carefully supervised both the surgery and the postoperative administration of the fluorouracil injections. I spent the next 2 months managing the persistent wound leaks and corneal toxicity I had induced. Things have gotten better since then. I have migrated away from a large fornix incision to a small limbal incision. Instead of retrobulbar anesthesia and a facial block, I use topical anesthesia and sub-Tenon's irrigation of additional anesthesia. I cannot recall the last time I used a superior rectus bridle suture for exposure. Surgical sponges moistened with mitomycin C (MMC) are applied to sclera posteriorly. My scleral flap is created with a micrometer diamond blade and a beveled micro blade. The dimensions of the scleral flap are much smaller than when I first trained. I use a small punch to create the ostium in peripheral cornea, or I can place a small aperture glaucoma filtration device through the sclera and eliminate the need for an ostium. The flap is closed tightly with planned suture lysis. Postoperative care is still rather intensive with planned suture lysis with elegantly designed laser lenses, titration of medications, and supplemental antifibrosis treatment based on the wound healing response. The theme is unchanged, but the myriad variations and evolution of technique have improved the intra- and postoperative course. Certainly, I believe we have enhanced what is. Yet, a beautifully performed trabeculectomy unleashes the paramount uncertainties of unpredictable wound healing and a lifetime risk of complications.

WHAT COULD BE

Why should not the goals of IOP-lowering surgery be the achievement of an effective, predictable, and technically reproducible procedure with rapid visual rehabilitation, excellent long-term control of IOP, and few early or late complications? I hope that describes what will be. How might we advance in that direction?

The subconjunctival space is a convenient target for the diversion of aqueous and is easily accessible from the anterior chamber. The surgical approach is straightforward. However, we still lack predictable techniques to modulate the wound healing response. If we could simply open conjunctiva, create aqueous outflow with modulated resistance, and close the conjunctiva in a watertight fashion with rapid and complete epithelial healing but limited subconjunctival wound healing, we might have a predictable pressure-lowering operation. The introduction of 5-fluorouracil and MMC have greatly enhanced our ability to achieve lower IOP but still in a highly unpredictable fashion. We are now plagued with fragile blebs with long-term risk of infection, encapsulated blebs with return of IOP to preoperative levels, or the occasional diffuse healthy bleb with excellent long-term control of IOP. Improved strategies for customized wound-healing modulation remain the greatest opportunity for evolutionary improvement of trabeculectomy. This would also invite the development of devices for active control of outflow to the subconjunctival space in response to continuous IOP monitoring.

The conventional outflow pathway is nature's solution for modulating IOP. This should remain a primary target for aqueous diversion. Several steps are potentially necessary for surgical success. Aqueous must exit the anterior chamber and enter Schlemm's canal. A strategy for bypassing the resistance of trabecular meshwork is appealing. We tried that; it is called goniotomy. Although goniotomy can work in pediatric glaucoma, it is not sufficiently successful in adults. A better approach is needed.

A contemporary effort is the development of surgical devices to eliminate or bypass TM resistance and allow aqueous direct access to Schlemm's canal. Accurate placement would seem essential, but, even then, Schlemm's canal must be a functional system in communication with the downstream outflow pathways. The segmental nature of Schlemm's canal might necessitate multiple bypasses. Is it possible to identify the functioning segments and recruit those for outflow?

A modern goniotomy can be performed with ablation of the trabecular meshwork. Yet, IOP does not approach the level of episcleral venous pressure in most patients who have this procedure. This suggests failure of outflow can reside further downstream. What is the nature of downstream failure? Can we rehabilitate collector channels and aqueous veins? These seem like opportunities for advancement.

The suprachoroidal space is another target for aqueous diversion. We tried that as well. It is called cyclodialysis. This was a highly unpredictable operation that could result in extremely low pressures and poor vision or sudden closure and very high IOPs. This target space has regained interest for an improved surgical approach. Several pilot studies have been initiated with devices to provide controlled access of aqueous to this space. Optimal or even acceptable devices need demonstrated utility. The wound healing in this suprachoroidal space is incompletely characterized. We need to understand this better. Yet, I believe the suprachoroidal space also remains a target worthy of further exploration.

Lowering IOP with trabeculectomy is effective. This is an unqualified statement, and glaucoma surgery is quite nuanced. I have often had conversations with colleagues who said, "I am comfortable with my glaucoma surgery procedure." I now interpret this statement to mean that the experienced glaucoma surgeon has developed a level of comfort with an operation that has many well-known shortcomings. The unpredictability of IOP control, slow and sometimes incomplete visual rehabilitation, and a lifelong potential for complications characterize our current state of IOP-lowering surgery. I often think the very best we now do is that the patient will be no worse, and we do not always achieve that goal. When faced with the alternatives of losing vision from glaucoma progression or undergoing trabeculectomy, it is not surprising that our patients are looking for another option. If we are honest, as glaucoma surgeons—so are we. I believe these needs will continue to drive our progress toward what will be.

LOOKING AT GLAUCOMA SURGERY

Joel S. Schuman, MD, FACS

We used to have weekly morning case rounds during my fellowship at Massachusetts Eye and Ear Infirmary. Whenever we discussed a patient who had intraocular pressure (IOP) uncontrolled on medications, one of the favorite questions asked by my glaucoma fellowship director, David L. Epstein, MD, was, "Why not give them the cure?" His point, of course, was that there was (and is) no cure for our patient with glaucoma. Surgery is a treatment for the disease, more potent but also more risky than medications or laser.

I have frequently thought about the need for improvements in surgical intervention. Notwithstanding that, given the complications associated with our traditional surgical techniques, we have done well with postoperative care. Having trained in the era of full-thickness glaucoma surgery in Boston at a time before the use of mitomycin C (MMC) in the United States, a time during which patients were routinely kept hospitalized postoperatively and when flat anterior chambers and choroidal effusions were commonplace, I did, and do, feel comfortable with my postoperative choices and ability to manage anything manifested by the patient.

Despite my knowledge and comfort with postoperative glaucoma management, I am extremely respectful of the risks attendant to glaucoma surgery. Although we almost always improve the patient's lot in the long run, there are still a few whose vision is compromised related to our intervention, even when everything goes perfectly intraoperatively. A sneeze, a cough, a slip on the stairs—suprachoroidal hemorrhage is forever an unwelcome guest who shows up at the worst possible time. The patient who calls with intense, aching pain and knows the minute that the pain began, is the one who is telling you that he or she has had bleeding into the suprachoroidal space.

Postoperative complications are an impetus for the current push toward better glaucoma operations. It has been more than 100 years that we have

Kahook M.
Essentials of Glaucoma Surgery (pp 403-404).
© 2012 SLACK Incorporated.

been bypassing the conventional outflow system one way or another. The surgery has gotten progressively more controlled intra- and postoperatively, going from full-thickness surgery to guarded filtration surgery, then later with the use of steroids and antimetabolites. We have even improved glaucoma drainage devices (GDDs) to the point where they are often considered a first-line surgical option, but we only recently advanced glaucoma surgery to focus on improvement of trabecular meshwork (TM) and Schlemm's canal (SC) inner wall outflow or removal or bypass of TM and SC inner wall.

Schlemm's canal surgery, including ab interno trabeculectomy, canaloplasty, and TM-SC bypass, is another step toward safety and control in glaucoma IOP reduction surgery. It is less risky than trabeculectomy or GDD implantation, but it is also less effective at IOP reduction. The trade-off of efficacy for safety may be acceptable in patients needing mid- to high-teens IOP, but patients requiring a very low IOP still need more invasive procedures like trabeculectomy or GDD.

Another aspect of the TM-SC bypass or removal procedures is actual surgical access to TM and Schlemm's canal. Perhaps the movement towards less risky and invasive surgery will have as a byproduct treatment of glaucoma through extended-release medication, cell-based or gene therapy applied directly in Schemm's canal or the TM.

Maybe, as such treatments emerge, Dave Epstein's suggestion to "give them the cure" will finally be said without irony.

Appendix A

SURGICAL SUPPLIES, INSTRUMENTS, AND IMPLANTS FOR THE OPERATING ROOM

Nathan M. Radcliffe, MD

TABLE A-1. SUTURE MATERIALS FOR GLAUCOMA SURGERY	
Suture	Purpose
10-0 nylon	Suture cornea
9-0 or 8-0 nylon	Secure tube or plate to sclera
7-0 silk	Traction suture
7-0 Vicryl	Tube ligation
8-0 or 9-0 Vicryl	Conjunctival closure
4-0 or 5-0 nylon	Tube occlusion/stenting suture

TABLE A-2. BLADES AND NEEDLES FOR GLAUCOMA SURGERY	
Instrument	Purpose
15-degree or No. 75 stab blade	Paracentesis
22-gauge or 23-gauge needle	Create ostomy for tube insertion
26-gauge needle	Create ostomy Ex-Press P-50 placement
Beaver blade (No. 57 or 69)	Outline scleral flap
Crescent blade	Dissect scleral flap
No. 11 BD Bard-Parker blade	Venting or "Sherwood" tube slits
1.7-mm keratome	Trabectome incision

Kahook M.
Essentials of Glaucoma Surgery (pp 405–406).
© 2012 SLACK Incorporated.

TABLE A-3. INSTRUMENTS FOR THE GLAUCOMA SURGICAL TRAY

Instrument	Purpose
Eyelid speculum	Retract eyelids
Kelly-Descemet punch	Excise trabeculo-Descemet's window
Jameson muscle hook	Expose and isolate rectus muscle
Cautery with thin "intraocular" tip	Hemostasis
Vannas scissors	Dissect conjunctiva and Tenon's capsule
Smooth-tipped conjunctival forceps	Retract conjunctiva and Tenon's capsule
Westcott or mini-Westcott scissors	Dissect conjunctiva and Tenon's capsule
Balanced salt solution on a 30-gauge cannula	Reform anterior chamber, pressurize eye
0.12 forceps	Manipulate tissue, suture scleral flap
0.3 or 0.5 forceps	Place glaucoma drainage device
Needle holder (small)	Close conjunctiva
Needle holder (large)	Tie 7-0 Vicryl tube ligature

Appendix B

DIAGNOSTIC AND PROCEDURAL CODES FOR GLAUCOMA AND GLAUCOMA SURGERY

Nathan M. Radcliffe, MD

TABLE B-1. CURRENT PROCEDURAL TERMINOLOGY (CPT) CODES FOR COMMONLY PERFORMED GLAUCOMA SURGERIES	
CPT	Procedure Name
66180	Glaucoma drainage device placement
67255	Patch graft
66185	Glaucoma drainage device revision
66170	Trabeculectomy with mitomycin C (MMC) (no prior conjunctival surgery)
66172	Trabeculectomy with MMC (prior conjunctival surgery)
66250	Revision of trabeculectomy
0192T	Ex-Press glaucoma filtration device placement
0177T	Transluminal dilation of canal; retained stent (canaloplasty)
0176T	Transluminal dilation of canal; without retained stent (viscocanalostomy)
66710	Ciliary body destruction, cyclophotocoagulation
66720	Ciliary body destruction, transscleral cryotherapy
68320	Conjunctivoplasty with extensive rearrangement
65820	Goniotomy
	(continued)

Kahook M.
Essentials of Glaucoma Surgery (pp 407–410).
© 2012 SLACK Incorporated.

TABLE B-1 (CONTINUED). CURRENT PROCEDURAL TERMINOLOGY CODES FOR COMMONLY PERFORMED GLAUCOMA SURGERIES

CPT	Procedure Name
65850	Trabeculotomy
65875	Goniosynechialysis
65930	Removal of blood clot from anterior segment
66680	Repair of ciliary body or iris
67015	Drainage of choroidal fluid
66984	Cataract extraction with intraocular lens (IOL) placement (standard)
66982	Cataract extraction with IOL placement (complex)
66985	Insertion of IOL without cataract removal

TABLE B-2. CURRENT PROCEDURAL TERMINOLOGY CODES FOR COMMONLY PERFORMED OFFICE-BASED GLAUCOMA PROCEDURES

CPT	Procedure Name
66821	Laser capsulotomy
66820	Laser hyaloidotomy
66762	Laser iridoplasty
66761	Laser iridotomy
66855	Laser trabeculoplasty (argon laser trabeculoplasty [ALT] or selective laser trabeculoplasty [SLT])
65800	Paracentesis (aqueous)
65815	Paracentesis (blood)
66020	Reformation anterior chamber
68200	Subconjunctival injection
67515	Sub-Tenon's injection
66030	Injection viscoelastic

TABLE B-3. International Classification of Diseases, Ninth Revision (ICD-9) Diagnosis Codes for Common Glaucoma Diagnoses	
ICD-9 Code	Name of Diagnosis
365.10	Open-angle glaucoma
365.89	Uncontrolled glaucoma
v45.69	Failed filter procedure
366.9	Cataract
365.20	Angle-closure glaucoma
365.02	Anatomical narrow angles
360.33	Hypotony
365.05	Ocular hypertension
997.99	Leaking bleb
366.53	Posterior capsular opacification
996.59	Complication of implant
363.71	Choroidal effusion
379.31	Aphakia

Appendix C

INFORMED CONSENT IN GLAUCOMA SURGERY

Nathan M. Radcliffe, MD

Informed consent is the term used to describe a process of communication between the physician and patient prior to a patient agreeing to undergo a medical intervention. Although a written consent form is typically signed to document this process, the communication itself is the focus of the informed consent process. The American Medical Association lists several important steps in the informed consent process[1] and notes that physicians are ethically and legally obligated to disclose or provide the following:

1. The medical diagnosis
2. The procedure's nature and purpose
3. The procedure's risks and benefits
4. Alternatives to the procedure (and their risks and benefits)
5. The risks and benefits of no intervention
6. An opportunity for the patient to ask questions

Additionally, the patient should demonstrate an understanding of the above material, which can be challenging given that not all patients with glaucoma will possess the appropriate health literacy to understand their glaucoma and what might be required to treat it.[2] In one study, only one-half of patients undergoing glaucoma surgery had a moderate understanding of their surgical problem despite over 90% of physicians reporting that they had taken enough time to explain the problem.[3]

Glaucoma surgery represents a unique paradigm in ophthalmology, and the process of informed consent in glaucoma surgery deserves special consideration. Whereas surgeries for cataract, corneal disease, and many retinal problems are usually performed to alleviate existing visual problems, glaucoma surgery is, on many levels, a prophylactic intervention designed to stabilize vision, or more to the point, to decrease the rate of progressive

Kahook M.
Essentials of Glaucoma Surgery (pp 411–414).
© 2012 SLACK Incorporated.

visual loss.[4] Many candidates for glaucoma surgery will be asymptomatic at the time that surgery is being proposed. Rarely will a patient undergoing a glaucoma filtration procedure see or feel better after the surgery, and patients will frequently experience a small amount of visual reduction or local ocular symptoms associated with the surgery to stabilize vision in the long run.[5]

Adverse outcomes often occur in glaucoma surgery. It is important that the informed consent process in glaucoma surgery include a frank discussion of the likelihood of complications. The surgeon and patient should consider whether, given a bad outcome, they would be able to look back and both agree that the possibility of the complication had been discussed and given appropriate consideration during the informed consent process. Any glaucoma surgeon performing a significant number of procedures will eventually have a patient who experiences severe vision loss in association with a glaucoma procedure. By carefully considering the risk profile of intervention and discussing all options in detail, both the patient and surgeon will be psychologically prepared for an adverse outcome should one occur.

When discussing the potential benefits of glaucoma filtration surgery, consider the highest-quality and most recent evidence. In the first 3 years of follow-up during the prospective Tube Versus Trabeculectomy Study, the cumulative probability of failure (intraocular pressure [IOP] above 21 mmHg or less than 20% reduction, hypotony, reoperation, or loss of light perception) was 15.1% in the tube group and 30.7% in the trabeculectomy group. Postoperative complications were common in both groups and occurred in 39% of the tube group and 60% of the trabeculectomy group, with roughly one-quarter of each group requiring reoperation for these complications.[6] Cataract worsening requiring cataract extraction is common following trabeculectomy and should be mentioned during the informed consent process.[7] Inflammation (uveitis), infection (early or late endophthalmitis), bleeding (hyphema and choroidal hemorrhage), as well as corneal decompensation and retinal detachment are additional potential complications to include. It is important that the patient understand that reoperation for any of the above complications is possible. Potential surgical augmentations, such as laser suture lysis, stenting suture removal, bleb needling, antifibrosis injection, or goniopuncture, should be mentioned at the time of the initial consent if the surgeon feels there is a reasonable likelihood that these procedures will be required and especially if the implied success rate includes the use of these enhancements.

The patient should be reminded that compliance with prescribed eye drops and postoperative visits is essential for the safety and efficacy of the procedure. Patients can sometimes frame the choice for surgery in terms of surgery *instead of* eye drops, and it is helpful to remind them that a successful surgery might include better IOP control on the same medications or similar IOP control with fewer medications. Similarly, patients can be unhappy following glaucoma surgery, even with excellent IOP control without medications in the case of bleb dysthesia. Finally, the possibility of rare, life-threatening systemic side effects should be disclosed, as should the potential for rare and sometimes unforeseeable side effects that have not been discussed.

CONCLUSION

In glaucoma surgery, it is important to provide a meaningful and extensive discussion of the risks, benefits, and alternatives of a proposed surgical intervention. By asking the patient to explain the diagnosis, proposed treatments, and potential complications in his or her own words, the surgeon will be able to assess the patient's understanding of the procedure and directly address any misconceptions. The possibility for adverse outcomes is relatively high in glaucoma surgery and should be addressed directly, and the patient should have a clear understanding that the glaucoma surgery is intended to preserve (not restore) vision. By providing the patient with appropriate expectations heading into surgery, the clinician can optimize the likelihood of both the surgeon and patient being pleased with the outcome, even in the most challenging glaucoma cases.

REFERENCES

1. American Medical Association. *Patient physician relationship topics: informed consent.* AMA Web site. Retrieved from www.ama-assn.org/ama/pub/physician-resources/legal-topics/patient-physician-relationship-topics/informed-consent.shtml
2. Muir KW, Lee PP. Literacy and informed consent: a case for literacy screening in glaucoma research. *Arch Ophthalmol.* 2009;127(5):698-699.
3. Kang KD, Abdul Majid AS, Kwag JH, Kim YD, Yim HB. A prospective audit on the validity of written informed consent prior to glaucoma surgery: an Asian perspective. *Graefes Arch Clin Exp Ophthalmol.* 2010;248(5):687-701.
4. Folgar FA, de Moraes CG, Prata TS, et al. Glaucoma surgery decreases the rates of localized and global visual field progression. *Am J Ophthalmol.* 2010;149(2):258-264.
5. Janz NK, Wren PA, Lichter PR, et al; CIGTS Study Group. The Collaborative Initial Glaucoma Treatment Study: interim quality of life findings after initial medical or surgical treatment of glaucoma. *Ophthalmology.* 2001;108(11):1954-1965.
6. Gedde SJ, Schiffman JC, Feuer WJ, Herndon LW, Brandt JD, Budenz DL; Tube Versus Trabeculectomy Study Group. Three-year follow-up of the tube versus trabeculectomy study. *Am J Ophthalmol.* 2009;148(5):670-684.
7. Wong TT, Khaw PT, Aung T, et al. The singapore 5-fluorouracil trabeculectomy study: effects on intraocular pressure control and disease progression at 3 years. *Ophthalmology.* 2009;116(2):175-184.

Appendix D

SURGICAL DICTATION EXAMPLES

Nathan M. Radcliffe, MD and Anna-Maria Demetriades, MD

The surgical dictation serves several functions. The operative note clearly lists the date of surgery, the patient's name and identification (medical record number), preoperative/postoperative diagnoses, surgeon and assistant(s), and the precise procedure(s) performed, including laterality. The type of anesthesia and concentrations of injected or applied topical anesthesia used are also documented. Any intraoperative complications are described. The model and details of any implanted materials (allograft or synthetic) and/or quantity of injected or applied pharmacotherapeutics (eg, duration and concentration of mitomycin C [MMC]) should be included, including serial numbers for implants if not carefully noted elsewhere. Some surgeons will begin the dictation by reiterating the risks, benefits, and alternatives of the surgical history or by providing a brief clinical narrative detailing the indications for the procedure.

In this section, we will provide examples of surgical dictations for commonly performed surgical procedures. In the interests of brevity, the dictations will be limited to surgical details, with our preferred template (Table D-1) given for the first procedure only. It should go without saying that the specific examples of procedures given here are just that, and the reader should refer to his or her training for the indications and alternatives for each procedure.

Kahook M.
Essentials of Glaucoma Surgery (pp 415–422).
© 2012 SLACK Incorporated.

TABLE D-1. FORNIX-BASED TRABECULECTOMY WITH MITOMYCIN C (TOPICAL)	
Date of Surgery:	_____/_____/_____
Preoperative Diagnosis:	Uncontrolled glaucoma _____ EYE (right/left)
Postoperative Diagnosis:	Uncontrolled glaucoma _____ EYE (right/left)
Surgeon:	_____
Assistant:	_____
Operation Performed:	Trabeculectomy with mitomycin C (0.4 mg/cc) _____ EYE (right/left)
Anesthesia:	Topical 1% lidocaine with monitored intravenous sedation
Complications:	None

Indications of Procedure: Uncontrolled intraocular pressure despite maximum tolerated medical therapy.

Description of Procedure: Informed consent was obtained from the patient, at which time the risks, benefits, and alternatives were discussed, and all questions were addressed. The patient was identified in the holding area, and the operative eye was identified as the _____ (right/left) eye.

The correct operative eye was confirmed and a single drop of tetracaine was applied to the eye. The eye was then prepped and draped in the usual sterile manner for ophthalmic surgery. A lid speculum was inserted. The patient was instructed to look down to infraduct the globe.

Topical 1% preservative-free lidocaine was subsequently applied to the superior conjunctiva. A superior limbal peritomy was created using non-toothed forceps and Vannas scissors, and 1% preservative-free lidocaine was injected into the subconjunctival and sub-Tenon's space. The peritomy was then dissected posteriorly, medially, and laterally with mini-Westcott scissors. The sclera was then devascularized with broad strokes of a No. 69 Beaver blade, using 0.12 forceps to stabilize the globe. A No. 75 blade was then used to create a 50% thickness trapezoidal scleral flap. This was extended toward the limbus with a No. 69 blade. Cellulose sponges soaked with 0.4 mg/mL MMC were applied beneath the conjunctiva and held in place for 2 minutes. A wide diffuse application was achieved, and all of the sponges were subsequently identified and removed. Copious irrigation with balanced salt solution was performed. Two interrupted 10-0 nylon sutures were then pre-placed through the scleral flap. A corneal paracentesis was created with a No. 75 blade, which was then used to enter the anterior chamber through the base of the scleral flap. A Kelly–Descemet punch was used to create a 0.75-mm sclerostomy, and a broad-based peripheral iridectomy was performed. The pre-placed nylon sutures were then adjusted for appropriate flow, tied, and the knots were buried. The conjunctiva and Tenon's fascia were then reapproximated to the limbus and tied in place with 4 interupted 10-0 nylon wing sutures, the knots of which were buried. Intracameral balanced salt solution was injected, an elevated conjunctival bleb was observed, and no leaks were identified. The intraocular pressure (IOP) by palpation was reconfirmed to be approximately mid-teens. 1% atropine ophthalmic solution was instilled, followed by a fourth-generation fluoroquinolone antibiotic. The eyelid speculum was removed, and the eye was shielded. The patient was brought to the recovery area in excellent condition, having tolerated the procedure well without any complications.

BAERVELDT GLAUCOMA DRAINAGE DEVICE WITH PATCH GRAFT

The patient was given a retrobulbar block under intravenous sedation consisting of a 1:1 dilution of 2% lidocaine and 0.75% bupivocaine. The correct operative eye was confirmed, a single drop of tetracaine was applied, and the eye was prepped and draped in the usual sterile manner for ophthalmic surgery. A lid speculum was inserted. A clear corneal 7-0 Vicryl traction suture was placed at the 12 o'clock position, and the globe was infraducted. Topical preservative-free 1% lidocaine was applied to the conjunctiva. A 3 clock-hour conjunctival peritomy was created using the Westcott scissors at the superotemporal limbus. A sub-Tenon's cannula was then used to deliver 1% lidocaine into the parabulbar and retrobulbar space through the peritomy. Hemostasis was achieved with gentle application of bipolar wetfield cautery. The Baerveldt 350-mm^2 glaucoma implant was inspected, and balanced salt solution was injected into the tube tip using a 30-gauge cannula to ensure patency. Tenotomy muscle hooks were used to isolate the rectus muscles, and the Baerveldt implant was placed under the superior and lateral rectus muscles, taking care to avoid the separation of any muscle fibers. The implant plate was secured to the globe approximately 8 to 10 mm posterior to the limbus using 2 interrupted 9-0 nylon sutures with the knots buried. The tube was ligated with a single 7-0 Vicryl suture and confirmed to be watertight by injection of balanced salt solution. The tube was trimmed with an anterior bevel, and a 23-gauge needle was used to tunnel into a deep position in the anterior chamber from an entry 2.5 mm posterior to the limbus. The tube was inserted into the eye and confirmed to be in excellent position in the anterior chamber and secured to the sclera using a 9-0 nylon suture. Two tube fenestrations were created using the Vicryl needle. A pericardial patch graft was trimmed to the appropriate size, placed over the tube's insertion and secured using several interrupted 7-0 Vicryl sutures. Conjunctiva and Tenon's fascia were secured at the limbus using interrupted and running 7-0 Vicryl sutures. At the conclusion of the procedure, the anterior chamber was noted to be deep and well formed, the tube was in excellent position, the IOP by palpation was confirmed to be approximately mid-teens, and no leaks or buttonholes were identified. A subconjunctival injection of Decadron and gentamycin was administered in the inferior cul-de-sac. The lid speculum was removed, Maxitrol ophthalmic ointment was applied, and a pressure patch and protective shield were placed over the eye. The patient was brought to the recovery area in excellent condition, having tolerated the procedure well without any complications.

LIMBUS-BASED TRABECULECTOMY WITH MITOMYCIN C (RETROBULBAR BLOCK)

The patient was given a retrobulbar block under intravenous sedation consisting of a 1:1 dilution of 2% lidocaine and 0.75% bupivocaine. After adequate anesthesia and akinesia were achieved, the patient was brought into the operating room. The operative eye was prepped and draped in the usual sterile manner for ophthalmic surgery. A lid speculum was inserted. A clear corneal 7-0 Vicryl traction suture was placed at the 12 o'clock position, and the globe was infraducted. The superior conjunctiva and Tenon's capsule were elevated and then incised approximately 10 mm posterior to the limbus, and a tangential incision was created approximately 6 mm in length, taking care to avoid the superior rectus muscle and associated blood vessels.

A No. 75 blade was then used to create a 50% thickness trapezoidal scleral flap, which was extended toward the limbus with a No. 69 blade. Cellulose sponges soaked with 0.4 mg/mL MMC were applied beneath the conjunctiva and held in place for 2 minutes. A wide diffuse application was achieved, and all of the sponges were subsequently identified and removed. Copious irrigation with balanced salt solution was performed. Two interrupted 10-0 nylon sutures were then pre-placed through the scleral flap. A corneal paracentesis was then created with a No. 75 blade, which was then used to enter the anterior chamber through the base of the scleral flap. A Kelly–Descemet punch was used to create a 0.75-mm sclerostomy and a broad-based peripheral iridectomy was performed. The pre-placed nylon sutures were then adjusted for appropriate flow, tied, and the knots were buried. An 8-0 Vicryl suture on a vascular needle was used to reapproximate the Tenon's capsule and conjunctiva in a running and locking fashion.

Intracameral balanced salt solution was injected, an elevated conjunctival bleb was observed, and no leaks were identified. The IOP by palpation was reconfirmed to be approximately mid-teens. 1% atropine ophthalmic solution was administered. The lid speculum was removed, Maxitrol ophthalmic ointment (neomycin and polymyxin B sulfates and dexamethasone ophthalmic suspension) was applied, and a pressure patch and protective shield were placed over the eye. The patient was brought to the recovery area in excellent condition, having tolerated the procedure well without any complications.

TRABECTOME AND CATARACT EXTRACTION

The correct operative eye was confirmed, prepped, and draped in the usual sterile manner for ophthalmic surgery. Topical tetracaine ophthalmic solution was applied and a lid speculum was inserted. A 1.7-mm clear corneal incision was made at the 3 o'clock position using a metal keratome blade. Preservative-free 1% lidocaine was then introduced into the anterior chamber, followed by viscoelastic. A goniolens was placed on the cornea, and visualization of the angle was confirmed. The Trabectome was then introduced into the anterior chamber, and the tip of the Trabectome was inserted into Schlemm's canal anterior to the scleral spur. Aspiration and ablation of the trabecular meshwork was thus performed in a clockwise direction for approximately 2 clock hours and redirected in an counterclockwise direction for approximately 1 clock hour. The trabectome was subsequently removed. Two clear corneal paracentesis incisions were made at the 7 o'clock and 11 o'clock positions using a No. 75 blade, and additional viscoelastic was introduced into the anterior chamber. A 2.75-mm keratome blade was used to enlarge the clear corneal incision through the prior Trabectome entry site. A bent cystotome needle and capsulorrhexis forceps were used to create a continuous curvilinear capsulorrhexis. Hydrodissection was performed using a flat 27-gauge cannula and balanced salt solution, and free rotation of the lens nucleus was obtained. Disassembly and removal of the lens was performed using standard chopping techniques with phacoemulsification. Residual cortical material was removed using bimanual irrigation and aspiration. The capsular bag was reformed with a viscoelastic and noted to be intact. An intraocular lens (IOL) with power + _____ D, serial number _____, was placed into the capsular bag. Residual viscoelastic was removed using irrigation and aspiration. The temporal clear corneal wound and paracentesis incisions were hydrated using balanced salt solution. The corneal incision was closed using a single interrupted 10-0 nylon suture and confirmed to be watertight without leakage. The lid speculum was removed, and a fourth-generation fluoroquinolone antibiotic was placed. The eye was shielded. The patient was brought to the recovery area in excellent condition, having tolerated the procedure well without any complications.

EX-PRESS GLAUCOMA DEVICE WITH MITOMYCIN C

Topical 1% preservative-free lidocaine was applied to the superior conjunctiva. A superior limbal peritomy was created with nontoothed forceps and Vannas scissors. 1% preservative-free lidocaine was then injected into the subconjunctival and sub-Tenon's space. The peritomy was subsequently dissected posteriorly, medially, and laterally with mini-Westcott scissors. The sclera was then devascularized with broad strokes of a No. 69 Beaver blade, using 0.12 forceps to stabilize the globe. Next, a No. 75 blade was used to create a 50% thickness trapezoidal scleral flap. This was extended toward the limbus with a No. 69 blade. Cellulose sponges soaked with 0.4 mg/mL MMC were then applied beneath the conjunctiva and held in place for 2 minutes. A wide diffuse application was achieved, and all of the sponges were subsequently identified and removed. Copious irrigation with balanced salt solution was performed. Two interrupted 10-0 nylon sutures were pre-placed through the scleral flap, and a corneal paracentesis was created with a No. 75 blade. The anterior aspect of the scleral spur was identified at the base of the flap, and a 26-gauge needle was used to enter the anterior chamber parallel to the iris plane. The needle was marked with a marking pen prior to insertion to facilitate identification of the entry site. The Ex-Press shunt was then placed in the newly created incision. The Ex-Press shunt tip was judged to be in a good position in the anterior chamber, and the back plate was flush with the scleral bed. A diagonal 10-0 nylon flap suture was then placed in each corner of the scleral flap. Balanced salt solution on a cannula was injected into the anterior chamber through the paracentesis, and steady flow was observed through the flap.

The conjunctiva and Tenon's fascia were then reapproximated to the limbus and tied in place with 4 interupted 10-0 nylon wing sutures, the knots of which were buried. Intracameral balanced salt solution was injected, an elevated conjunctival bleb was observed, and no leaks were identified. The IOP by palpation was reconfirmed to be approximately mid-teens. 1% atropine ophthalmic solution was administered, followed by a fourth-generation fluoroquinolone antibiotic. The eyelid speculum was removed, and the eye was shielded. The patient was brought to the recovery area in excellent condition, having tolerated the procedure well without any complications.

AHMED VALVE IMPLANTATION WITH PATCH GRAFT

Following initiation of IV sedation and topical application of tetracaine and betadine ophthalmic solution, retrobulbar anesthesia was induced with a 4-cc injection of 1% lidocaine and 0.75% bupivacaine mixed in a 50-50 concentration. The _____ (right/left) eye was then prepped and draped in the usual sterile ophthalmic manner, and a lid speculum was applied.

Using Westcott scissors and nontoothed forceps, a conjunctival peritomy was created in the superotemporal quadrant. Blunt dissection was performed between Tenon's fascia and the sclera to expose the bare sclera between the superior and lateral rectus muscles. A muscle hook was then used to identify the superior and lateral rectus muscles. Balanced salt solution on a 30-gauge cannula was then used to "prime" the silicone Ahmed FP7 valve, demonstrating its patency and ability to provide resistance to balanced salt solution. The plate was then inserted between the superior and the lateral rectus muscle over the bare sclera approximately 8 mm posterior to the limbus. Using 8-0 nylon, the valve was sutured to the sclera through the plate's anterior suture holes. The tube of the valve was then laid flat on the cornea and cut with Westcott scissors in a bevel-up fashion to allow several millimeters of tube tip in the anterior chamber following insertion. A corneal paracentesis incision was then created inferotemporally. A 23-gauge needle was then inserted 2 mm posterior to the limbus and tunneled into the deep anterior chamber parallel to the iris plane at the 12 o'clock position. Using Kelman–McPherson tying forceps, the tube of the Ahmed valve was inserted into the anterior chamber, which was reformed and repressurized using balanced salt solution. The tube was then secured in position using a 10-0 nylon horizontal mattress suture. An approximately 4- × 4-mm sheet of pericardial patch graft was then furnished to cover the tube over its limbal insertion and posteriorly. The pericardial patch was sutured into place with 2 8-0 Vicryl interrupted sutures. Conjunctiva and Tenon's capsule were then reapproximated to the limbus using 8-0 Vicryl interrupted wing sutures. A subconjunctival injection of Decadron and gentamycin was administered in the inferior cul-de-sac. The lid speculum was removed, Maxitrol ophthalmic ointment was applied, and a pressure patch and protective shield were placed over the eye. The patient was brought to the recovery area in excellent condition, having tolerated the procedure well without any complications.

Appendix E

COMMONLY USED LASER SETTINGS

Nathan M. Radcliffe, MD

TABLE E-1. LASER SETTINGS FOR COMMONLY PERFORMED GLAUCOMA PROCEDURES

Procedure	Time (s)	Power	Spot Size (microns)	# of Applications
Iridoplasty	0.5 to 0.7	240 mW	500	24
Argon laser suture lysis (tube ligature)	0.02	1000 mW	50	As few as possible
Vicryl laser suture lysis (tube ligature)	0.5	500 mW	50	As few as possible
Argon trabeculoplasty	0.1	780 mW	50	56/180
Selective trabeculoplasty	n/a	0.6 to 1.0 mJ	n/a	40 to 60/180 75 to 100/360
Argon iridotomy	0.02	400 to 1500 mW	50	As few as possible
YAG iridotomy	n/a	1.2 mJ and up	n/a	As few as possible

Kahook M.
Essentials of Glaucoma Surgery (pp 423–424).
© 2012 SLACK Incorporated.

Financial Disclosures

Dr. R. Rand Allingham has no financial or proprietary interest in the materials presented herein.

Dr. Ramesh S. Ayyala has a patent pending on a slow release drug delivery system. He is a consultant for iSciences Interventional, and recieves research support from New World Medical. He is president of Meditred.com. The chapter was supported by a Tulane Glaucoma Research Grant.

Dr. Amy Badger-Asaravala has no financial or proprietary interest in the materials presented herein.

Dr. John P. Berdahl is a speaker for Alcon and Allergan, and a clinical investigator for Alcon, Glaukos, Calhoun, and Avedro.

Dr. Gabriel T. Chong has no financial or proprietary interest in the materials presented herein.

Dr. Nathan Congdon has no financial or proprietary interest in the materials presented herein.

Dr. Anna-Maria Demetriades has no financial or proprietary interest in the materials presented herein.

Dr. Jonathan A. Eisengart has no financial or proprietary interest in the materials presented herein.

Dr. David L. Epstein is on the board of directors and is a shareholder with Aerie Pharmaceuticals. He holds a stockolder agreement with Glaukos Corporation. He also receives grant support from NIH, NEI, and Research to Prevent Blindness.

Dr. Malvina B. Eydelman has not disclosed any relevant financial relationships.

Dr. Robert D. Fechtner has no disclosures relative to his chapter, but is supported in part by Research to Prevent Blindness.

Dr. David Fleischman has no financial or proprietary interest in the materials presented herein.

Dr. James A. Fox has no financial or proprietary interest in the materials presented herein.

Dr. Douglas E. Gaasterland has been a medical advisor for IRIDEX Corporation, and also holds stock and recieves royalties from them.

Dr. Preeya K. Gupta has no financial or proprietary interest in the materials presented herein.

Dr. Ben J. Harvey has not disclosed any relevant financial relationships.

Dr. Leon W. Herndon is on the Glaucoma Advisory Board for Alcon.

Dr. Michael B. Horsley has no financial or proprietary interest in the materials presented herein.

Dr. Nauman Imami has no financial or proprietary interest in the materials presented herein.

Dr. Denise A. John has no financial or proprietary interest in the materials presented herein.

Dr. Suzanne Johnston has no financial or proprietary interest in the materials presented herein.

Dr. Malik Y. Kahook is a consultant for Alcon, Allergan, Merck, Glaukos, Ivantis, Genentech, and the Food and Drug Administration. He has received research support from Allergan, Alcon, Merck, Genentech, Actelion, and the State of Colorado. Dr. Kahook has ownership interest and patents licensed to ShapeOphthalmics, ShapeTech, and Innovative Laser Solutions.

Dr. Mahmoud A. Khaimi has not disclosed any relevant financial relationships.

Dr. Anup K. Khatana is a speaker and consultant for IOP Inc, and an investigator for Transcend Medical Inc.

Dr. R. Lee Kramm has no financial or proprietary interest in the materials presented herein.

Dr. Dennis S. C. Lam has no financial or proprietary interest in the materials presented herein.

Dr. Danielle M. Ledoux has no financial or proprietary interest in the materials presented herein.

Dr. Richard K. Lee has no financial or proprietary interest in the materials presented herein.

Dr. Christopher K. S. Leung has not disclosed any relevant financial relationships.

Dr. Richard A. Lewis recieves support from Alcon, Allergan, Merck, Aerie, Santen, iScience Interventional, Ivantis, Aquesys, and Glaucos.

Dr. Marlene R. Moster recieves support from Alcon, Allergan, Merck, Solex, BD Medical–Ophthalmic Systems, iScience Interventional, Ista Pharmacueticals, and Genentech.

Dr. Sayoko E. Moroi has investigator-initiated clinical research support from Merck.

Dr. David C. Musch is a chair on the Data & Safety Monitoring Board for Ivantis Inc. He is a consultant to AqueSys Inc, Glaukos, and InnFocus LLC. He recieves grant support from NEI/NIH: EY20912 and Pfizer Corporation.

Dr. Mina Pantcheva has no financial or proprietary interest in the materials presented herein.

Dr. Kathryn L. Pepple has no financial or proprietary interest in the materials presented herein.

Dr. Nathan M. Radcliffe has served as a consultant or speaker for Allergan Inc, Alcon Laboratories, Ophthalmic Imaging Systems, Carl Zeiss Meditec, Merck, and Iridex.

Dr. Marcos Reyes has been a consultant for Alcon.

Dr. Douglas J. Rhee has no financial or proprietary interest in the materials presented herein.

Dr. Robert Ritch has no financial or proprietary interest in the materials presented herein.

Dr. Matthew Rouse has no financial or proprietary interest in the materials presented herein.

Dr. Travis C. Rumery has no financial or proprietary interest in the materials presented herein.

Dr. Sarwat Salim has no financial or proprietary interest in the materials presented herein.

Dr. Thomas W. Samuelson is a consultant for Alcon, AcuMems, Allergen, AMO, AqueSys, Endo Optiks, Glaukos, Ivantis, Merck, Ocular Surgery News, QLT, Santen, and SLACK Incorporated.

Dr. Fiorella Saponara has no financial or proprietary interest in the materials presented herein.

Dr. Steven R. Sarkisian Jr has no financial or proprietary interest in the materials presented herein.

Dr. Joel S. Schuman has no financial or proprietary interest in the materials presented herein.

Dr. Leonard K. Seibold has no financial or proprietary interest in the materials presented herein.

Dr. Robert Stamper has no financial or proprietary interest in the materials presented herein.

Dr. Joshua D. Stein has no financial or proprietary interest in the materials presented herein.

Dr. Tiffany N. Szymarek has no financial or proprietary interest in the materials presented herein.

Dr. Clement C. Y. Tham has no financial or proprietary interest in the materials presented herein.

Dr. Stephen P. Verb has no financial or proprietary interest in the materials presented herein.

Dr. Elizabeth T. Viriya has no financial or proprietary interest in the materials presented herein.

Dr. David S. Walton has no financial or proprietary interest in the materials presented herein.

Dr. Jennifer Somers Weizer has no financial or proprietary interest in the materials presented herein.

Dr. Joseph R. Zelefsky has served on the speakers bureau for Allergan and Alcon.

Dr. Jeffrey M. Zink is a subinvestigator for COMPASS trial, a site investigator for the Primary Tube vs Trabeculectomy Trial, and has been a speaker for Merck.

Index